Praise for Tracy Gaudet
and
Consciously Female

"Dr. Tracy Gaudet is the sort of doctor that every woman wants. Her unique approach to women's medicine blends the wide expertise of an integrative-medicine physician with the deep insight and personal understanding only one woman can offer another. In *Consciously Female*, she shows us how to untangle the net of mind, body, emotions, and spirit and weave it into a fabric far stronger than we have ever dreamed. If you are a woman, you owe it to yourself to read this one."
—Rachel Naomi Remen, M.D., author, *Kitchen Table Wisdom* and
My Grandfather's Blessings

"A veritable cornucopia of wise and practical information and compassionate guidance from a physician who practices what she preaches and is a highly respected advocate of a truly integrative medicine. *Consciously Female* may be the ally, friend, and expert you so sorely need and miss in today's rapidly changing medicine. It is a specific and scientifically based prescription for optimizing health and well-being, a true gift to women of all ages, and a source of comfort and reassurance that honors the universe of the feminine in matters of soma, psyche, and relationship, including importantly, with yourself . . . consciously."
—Jon Kabat-Zinn, Ph.D., author, *Coming to Our Senses: How We Can Use Mindfulness to Heal Ourselves and the World*

"This book is about waking up, becoming conscious of not only our body but our mind and spirit as well. It is about using deep intuition along with rational discernment in making smart choices about our health. Let us be grateful for the blessings of scientific medicine, but let us also honor the consciousness, soul, and spirit that lie at the heart of Dr. Gaudet's elegant medical vision."
—Larry Dossey, M.D., author, *Healing Beyond the Body, Reinventing Medicine,* and *Healing Words*

"Tracy Gaudet has written an inspiring guide to health and the healing journey. It's a fabulous book—intelligent, alive, and practical. She shows how a new medicine is not just adding new drugs or herbs or treatments: it depends on a deeper understanding of healing and of being human. She is pointing to the direction we now need to take in medicine. It's *the* book to give to the women you care about most in your life."
—John Tarrant, Ph.D., author, *The Light Inside the Dark: Zen, Soul and the Spiritual Life*

Consciously
Female

How to Listen to Your Body and
Your Soul for a Lifetime of Healthier Living

Tracy W. Gaudet, MD,
with Paula Spencer

 Bantam Books   New York Toronto London Sydney Auckland

This book is designed to help you make informed choices;
it is not meant to replace consultation with
a physician or other licensed health care provider.

CONSCIOUSLY FEMALE
A Bantam Book

PUBLISHING HISTORY
Bantam hardcover edition published April 2004
Bantam trade paperback edition / January 2005

Published by
Bantam Dell
A Division of Random House, Inc.
New York, New York

Grateful acknowledgment is given for permission to reprint from the following:

Bill Holm, "Advice" in *The Dead Get By with Everything*
(Minneapolis: Milkweed Editions, 1990). Copyright © 1990 by Bill Holm.
Reprinted with permission from Milkweed Editions.

Illustrations on pages 218, 219, and 363 are reproduced from *Clinical Gynecologic
Endocrinology and Infertility* by Leon Speroff, 6th edition, 1999. Reprinted by permission.

Illustration on page 221 is reproduced from *Comprehensive Gynecology, 4th edition,*
Stenchever, et al, p. 116, copyright © 2001 by Mosby, with permission from Elsevier.

Book design by Ellen Cipriano

Library of Congress Catalog Card Number: 2003065248

ISBN: 0-553-38186-5

www.bantamdell.com

Printed in the United States of America
Published simultaneously in Canada

BVG   10   9   8   7   6   5   4   3   2   1

To my passionate, committed, and loving husband, Rich Liebowitz, and
To the love of my mom, my dad, Hexi, and Noodle

Acknowledgments

The greatest blessing in my life has been the extraordinary individuals whom I have had the opportunity to know, to learn from, and to grow with. Each has influenced my life, my career, and the creation of this book—some directly and others indirectly. Attempting to capture this on paper is a daunting task indeed.

To start, I would like to acknowledge my family: my mom, Mary Louise Williams, who was the embodiment of unconditional love, with a sharp intellect and clever wit; my dad, Earl Kenneth Williams, who taught me the power of determination, hard work, and ingenuity; my sister, Wendy Williams, with whom I have grown through our many shared life experiences; my beautiful niece, Jessica, whose depth and honesty I cherish. My greatest support has been my incredible husband, Rich Liebowitz, who is passionately committed to our path together and whom I am blessed to have as my life partner. At long last our relationship has the chance to outlive the process of this book! And along with Rich, I have been blessed by his wonderful children, Corey and Josh; his mother, Edie, and her husband, George; and his brother, Ron, and his wife, Jessica.

The path of my life has been guided all along the way by inspiring teachers and friends: Todd Welch, Kelly Guthrie Bruneau, and Virginia McCabe Keeler—the deep friendships we shared in our teens were profound gifts that taught me the mysteries of soul mates; the Reverend

John Robertson, who was always there for my family and for me; Mark Gaudet, who joined with me in this journey and with whom I have learned and loved so very much; Debbie Kredich, my medical school advisory dean, and my friends Katharine Liu and Michael Battistone, who were always there to support me. My many thanks to all the people at the University of Texas Health Sciences Center in San Antonio who helped me form the foundation of who I am as a physician: the nurses on Labor and Delivery; the midwives, especially Jan Olsen; my fellow residents, most notably Barbara Schroeder, Shannon Turner Abikhaled, Julie DaVolio Novak, Mark Funk, and Animesh Agarwal; my dear friend Elly Xenakis and her father, Phrixos, who "adopted" me into their family when it felt like I had lost my own; Craig Witz, my first chief resident, friend, and doctor, who taught me about the finer points of female anatomy; Carann Easton, with whom I went to my first alternative medicine conference; Karin Brewer; the faculty who supported my learning, my growth, and my leaving to go to Arizona, particularly Carl Pauerstein, Oded Langer, and Robert Huff; and Chris Northrup, who taught me and mentored me while I was still a resident and who has supported me each step of the way since.

Many talented and passionate people dove into the unknown with me and helped to create the Program in Integrative Medicine at the University of Arizona: Dean James Dalen, who had the courage and vision to support the program, and his wife, Priscilla, who shared his personal caring and support; Joe Alpert, who took a chance and hired a young ob-gyn faculty member in his Department of Medicine to lead a controversial new program; Andy Weil, who, along with his willingness to share the breadth of his knowledge, gave me the freedom to create and the opportunity to lead; Sue Fleishman and David Rychener, who *were* the program in the beginning; Colleen Grochowski, who joined us early on as we pulled it all together and who became a wonderful friend; Sharon Scott, who was always there, personally as well as professionally, with passion and loyalty; Roger Kirkpatrick, who guided us in many ways and who became a wonderful partner in my life journey; John Tarrant, who created the "container for change," in which the fellows as well as the faculty learned to embrace their own woundedness and see the light inside the dark, and who blessed me personally with his deep friendship, presence, and poetry; the first class of fellows, Russ Greenfield, Karen Koffler, Wendy Kohatsu, and Robbie Lee, who were true pioneers and great colleagues, and all of the fellows who followed. I also need to thank the many faculty members who helped to build the curriculum and my learning: Marilyn Ream, Roxanne Whitelight, Ruth Langstraat, Dan Shapiro, Carol Locust, Harmon Myers, Cindy Thompson, Christy Allen, Margo Parker, Ilene Spector, Francis Brinker, Jeff Beeley, Steve Gurgovich, Kathy Grant, Susan Phillips, Marty Hewlitt, Donna Swaim, Gary Schwartz, Linda Russek, John Misiaszek, Jim Gallaway, and Nancy Koff. Thanks, too, to the other members of PIM, who gave from their hearts because they believed in the vision; other key people who helped along the way, especially Gail Patrick, Pat St. Germaine, Fayez Ghishan, Lyle Bootman, Sy Reichlin, John Duval, Francisco Garcia, Nikki Rogers, Jane Barth, and Barbara Raney; Alice Ferrell, who was a tremendous assistant and friend; Patty Popp, Marlene Callaghan, and Mary Helen Kaiser, who donated their time and talent to support us and were the first of many volunteers; my other friends who supported me limitlessly, Mary Koopman, Linda Freidman, Sabine Weil, Alice McKittrick, Barbara Anderson, Rosemary and Rod Parrish, Nancy Lowe, Kathy Reed, Joyce Rychener, Chris Grochowski, and Ted Koff; Richard Baxter and David Thorne, who each helped me broker the chaos, the politics, and the insanity, and helped me to remember what Rumi says: "There are many ways to kneel and kiss the ground"; Pat Blessington, whose wonderful work with me as a Jungian and a friend helped me to grow and learn through the challenges; and Barbara Prested, whose gifted hands and heart replenished my body and soul.

I have often said that the University of Arizona was the perfect place to pioneer integrative medicine, and that Duke University is the perfect place for its next stage of development. This has also been paralleled in my own personal and professional growth. Sincere gratitude to: Ralph Snyderman, the chancellor of the Duke Health System, who possesses the courage and the insight to challenge the existing health care system, for his support of my work; Gary Stiles, who has met the field of integrative medicine with an open mind and heart and has facilitated the growth and development of the Duke Center of Integrative Medicine (DCIM); Jean Spaulding, for spearheading Rich's and my recruitment to Duke; Charles Hammond, who began mentoring me when I was a medical student and continues to this day, sharing his wisdom and experience; my friends and colleagues at DCIM, Sam Moon, Linda Smith, Larry Burk, Jeff Brantley, Ruth Quillian, Marshall Adesman, and the rest of our team, with whom it has been great doing this work together. To the many leaders in the field at Duke, including Diana Dell, Mitch Krucoff, Susie Crater, Redford Williams, Harold Koenig, Richard Surwit, Paul Vick: thank you for your work and your support. To my colleagues in the Consortium of Academic Health Centers in Integrative Medicine, it's great to know that we're all in it together, and enjoying it along the way. Also thanks to Joseph DeNucci, a partner and friend in the vision; my friends Steve and Jodie Forrest, for the fun and the love, and, Steve, for all that I have learned from you and with you; Christy Mack, chair of the National Advisory Board for the Duke Center of Integrative Medicine, whose friendship has been inspirational and whose vision and commitment have moved the entire field forward; and John Mack, who always keeps me guessing (and smiling).

My deep appreciation goes also to the many individuals whose work and generosity in philanthropy have helped to change the world, including: the Congdon family, whose gift allowed me three transformative years at Dana Hall School; the Ungerleiders; the Martoris; the Zuckermans; the Colbys; Peter Lewis; the Georges; most of all the Macks; and Diane Neimann and the Philanthropic Collaborative in Integrative Medicine, for their pioneering effort.

An amazing cadre of individuals have guided me with their teaching, their mentorship, and their friendship, among them: John Kabat-Zinn, Larry Dossey, Cheryl Richardson, Rachel Remen, Saki Santorelli, Dean Ornish, Joan Borysenko, John Astin, Steven Petrow, Rosalyn Bruyere, Kevin Ergil, Clyde Evans, and Carol Aschenbrenner.

I also would like to acknowledge the many people who helped this book become a reality: Louisa Kasdon Sidell, whose early collaboration and hard work got the ball rolling; Robin Michaelson, who believed passionately in this project; Beth Rashbaum, whose skill and commitment are evidenced throughout the pages of the book; Paula Spencer, whose incredible talent captured the essence and all of the nuance of my message; Doe Coover, my agent, who shepherded this book through its many stages (as well as me through mine)—her help and guidance were invaluable; Greg Hottinger, friend and awesome nutritionist, who contributed his wealth of knowledge; Lynn Willeford and Gwyneth Cravins for the generosity of their time and energy; and the women in both Arizona and North Carolina, who gave of their time and of themselves to participate in Consciously Female groups. Your contributions helped bring the Consciously Female process to life: Lana Barker, Christine Stamm, Erin O'Meara, Mimi Griffis, Kimberly Lorenz, Nancy Lowe, Diane Katz, Mary Koopman, Barbara Prested, Sharon Criss, Carolyn Cooper, Ruby Moon, Glaeshia O'Rourke, Tracey Koepke, Jennifer Mungle Terry, Michele Lewis, and Laura Wood.

Finally, my deepest gratitude to my patients. You have honored me by sharing the most intimate aspects of your lives. I have no better teachers. Thank you.

—T.G.

My deepest appreciation also goes to Beth, Doe, and Robin for connecting me with Tracy and this project; to Beth (yes, doubly!) and Stacie Fine for their editorial help; to those aforementioned who helped provide the rich source material and interviews; and to the patient souls I am most conscious of every single day, my George and our Henry, Eleanor, Margaret, and Page.

—P.S.

Contents

Chapter 3: Health Care a Woman Can Love

Part Two: The Consciously Female Tool Kit:

Chapter 4: Commit: Tools 1–5

Chapter 8: Living the Conscious Life

    • The Feedback Loop.

    • Five-Center Balance.

    • Centers of Wellness Basics. *The Movement Center. The Nutrition Center. The Mind Center. The Spirit Center. The Sensation Center. Sheila's Story: Beginning a Plan.*

Chapter 9: The Cycling Pathway

    • What's Happening Now: The Primal Cycle. *Lindsay's Story: No Tick, Tick, Tick? No Problem.*

    • Landmark: PMS. *Rhiannon's Story: "I'm Not Myself Half the Time!"*

    • Landmark: Contraception Choices. *Jenny's Story: Changing Contraception Needs.*

    • Landmark: Unplanned Pregnancy. *Rita's Story: "More Ready Than I Thought." Anya's Story: Reversal of Impulse.*

    • Centers of Wellness Modifications for Cycling.

Chapter 10: The Fertility Pathway

    • What's Happening Now: Before Conception to After-Delivery

    • Landmark: The Baby Question. *Meredith's Story: It's Time—Isn't It?*

    • Landmark: Outside Fertility Help? *Hanna's Story: Choosing Support. Rachel's Story: Getting Off the Conveyor Belt.*

    • Landmark: Pregnant! *Cicely's Story: To Amnio or Not to Amnio?*

    • Landmark: Labor and Delivery. *Jo's Story: "I Can't Do It!" Helen's Story: Something Beautiful to Watch*

    • Landmark: Postpartum.

    • Landmark: Miscarriage. *Wendy's Story: A Farewell Ritual.*

    • Centers of Wellness Modifications for Fertility.

Chapter 11: The Transition Pathway

From perimenopause to menopause, as the reproductive system winds down 323

Chapter 12: The Transformation Pathway

After menopause, the second half of a woman's life 361

Foreword

Andrew Weil, MD

It is no secret that conventional medicine often neglects the needs of women. Although women are more likely than men to seek professional help for health problems and are also more proactive than men in matters of diet and self-care, physicians often dismiss their complaints, pay little attention to their special health risks, and ignore the very significant differences in men's and women's responses to pharmaceutical drugs and other treatments.

The recent reversal of policy on universal hormone replacement therapy for menopausal women should be a shocking case in point. For years, doctors pushed horse-derived estrogen and synthetic progestin on women at midlife, in the belief that this treatment not only cured menopausal symptoms but also lowered risks of heart attacks, osteoporosis, and other serious diseases. They even made women who resisted the prescriptions feel foolish for not agreeing to take "scientific" treatment. In fact, the risks of hormone replacement—especially increased incidence of cancer—were well known, but evidence for the assumed benefits was simply not there. It was the women who resisted who made the right choice. The rise and fall of hormone replacement therapy should become a case study of the mismanagement of women's health. I hope that future generations of doctors and patients will look long and hard at it to see why it happened.

One reason, of course, is that until relatively recently most physicians were men. Today equal numbers of men and women enter medical training, but I doubt that many of those women are able to continue to think like women and make use of their intuitive knowledge of their bodies by the time they finish.

The appearance of books on women's health written by female physicians is an even more recent phenomenon, part of the larger self-help movement that women are so active in. *Consciously Female* is one of the best examples of this kind of work. I am pleased to be able to introduce it to readers, especially because Dr. Tracy Gaudet is a colleague and friend who helped me create the Program in Integrative Medicine at the University of Arizona.

Integrative Medicine is healing-oriented medicine that takes account of the whole person (body, mind, and spirit), as well as all aspects of lifestyle. It emphasizes the therapeutic relationship and makes use of all appropriate therapies, both conventional and alternative. This will, I am sure, be the mainstream medicine of the future, but it is also the kind of medicine that women need now.

Women need doctors who will partner with them and empower them in their journey to optimal health, not paternalistic, authoritarian figures who just hand out drugs. They need doctors who understand that the body can heal itself if given a chance, who value natural remedies, and who know when and when not to use more drastic interventions. They need doctors who know that moods and emotions affect the physical body and who include spirituality in the total picture of health and well-being.

Tracy Gaudet is such a doctor, and she and I have been working to train others. Eventually you will be able to find the kinds of doctors you need and want. In the meantime you must seek out reliable sources of information and learn to take more responsibility for your own health. This book is such a source. It is full of general advice about a philosophy of healthy living that I agree with and specific advice about a variety of health concerns, from menstrual cramps to pregnancy. Tracy illustrates her points with numerous case histories from her own experience as a woman and as a physician specializing in women's problems. You will find it easy to read, gently inspiring, and reassuringly informative.

Tracy Gaudet and I are both proponents of *mindfulness*—bringing more conscious awareness to every moment in order to live life more fully and more competently. Mindfulness is the key to mastery of any skill or challenge, from driving a car to cooking, managing relationships, and, certainly, managing the body through the different stages of life. Being Consciously Female is simply being mindful of your body: learning about it, understanding its needs, paying attention to the messages it sends you. I can think of no better way to undertake the process than to let Dr. Tracy Gaudet lead you through it.

Introduction

What if you woke up every morning feeling that your body and soul were centered, rather than scattered? What if you viewed each menstrual period as an opportunity instead of a curse? What if instead of simply getting through tumultuous phases of your reproductive life such as pregnancy and menopause, you found a deeper way to get into them—and get more out of them? What if you could make decisions about your health and healing that were uniquely suited to your physical and emotional needs, your place in life, and your very sense of yourself?

What if you could work *with* your female physiology instead of feeling that your physiology is working against you?

To be Consciously Female is to be and to do all of these things. To be Consciously Female is to live your life in tune with the realities of your woman's body and all that it entails—its reproductive system, its hormonal shifts, its menstrual cycles, its seasons of fertility, and the changes it undergoes when fertility ends. To be Consciously Female is to actively access what's happening to you, body and soul, and to nourish yourself accordingly.

It sounds straightforward, and it is. Yet women today are often checked out of this level of intimacy with themselves. We're *unconsciously* female. And we pay a high price for our obliviousness.

My goal is to show you a process by which you can reframe and reclaim what it means to live in your female body, and to be conscious of all that means for you on a daily basis. Living a Consciously Female life means constructing a personal framework for your health and healing that can change and evolve through all the cycles and seasons of your life. Any woman can learn these techniques and apply them to her own unique situation. All it takes is a willingness to open up to a new way of thinking.

PERSONALLY CONSCIOUS

I didn't set out to develop a process for women to reclaim their consciousness about themselves and their wellness. Initially, I did it just for me.

I used to be as out of touch with my body as any woman. But a series of personal experiences led me to transform the way I regarded my own well-being. As I combined these new insights with what I knew from my medical training, I began to see that an entirely new approach to my health was in order. Later I shared these insights with colleagues and patients. That's how the Consciously Female way of life evolved.

Two women, in particular, started me on this journey. The first was a nurse working in Student Health when I was a first-year medical student. She found me in the examining room doubled over with horrific menstrual cramps. I'd suffered from them for years. Each period was so bad that, without prescription-strength pain relievers, I literally would take to my room for two days until the pain and resulting nausea, vomiting, and diarrhea faded. To cope, I had learned it was best to pop something like Motrin at the first twinge—my idea of preventative medicine! But that particular month I'd been so caught up in med school, studying for a big exam, that I completely lost track of my cycle. The first pains struck as I was heading to the exam. By the time I finished the test, things were so bad that I went straight for the clinic.

The nurse I saw dispensed pain medicine. As it began to take effect, the nurse surprised me by settling by my side instead of dismissively shooing me off. Gently she began asking questions: Was I under a lot of stress, and did that seem to make my cramps worse? Or was I in more pain when I was really tired? Did eating certain foods seem to make a difference? Did exercise? Were my cramps always bad at the same point in my cycle?

Sheepishly I answered over and over, "I don't know." I had never observed a single thing. I had never even thought about it! All my focus had always been on just getting through those two days of misery.

The irony wasn't lost on me: After four years of college and almost a year of medical school, all I had learned to do for my major menstrual discomfort was to take a pill. I had never been taught anything about how diet, exercise, sleep, or my mental state could affect what was happening to my body. I simply thought of the cramps as if they were some nasty invasive force, quite apart from me, to be endured for a few days every four weeks until they retreated.

The next month, not sure what I was looking for, I began jotting down my eating and exercise habits and what was going on in my life when the cramps struck. Nothing revealed itself. Not yet. I kept at it, though—and within several cycles, sure enough, the interplay between my lifestyle and my periods became very clear. When I was either emotionally or physically depleted—before exams or in the middle of a particularly demanding rotation, when sleep was erratic or just plain hard to come by—my cramps were most severe. When I was able to take better care of myself—say, thanks to a break between rotations—my periods seemed less painful.

I know it sounds basic. Nevertheless, it had taken me more than a decade to notice this connection. What else, I wondered, was my body telling me that I had not been attuned to hearing?

A few years later, near the end of my residency at the University of Texas Health Sciences Center, San Antonio, I decided to attend a conference being offered by Dr. Christiane Northrup at a coastal island retreat in Canada. Because she was a pioneering ob-gyn who specialized in holistic medicine, I figured she could bring some cutting-edge insights into my chosen field. But to tell you the truth, I was so burned out that I was mainly thrilled with the prospect of going to a remote and beautiful place to unwind. So I was in more of a vacation mode than a learning one as Chris clicked through her carousel of colorful slides.

Then one image grabbed me. It was a circular chart showing the concurrence of the menstrual period within the lunar cycle. Chris described the first half of the cycle—from the first day of menstruation until ovulation, also known as the follicular phase—as a time when women are more energetic and upbeat. We're more receptive then to others and to new ideas, she said, more "fertile" in every sense of the word. In contrast, she characterized the second half of the cycle (from ovulation to the start of your period, the luteal phase) as a more personal and reflective time, a time of looking back on what's come before and determining what needs to be readjusted. We turn inward.

In other words, during our menstrual cycles we wax and wane, like the moon. What a revelation! (She went on to explain how the moon and the tides are thought to be connected to other biological and emotional rhythms as well.) It made perfect sense to me. As Chris details in her book *Women's Bodies, Women's Wisdom,* "When we routinely block the information that is coming to us in the second half of our menstrual cycles, it has no choice but to come back as PMS or menopausal madness, in the same way our other feelings and bodily symptoms, if ignored, often result in illness."

Or to come back as wrenching menstrual cramps, I realized. I had never thought of the second half of my cycle as a time when I had access to my inner voice, the insistent whisperings about the difficult issues of my life, from my stressful medical training to my relationships and dreams. Like most women, I had always dismissed such restless ruminations as just the moodiness wrought by my period. Now I wondered if, rather than sitting out a few days of my life until the gloom passed, I shouldn't be listening more carefully. Maybe my menstrual "moodiness" was actually my opportunity for greater emotional honesty.

After that conference, I tried to fold this new perspective into my ongoing observations about my cycle. How did I feel just as my period hit? Did my energy level change throughout my cycle? What was on my mind? It was true, I observed, that I felt more depressed and overwhelmed by the circumstances of my life in the week or so preceding my period. Always an introspective person, I found that I wrestled even more with my thoughts as P-day neared.

Dr. Northrup's presentation and my own experience taught me that my menstrual cycle offered a time of heightened access to the very heart of my life. I learned not to dismiss the moodiness, not to wait out the sadness and the irritation, but to value these bleaker moods as authentic messages from my unconscious. Gaining that insight was an extraordinary turning point in the development of my consciousness as a female. If I listen carefully, I've learned, I can hear my inner self. Since then I've rarely experienced a cycle without being at least somewhat eager to learn where my thoughts will take me during that phase.

As I continued to observe my own menstrual cycle from every angle—physically, hormonally, behaviorally, emotionally—it was like watching a thousand seemingly random pointillist dots swim into focus as a beautiful Impressionist painting. It wasn't me vs. my menstrual cycle anymore, or me vs. the pain. It was all me.

From that kind nurse at Student Health, I learned to better read the interface between my body and my outer life. From Chris Northrup, I learned how to better read the interface between my body and my inner life—something I've come to think of as my female soul.

PROFESSIONALLY CONSCIOUS

My personal odyssey has naturally informed and shaped my professional life. I had not originally intended to become a physician. Although always interested in a health profession, I first studied psychology and sociology. The intense cramming and the punishing shifts involved in a medical education had always struck me as fairly unhealthy. The system seemed to beat out of people the very qualities that seemed essential for a healing profession—compassion, listening, the human aspects—all of which were instead delegated to the "ancillary" staff, like nurses. I was perplexed how such a system could produce people who were supposed to be facilitating healing in others. Like many would-be doctors, I wished it could be different. Ultimately, I realized that if I wanted to have an impact on the system, I needed to be a product of it to have credibility. So I began my medical training with the idea that I would one day work toward helping transform physician education.

I chose obstetrics and gynecology as my specialty because it affords a physician the opportunity to be present at birth. There is nothing more intense and real than witnessing and aiding the amazing transitions at each end of the life spectrum. Conception, gestation, and childbirth are pure miracles to me. Yet they are also fraught with challenge for a physician. Because the expectations are only positive and are so high, when things go wrong in obstetrics, they tend to go very wrong. The decisions can be extremely difficult and ethically charged. Ultimately, I felt it was a field where my interpersonal skills and my interests in counseling, psychology, and sociology would be put to good use. It's a field where the whole-person perspective is critical. And it's a rapidly changing field where we know we don't have all the answers, which means the door is open to looking at new approaches.

I was deep into my training when, during my residency, I first heard about a proposed Program in Integrative Medicine at the University of Arizona. An evolving approach to practicing medicine, Integrative Medicine (IM) seemed completely aligned with my own beliefs. These include the idea that there is a powerful interrelationship between the mind, body, spirit, and community in the interplay of both health and disease; that the best of conventional medicine should be used in combination with the best of complementary and alternative therapies; and that the physician should work in partnership with the patient. The Arizona program was the brainchild of Andrew Weil, MD, the Harvard-trained general practitioner (and popular author-educator) who wanted to teach other physicians about this revolutionary approach to health care and healing. Later in this book I will tell you more about integrative medicine, but for now, let me just say that the ideas for Andy's program resonated deeply with me. I had begun pursuing similar ideas during my residency, and although I had great support for doing such work in San Antonio, I always felt like a bit of a lone wolf. Now, it seemed, I was picking up the scent of a like-minded pack.

A series of events followed that I can only describe as amazingly serendipitous—and resulted in my becoming not a fellow (participant) in the University of Arizona's Program in Integrative Medicine but its founding medical director and later its executive director. It started with my attending a weeklong retreat on integrative medicine that Andrew

Weil was leading in Montana. Before I applied for the Arizona program, I wanted to reassure myself that Andy Weil, whose books I hadn't yet read, wasn't some quack. As the participants, most of them his enthusiastic fans, went around the room introducing themselves, I felt like the only health-conscious American unfamiliar with him. Of course it quickly became apparent Andy was 100 percent on the level and a visionary—no quack. During the week, I asked him more about his planned IM program, but was stunned to learn that I was not eligible to attend because I was an ob-gyn. The program was open only to specialists in internal medicine and family medicine, on the rationale that these are the two types of medicine considered most consistent with a patient's overall primary care. I argued that for many women, an ob-gyn *is* the primary care physician. Following that retreat, I chose to remain on the faculty in the Department of Obstetrics and Gynecology at the University of Texas after finishing my residency, but an interesting dialogue had been launched between me, Andy, and the fledgling program staff, which continued informally even after I finished my residency.

Meanwhile the national search for a director of the Arizona program had stalled when it became apparent that the senior-level candidates being interviewed were more likely to reproduce what they already knew (which was, after all, their expertise) than to invent a new kind of wheel (which was what was needed). Though fascinated by the prospect of the integrative medicine program, it never occurred to me to apply as director, because I was not a senior-level academic—and there was that sticking point of my being an ob-gyn! Here's where the serendipity kicks in. Around this same time I had booked a cheap ticket to Tucson thanks to an airfare war; all the previous months' talk of the program had piqued my traveler's interest in a state I'd never seen before. Since I was going to be there, I checked in with Andy Weil. That vacation turned into a job interview—and I've never looked back.

Both in Arizona and in my current position as the director of the Duke Center for Integrative Medicine at Duke University in Durham, North Carolina, I fulfill two dreams: teaching doctors a new way to practice while working to change the system, and teaching patients a new way to approach their health and healing.

One of my great joys in being an ob-gyn is that I am privileged to see women at all stages of the female life cycle, from the onset of puberty and the awakening of sexuality through menopause and beyond. Together, my patients and I watch each new life grow, from the insistent whoosh of a fetal heartbeat to that always thrilling instant when the baby wriggles through the birth canal to greet the world. I counsel women through the perplexing array of options in perimenopause. And I hold their hand when infertility, cancer, and other frightening problems throw snags into their hopes and dreams. This vantage point has given me a unique gift. I have been able to get a glimpse of the challenges that may be in store for me, and I have been able to take some vivid retrospective glances as well. Working with patients of all ages has made me keenly conscious of the whole spectrum of female life and my place in it. That knowledge informs the way I deal with medical decisions, the way I consider my fertility, and the way I feel about myself. I have witnessed firsthand the gathering degrees of self-awareness a woman can accumulate as she progresses through the stages of her reproductive life. Above all, my experience has shown me the usefulness of such a broad perspective on my life, one I would like every woman to benefit from.

My work has also allowed me to observe the remarkable differences between a woman approaching a given situation consciously and one who does not. I've seen the otherworldly flow of a laboring woman in sync with the dramatic, minute-to-minute changes her body experiences during labor, and the struggle of a woman who is fighting them. Whether a woman is a perimenopausal forty-something weighing her options for hormone replacement therapy or a fifty-year-old absorbing a diagnosis of breast cancer and trying to find healing while the bottom has dropped out of her world, she is better able to make clear, informed decisions that she feels good about, if she can tune in to what both her body and her soul are telling her. She is better equipped to work in partnership with her physicians, as opposed to having things "done to" or "done for" her. She is more apt to come out the other end of her experience—whether it was joyful, painful, sorrowful, or frightening—with inner satisfaction and a calm confidence about where it has taken her. This process is no big mystery. Its potential already rests within you.

HOW THIS BOOK CAN HELP YOU

I hope this book will inspire and challenge you. The material is divided into three parts, each with a slightly different route toward that goal.

Part One, "Ready, Set, Reframe: A New Way to Think About Health and Healing," lays the groundwork. I'll describe my Consciously Female philosophy in detail and make the case for how it can dramatically enhance your well-being. I'll explain what exactly I am asking you to be conscious of (Chapter 1: "The Body and Soul Reunion"). Then I'll show you the price of remaining unconscious (Chapter 2: "Consciousness in Action"). And since engaging with the health care system is a big part of health, I'll draw a picture of what it looks like to be a Consciously Female patient, from my dual perspectives in ob-gyn and in the exciting, emerging field of integrative medicine (Chapter 3: "Health Care a Woman Can Love").

Part Two, "The Consciously Female Tool Kit: How to Tune In to Yourself Every Day," is the book's practical centerpiece. Being a conscious female is largely a matter of process, of having the tools to obtain greater consciousness. In this section, I provide the specific tools you can use to access this information. You can use them to help you make any kind of decision in life. This is my favorite part of the book because I find that these techniques are new and life-changing for many of my patients. Use the first chapter in the section, "Commit: Tools 1–5" (Chapter 4) to launch your program. Then learn in the next chapters the various techniques I teach women at Duke and, indeed, use in my own life. These include exploring your history, observing your body and your soul, and using dialoguing and imagery techniques to readily access what's "on your soul" (Chapters 5–7). Some of these techniques may strike more of a chord with you than others. That's fine. Experiment with them. Ideally, you'll use bits and pieces from each chapter. Give them time to take root and try sticking with them even if you're skeptical at first. Eventually you'll learn what seems to work best for you.

Part Three, "The Consciously Female Life: How to Make It Real at Every Age and Stage" brings it all together. I'll explain how any woman can construct a conscious life plan by using the Feedback Loop and understanding her five pivotal Centers of Wellness (Chapter 8, "Living the Conscious Life").

The chapters that follow illustrate the Consciously Female approach to specific issues that arise during the different phases of a female life. No matter what your age, if you are past puberty, you will be on one of the pathways described in this last section: Cycling, Fertility, Transition, or Transformation (Chapters 9 to 12). These are the pathways that mark a woman's life. Their titles refer to a woman's hormonal and reproductive-life status, and they also signal the shifts that occur at the soul level as she progresses through her life. These pathways are not necessarily linear—you may travel back and forth between the first two during the course of your adult life. Within each pathway are key issues that I call Landmarks, experiences that are common to many or most women. They're akin to the "touchpoints" described by Harvard pediatrician T. Berry Brazelton, MD. He coined that word to describe the universal, predictable turning points that occur just before a surge of rapid growth in a child's development. These touchpoints, he said, become a window through which parents can view a child's learning. So I think it is with a woman's landmarks—those passages of development that can serve as opportunities to understand ourselves more deeply.

Throughout the book I've included the voices and examples of many of my patients. Often the best way to understand a concept is to see it in action and to hear how another person has used it to change her own life. To respect their privacy, I have not included real names and have changed many identifying details, but the spirit of their stories and the breadth of their experiences stand true.

What this book doesn't contain are a lot of edicts about how you should conduct your life. I've included ample explanations and advice, but my overall mission is not to simply present yet another woman's health guide. Rather, I want to arm you with a new way of thinking and a head start on applying it to your own unique life situations. A Consciously Female way of life is what I myself have embraced. I use its principles and practices every day in trying to get a better grip on who I am, how I'm feeling, and where I'm heading.

Many of the ideas in this book can be applied to men, too, of course. I've chosen to focus on women in large part because their health is my specialty. But also I firmly believe that the unique cycles of a woman's life afford her special opportunities to connect her physical experiences with her core self—and that she can derive special benefits from doing so.

Above all, I want to help you realize that the changes that come with being a woman—the small daily ones and the bigger monthly ones, the life-passage kind and the life-changing kind—are not just happening to your body. They are happening to you. *They are you.*

Consciously Female

Someone dancing inside us
has learned only a few steps;
the "Do-Your-Work" in 4 /4 time,
and the "What Do You Expect" waltz.
He hasn't noticed yet the woman
standing away from the lamp,
the one with black eyes
who knows the rumba,
and strange steps in jumpy
rhythms from the mountains of Bulgaria.
If they dance together,
something unexpected will happen.
If they don't, the next world
will be a lot like this one.

—BILL HOLM, "ADVICE"

Part One

Ready, Set, Reframe:

A New Way to Think About
Health and Healing

Chapter 1

The Body and Soul Reunion

What does it mean to be Consciously Female?

"I think that I will spend about half my life feeling like I am not myself. If you count the week or so every month before my period, when I am less than efficient, then throw in pregnancy, nursing, and recovery, and top it off with that whole perimenopause and menopause part, it really adds up. My question is—if I am not myself for so much of my life, who am I really?"

You are yourself. Every week of the month. Every month of the year. Every year of your life.

Let me show you how to embrace that reality.

Let me show you ways to work *with* your female physiology instead of feeling that your physiology is working against you.

Let me show you how to enjoy better health and a more fulfilling life by changing the way you take care of yourself—at every stage of womanhood, from your first menstrual periods through the last ones, and beyond.

As a woman's doctor—and as a woman—I am all too familiar with the complicated relationship we have with our well-being. We know it's important to eat right, exercise, get plenty of sleep, and so on, but we have trouble making the time. We yearn to be well yet ignore symptoms of problems. We nurture everybody else before ourselves. We depend on our strength even as we do nothing to build or maintain it. We find it easier to criticize, complain about, and obsess over our bodies than to admire, celebrate, or feel pride in them We dream about balance and rush to the next item on our to-do list.

Meanwhile, our energy levels, moods, appetites, and desires can fluctuate by the hour or the minute. Heck, even our waist size seems to change from one day to the next. A never-ending parade of female issues continually disrupts the brief periods of peace. PMS, irregular cycles, birth control decisions, pregnancy scares, pregnancy losses, pregnancy itself, postpartum weepiness, infertility workups, hot flashes, HRT decisions, yeast infections, lumps that show up on breast exams or abnormalities that appear on mammograms, problem Paps, cancer scares—you name it. Our reactions range from mild annoyance at each inconvenience to outright anger at the rude interruption in our lives. Sometimes we feel betrayed by our bodies. Sometimes we choose not to notice. Mostly we grit our teeth and wait for each "glitch" to pass and return us to our "real" self. Whoever that is.

We overlook the key fact that all of these experiences are real. The ups and the downs, the highs and the lows, the light moments and the dark ones. It's all authentic. It's all part of you.

It *is* you.

Unfortunately, the ordinary facts of femaleness have somehow become divorced from women's everyday lives. Our society may have more knowledge about the human body than at any time in history, for example, but many of my patients are surprisingly unfamiliar with their own anatomy, let alone the hormonal and reproductive rhythms that are such huge parts of being female. A woman's daily rhythms can blur by. We're almost too busy to eat or sleep, let alone respond to the more subtle messages our bodies and souls are communicating. Monthly rhythms get jangled, too. If I were to ask where you are in your cycle on this day, could you tell me? Periods are practically a relic of the past for the many women who choose to erase them altogether by continuously taking the Pill.

And the broader passages of a woman's life cycle are similarly downplayed, taken for granted, or ignored. Perspectives on fertility often amount to wishful thinking. Labor can be scheduled in advance and induced, its pain drugged completely away, all with an eye to convenience as much as medical prudence. For too many women I treat, menopause looms as a synonym for old age, despite the fact that it usually happens during one's forties or fifties—closer to the middle of life, considering that the average American woman's life expectancy is approaching eighty. Part of the widespread dismay over the findings linking one type of hormone replacement therapy with increased risks of coronary heart disease, breast cancer, and dementia, I think, was caused by women's perception that they were losing a magic bullet to offset the upsetting effects of aging.

I'm not saying that every medical advance is unwise, or that every aspect of each female passage is a thrill. But I believe that we are giving far too much away. We have made a huge part of what and who we are unconscious, and in so doing, we are not living the healthiest or most fulfilling lives that we can.

Our female souls have become disconnected from our female bodies.

UNCONSCIOUSLY FEMALE

What fascinates me is that this lack of awareness isn't limited to patients at a particular stage of life. It's as true of women just past puberty as it is of women well past menopause. It doesn't matter if they are healthy or sick, married or single, straight or lesbian, infertile or fertile. I see the same disconnect cutting across all economic groups, all levels of education, all races, and all kinds of professions. These are women who are smart, beautiful, accomplished, happy. Yet something vital is missing from their lives.

That missing element is consciousness, a nonjudgmental awareness of who you are and an ability to listen to the insistent murmuring of how you feel, inside and out. Your physical self, your body, is one dimension of you. Another, deeper dimension is your inner self or your soul—the essence of who you are as a human being. Your soul is the "you" that you encounter when you look past the immediate surface to encounter your feelings, dreams, fears, and instincts. Your soul is your inner voice. And your soul, as I'll show you, has needs that must be tended, just as your body does.

Optimal health requires being attuned to what both body and soul are telling you. A balance between the two—body and soul, equally nurtured, functioning in concert—is my definition of true wellness. When they are in sync with each other, your health can't help but benefit as a result.

The job of finding that balance rests with you. No one else can listen to you in the way that you can hear yourself. Your tears, your tension headaches, your laughter, and your energy surges—all are worthy of your close attention. Emotions, desires, and "gut feelings" are information about your state of being that are as valid and useful as your physical symptoms or your medical test results. Understanding all this data and using it to improve your daily living begins with a commitment to embracing it. If you don't value your sensations as messages, who will?

The irony is that it is the very same experiences that vex a woman so much that are her biggest picture windows into this consciousness. Menstruation. Pregnancy. Postpartum. Perimenopause. Menopause. Each experience we have been conditioned to view as a bother, a *distraction* from our everyday lives, is actually quite the opposite. The intrinsic nature of being female is cyclical: monthly (because of menstruation) and across the arc of a reproductive life. These rhythms allow us to access our inner realities in a profound, enthralling way—if we allow ourselves to pause and pay attention to them.

It's great to be female. It's even greater to be Consciously Female.

Annie's Story ⌒

From the time she wakes her family up in the morning until she makes the rounds locking doors and turning off lights at night, forty-one-year-old Annie feels dogged by a sense that there is something else more important she is supposed to be doing. "I get up before my husband and my kids, shower, dress, put on makeup," she says, "and that is probably the last time that I think about myself all day." By the time she drops her youngest child off at nursery school, her heart has already begun racing. She's always nearly late for work. Eight or nine hours of meetings, phone calls, e-mails, and deadlines later, she climbs back in her car to retrace her rushed, multitasked morning in reverse.

One day Annie showed up in my office complaining of a persistent burning sensation whenever she went to the bathroom. It turned out to be a severe urinary tract infection, which had probably worsened because she'd ignored the burning for three or four days before calling my office. I asked how often she drank water or other liquids and how often she urinated in a typical day. Annie looked embarrassed. "Do you know what?" she admitted. "I don't have time to go to the bathroom! I almost never leave my desk at work, and then I race home, start dinner, and figure out who has to be where. In fact, I cut way back on drinking fluids just so I don't need to be bothered going. I'm so busy that I resent the time it takes to pee!

"I used to think it was pretty humorous that the only time all day that I could manage to get to the bathroom was when my bladder woke me up at three A.M.," she added. "It's not so funny now."

Your physical needs don't get much more basic than water, food, and sleep (and next maybe sex). When you get to the point where you're not even allowing yourself the most fundamental bodily functions—in essence, tuning them out—that's pretty scary. On a physical level, it's simply not healthy. Beyond the UTI, Annie's practices were putting her at risk of dehydration and kidney stones. Her habits are troubling in another way, too. Neglecting to properly hydrate and void—elemental biological acts—reveals a deep disconnect with one's needs. If those things are missing, you have to wonder what else is missing. Later, in Chapter 3, I'll discuss five Centers of Wellness that every woman needs to stoke every day: mind (specifically, the intersection of your mind and your body), movement (including exercise and your body mechanics), nutrition (what you eat, or don't), spirituality (meaning a sense of meaning, purpose, and connectedness), and sensation (sensuality and sexuality, or pleasure that is carnal, tactile, visual, and so on). You can be sure that if you're at the point where you don't even have time to tend to your bowels and bladder, then the other foundations of a balanced life of good health, such as spiritual nurturing and sensual pleasures, probably flew out the window a long time ago.

What's more, people like Annie who ignore their physical needs also miss their physical symptoms. Ideally, she would have taken care of herself so that she never developed an infection in the first place. But even if Annie had good self-care practices but was nevertheless prone to recurrent UTIs, had she been more Consciously Female she might have noticed the earliest symptoms, such as the first burning sensations or the need to urinate more frequently than usual. She might then have self-treated—for example, by drinking added fluids as well as cranberry juice, a proven way to curb the ability of bacteria to stick to the cells of the urinary tract. Unfortunately, patients who ignore their symptoms also tend to be patients who postpone entering the health care system—as Annie did—until their problems are more severe.

Our bodies and souls are constantly talking to us. They generally speak in insistent whispers. If we don't take the time to listen, they begin to shout.

Laurie's Story

It was close to nine o'clock on a summer night, and Laurie, a thirty-two-year-old ob-gyn resident, was getting ready to perform a cesarean section on a patient. It was a routine operation and all went well; both mother and child were fine. The only thing out of the ordinary, in fact, was that a scant three hours later, the doctor herself gave birth to her own firstborn! Now, granted, not all contractions hurt. And not every first-time mother experiences a protracted labor. But no labor—not even a quick one—happens without a considerable number of gradual physical changes working in concert in the mother-to-be's body. It hardly seems reasonable for a woman—even a highly trained and disciplined professional like Laurie—to acknowledge nothing out of the ordinary going on in her own body while preparing for so remarkable an event as imminent childbirth. What does that say about her level of self-awareness? As a friend of mine observed, "She had the event. But did she have the experience?"

Perhaps Laurie had adapted too well to the traditional, vaguely macho model of medicine, which holds that a physician's responsibility for patient care should be unimpeded by personal conditions such as illness, fatigue, or having something else on your mind—or wedging its way into your birth canal! But she had so effectively tuned out the ruckus of her body and soul that I suspect she would have been equally oblivious had she been watering the lawn in her backyard instead of performing major surgery in those hours before giving birth. I fear that Laurie, by living this day like any other, lost contact with a miracle. More than being an astounding biological feat, childbirth is also an amazing opportunity to gain unparalleled insights into one's body, one's strength, one's relationships, and even one's sexuality.

Many of my patients report a new awareness of their physical power and grace after delivery, for example. "I can't believe I did that" is a popular refrain—one that's uttered with a fair amount of astonished pride. Mindfulness in labor has not been formally studied. But I often see its benefits in action in women who have had Lamaze-style childbirth training. Lamaze, which highlights disciplining the mind along with relaxation, imagery (finding a focal point), and breathing management, is one proven method that helps women focus on the experience at hand, with better outcomes as a result: Women who take Lamaze classes generally use fewer medications, have a lower rate of forceps deliveries, and express more positive attitudes toward childbirth both during delivery and afterward. The effects are even more dramatic in laboring women who are already skilled in meditation and other mindfulness techniques. When I walk into the birthing room of such a woman (and in my practice I work with many who use such skills routinely in their daily lives), the sense of calmness is palpable. From the outset, they're very centered and approach labor as an opportunity to delve deeply into what is, after all, one of life's seminal events. Needless to say, they almost invariably report very positive birthing experiences and, often, transformative personal experiences as well.

Giving birth is so unique for every woman that it is impossible to say that you can expect this or that. But I can say that if you are willing to engage, you will be surprised. You will learn things about yourself. This is true not only of labor, but of any event or transition in your life.

HOW DID WE GET HERE?

So what accounts for this rampant lack of consciousness among women about the state of their bodies and their souls? Why the collective tune-out? I think it's the by-product both of our conditioning and of our times. Let's look at four main threads that have brought us to this dis-connect.

Preoccupied Unconsciousness

First of all, it's easy to fall into unconsciousness *because we are driven to it.* Our culture and our daily demands conspire to claim every waking hour. Can you relate to that? I sure can. When I was in third grade, I clearly remember my teacher, Mrs. Jackson, promising that the age of technology would blossom in my lifetime. In the future, she predicted, everyone would work only three- or four-day weeks. Thanks to the wonders of our age, we would be freed from the drudgeries of office work and paperwork just as labor-saving gadgetry had freed our grand-parents from hours toiling over coal stoves and washboards.

Well, ha! Instead, the opposite has happened: We are plugged in to our work all the time. And this transformation has been so swift and complete that many of us can't remember another way. Once not so very long ago, if you couldn't reach someone by phone, you called back later; now we have call waiting, pagers in our pockets, and cell phones to plague us as we walk down the street or drive across town. Once you could look forward to long plane rides for R&R; now your laptop is ready to go as soon as the jet reaches a comfortable cruising altitude. E-mail, faxes, and FedEx can follow you to the ends of the earth. Don't even get me started on the "wonders" of instant messaging and personal digital assistants. The World Wide Web is well named, all right—we're all caught in it!

We overlook the fact that we are human beings, not human *do*-ings. One of my favorite health care commercials, for mammograms, cap-tured this perfectly. It showed quick cuts of a series of busy women, at work, tending children, on the phone, who kept saying over and over,

"I have to cancel" and "I don't have time." *I'm too busy for my own good* is the spot-on message. Like probably every woman who saw that commercial, I could identify with the impulse to postpone a screening test—and I'm a doctor! What woman hasn't been caught off guard without tampons in the bathroom cabinet on the day her period starts, or away on a trip some Sunday night when her new birth control pill series is supposed to start but she forgot to pick up the prescription refill? I can assure you that you have plenty of company if you're too busy to track your cycles on paper or if you rely on your doctor to remind you when your next Pap and mammogram are due. (Unfortunately, unlike dentists, most don't!)

It's not just our physical selves that suffer from overload. Ironically, the Information Age is the Age of Unknowing when it comes to having a real understanding of who we are in our own skins. As the pace of everyday life steps up, opportunity for contemplation and introspection gets squeezed out. And yet they're absolutely essential. Consciousness requires time. Not necessarily a great deal of time on any given day (later I'll show you quick ways to begin to acquire it), but it does demand a commitment. Nevertheless, many of us feel too stretched to devote even a few precious moments of each day to our interior lives—not realizing that doing so would help energize us, rather than being yet another burden.

On top of technology overdrive and a hurried culture, the very nature of being mothers and caregivers can get in the way of listening to one's self. The so-called sandwich generation—women at midlife with children at home plus aging parents—is especially vulnerable. But relationship nurturing is expected of females throughout their lives. Most women are programmed to ask others, "What do you need?" Other, equally important questions such as "What do *I* need?" and "What am *I* feeling?" slip beneath the radar. A new mother knows when her baby has been fed, changed, rested, stimulated, and vaccinated even better than she knows these things about herself. As the baby grows, so does the range of details for which she is responsible—discipline, wardrobe, education, checkups, child care, sleep schedules, school paperwork, and on and on. Her own needs are pushed aside. If it's not children absorbing your attention, it's your partner, your aging parents or grandparents, your siblings, your pets, your troubled girlfriends, maybe your office "family." In a family system, women are typically the "kin-keepers," nurturing and sustaining extended-family relationships by doing everything from sending all the birthday cards on time to organizing the annual reunions. And if, like me, you're not very adept at this role, you suffer the consequences of guilt, occasional hurt feelings or disconnection, and way too few family get-togethers!

Inattention to one's self is partly a function of time, of course. But inattention is also a function of guilt. Many mothers, for example, don't focus on themselves because they think it's selfish to make self a priority. Nothing, of course, could be further from the truth! The life coach Cheryl Richardson urges her clients to create an "absolute yes" list of the priorities that most require their attention. "Almost never do women put their own self-care on the top of that list," she told me. "But that's absolutely what needs to be number one." By nurturing yourself you do your whole family system a favor because you are in better overall condition to handle those responsibilities. Think about it. You aren't inclined to feel patient and loving, at least not continuously or happily, if you are depleted yourself. By making yourself a top priority, you also model for your children and your partner a great gift—the practice of "extreme self-care," as Cheryl calls it. Self-nurturing as a primary family value is not about being selfish, it's about being self-*ful*. To be self-ful means to be helpful to yourself so that you can help those you love. Everyone wins.

Medicalized Unconsciousness

A second reason we find ourselves unconscious is *because we can be.* At every stage of female reproductive life, a huge medical armamentarium exists to cure what ails us. Think for a moment about all the hallmarks of female life that a twenty-first-century woman can gloss over nowadays. Don't want to bother with menstruation? Now you can skip that week of placebo pills, start in on the next pack, and go for months without ever getting a period! Sick of fiddling with diaphragms and worrying about getting pregnant? You can slap on a patch and forget about birth control, or pop some emergency contraception should you goof. Don't want to be hamstrung by your biological clock? A young woman can choose to have her eggs harvested and stored away for fertilization at some later convenient date. Unable to conceive? Mind-boggling advances such as hormone therapy and in vitro fertilization have become routine; sperm donors, artificial insemination, and surrogate mothers mean that thousands of women who might have gone empty-nested now have cradles to rock. Worried that your due date is perilously close to a big family event you don't want to miss? You can select in advance the day of your baby's birth, by induction or scheduled C-section. Starting to experience the telltale signs of menopause (or hoping to avoid them altogether)? Here's your HRT. In short, we can breeze with a minimum of inconvenience through many experiences that were once practically the definitions of being a woman. Many women today spend more of their lives in a chemically altered state than not.

No doubt these advances often ease a woman's way. Yet I embrace many of the new technologies with a conflicted heart, for they come at a cost that is often ignored. Let's look at childbirth, for example. I wouldn't want a pregnant woman to be so wild with pain that she could not tend to the task at hand of pushing out her baby. And I wouldn't skip a C-section under emergency anesthesia for all the world if it meant saving the life of a newborn whose blood supply was suddenly at risk of being cut off by a prolapsed umbilical cord. Yet I also feel women have come to expect the medicalization of childbirth as a matter of course. Rather than their hoping for a natural experience and having to be gently advised that sometimes interventions are necessary, the opposite has become true. The typical obstetrics patient walks through her doctor's door expecting as many tests, drugs, and monitors as technology can give her. Many women, in fact, expect a pain-free delivery: "If I don't have to feel any pain when I'm in surgery," they reason, "why should I in ordinary labor?"

But precisely because childbirth *is* an "ordinary" event (I prefer "natural"), I'd argue that the pain of labor is not the equivalent of pain from an injury. The pain of surgery or an injury is a sign that something's wrong. The pain of contractions, on the other hand, is a sign of something going *right*. It's constructive, the evidence of work that your body is undertaking to achieve delivery. (There's a good reason it's called "labor.") What's more, having some awareness of the pain directs you in where and how to push. When women are given epidurals so dense that they are left with no sensation, they are unable to push effectively. The result is that they have longer labors and need more interventions such as forceps or vacuum delivery. Of course I'll do all I can to help a woman have a healthy baby. But we seem to have lost sight of the fact that birth is a normal, natural process experienced by women throughout the ages.

Or let's look at the routine way we "tame" the body's roller-coaster hormonal gyrations. The natural fluctuations of estrogen and progesterone, which admittedly can be dramatic, are frequently smoothed out so that a woman can experience daily life at a more even keel, relatively free from crying jags, cramps, feelings of dragginess, and so on. PMS, for example, is treated with everything from birth control pills to vitamin B_6 to Prozac—which was rechristened Serafem just for this female purpose. (Prescribed cyclically, antidepressants seem to work on a different mechanism than they do for depression.) We can similarly medicate away the mood swings and other effects of impending menopause, or at least make them more bearable. With this strategy of smoothing the disruptions away, only the most extreme peaks and valleys will manage to break into a woman's life. She'll be unconscious of all but the more intense episodes of PMS. She'll notice only the most extreme hot flashes brought on by depressed levels of estrogen. All to the good? Not exactly. The more subtle hills and dips of our hormonal fluctuations will also be muted. A woman may lose the blues before her periods, sure, but she also misses those bursts of dynamic energy that can come with the first half of her cycle. She risks flattening the experience of perimenopause and menopause so that she misses the amazing revelations that introspection and reevaluation often bring at the juncture between the two halves of a woman's life.

Again, I'm not saying that we *shouldn't* treat the symptoms of hormone shifts. I am totally supportive of a woman choosing to use appropriate modern advances—that is, so long as she has made her decision consciously. But conventional medicine is too quick to step in with remedies that may or may not be best for a given individual. Many cause a woman to miss out on as much as she gains. Of course, you can just as easily pursue alternative therapies without being fully conscious of how you feel about them, and wind up similarly removed from your best possible state of well-being. The key—whether you decide to take hormonal supplements or not, whether you choose an epidural or not, whether you try acupuncture or not, whatever health strategies you pursue—is to be fully aware as you make your decision, and to make the decision that feels best for *you*.

Willed Unconsciousness

Here's another basic but perhaps surprising reason we are unconscious: *because we want to be.* So many of the physical aspects of being female are problematic for many women that it can seem easier to look the other way. Consider the negative characterizations given to perfectly natural occurrences—our periods are a "nuisance," and the pain of child-birth is deemed a "curse," God's punishment for Eve's betrayal in the Garden of Eden. From the messiness of menstruation to the myriad of symptoms that make up PMS, is it any surprise that our periods are grimly referred to as *"that* time of the month"? Pregnancy, even when it's a cherished experience for a woman, nonetheless rocks her body with one seismic shift after another—nausea, skin changes, weight gain, swelling breasts, a revised center of gravity—and sometimes culminates in pain unlike anything she's encountered before. Indeed, nearly every aspect of your reproductive life, whether it's becoming a mother or choosing birth control, contemplating abortion or coping with infertil-ity, getting your first period or having them no more, rocks not just a woman's body but her very being. The ripples can be felt for years to come. Given the seemingly unpleasant sides of a woman's physicality, many opt not to get too close. I call this the Grit Your Teeth and Just Get Through It (GYT&JGTI) approach. And no, I don't recommend it.

All of those experiences are just the normal givens, the predictable effects of being born with a female reproductive system. When things go awry a woman encounters feelings she'd prefer to ignore. The alarm a woman feels when she discovers a breast lump, for example, is only the first stage of an emotional journey that may or may not end with the loss of one of her most visible symbols of femininity. No wonder many women put off going to a doctor to have it examined. A miscarriage never fails to stir a woman's emotions, whether the pregnancy was wished for or not. A loss has occurred, and the feelings of self-blame, lost dreams, and physical betrayal are often overwhelming. Even less frightening, less dramatic disorders tend to fall into the category of things we'd rather not dwell on. Your periods suddenly grow erratic and you have no idea why. You develop a yeast infection and you've got ferocious itching in places you can't even scratch easily. You get the picture—you GYT&JGTI.

Every day I see women who are one step or twenty steps removed from the things happening to their bodies. It's an understandable impulse to avert our eyes from the things we fear, dread, or simply don't like. But remember: These are not distant "things." They are happening to and within you. It's never in your best interest to play ostrich.

Let me make one clarification here: I'm not suggesting that you need to be hypersensitive to your femaleness every waking second of the day. There are times when it is very useful to possess the skill of "going unconscious," of purposely tuning out for a short period. This is also known as compartmentalizing. I call it "pushing the hold button." If you are not in a time or situation in which you can fully and consciously address the situation—you are at work and get your period when you were hoping to be pregnant, or you miscarry when your home is full of family at Thanksgiving—you might consciously choose not to deal with the matter at that moment. It's not blindness; it's a great self-protective skill. You can consciously set aside time later to examine your experience. Choosing a time that is right and safe for you to explore what's going on within your body and soul is an appropriate and healthy response.

Politically Driven Unconsciousness

Finally and not least, we have disconnected from our femaleness *because we think we should.* Around the late 1960s and 1970s, it began to be considered politically disadvantageous by many women to lay claim to our femaleness, our differentness. The goal, after all, was for men and women to receive equal treatment and equal opportunities. In the early days of feminism, women often chose to neutralize gender so that it could not be used against them—for example, so that they couldn't be deemed unfit for serious responsibilities because their cycles made them moody and "irrational" at certain times of the month. Those were the days of "dressing for success," when floppy bow ties, trousers, and man-tailored power suits aided the goal of looking, and in turn acting, as much like men as possible. At the same time, medical advancements such as the Pill allowed women to gain control of their reproductive ability—erasing one of the primary differences between the sexes, the vastly unequal consequences of unprotected intercourse. Similarly, practices such as taking birth control pills to lessen bleeding or PMS symptoms and taking estrogen to vanquish hot flashes came to be seen as boons. All the better for a woman to appear as unflappably interchangeable with her male counterparts as possible.

Concealing the differences between the sexes was surely an effective strategy to help women gain a more equal footing in a male-dominated society. But now that we have our proverbial seat at the table, I think it's time to reevaluate. When I made that statement at a recent workshop, a sleek, sharply dressed woman in her late fifties rushed up afterward to excoriate me. "Don't you realize that by saying things like that you're going to undo everything we fought for in the feminist movement?" she chastised. "Do you want to send us back to the days when people said a woman couldn't be president because what if she had to make a decision about war and it was *that time of the month?*" I was taken aback. That line of thinking had never crossed my mind. My point is that we are already, by and large, on equal footing with men in today's society. We have earned that seat at the table and it's great. Now we are ready to bring the rest of ourselves to the table.

Women need to be conscious of who they really are, in the boardroom, in the bedroom, anywhere. The importance of that idea is underscored by some recent findings of economist Sylvia Ann Hewitt. She studied ten prominent women in the "breakthrough generation," women who broke past barriers to become powerful figures in fields previously dominated by men. Unexpectedly, Hewitt discovered that none of her ten chosen subjects happened to be a mother. She assumed this had been by design, until she probed deeper. "None of these women had chosen to be childless," Hewitt writes in *Creating a Life,* the book that her study evolved into. "No one said, 'I sat down at age 30 and decided that motherhood was not for me,' [or] 'I planned on devoting my life to building a huge career. I wanted celebrity/power/money—children were an easy trade-off.'...Rather, they told haunting stories of feelings that were crowded out of their lives by high-maintenance careers and needy partners." One woman described her childlessness as "a creeping nonchoice." What struck me about the women in Hewitt's book—and the millions of other women she says have lived or are living a similar pattern—is their sheer unconsciousness regarding this central female experience. The women admitted they had never consciously examined their feelings about motherhood, never weighed their inner feelings and their career realities in order to arrive at decisions they felt comfortable with, whether the choice was childlessness or children. Instead, they had filed away the reproductive aspect of their femaleness, and then, when it was too late, struggled to come to terms with the consequences of their nonchoice.

I would like to remind women that being conscious means that there is always the opportunity to make the choices that will serve you best—and then to reevaluate and remake them if your circumstances change. If choices are made in a timely, conscious way, they can evolve with our changing needs.

I would like women to be able to use the tools that have liberated us, such as hormone supplements and birth control, not in knee-jerk fashion to flatten out every peak and valley of our femaleness, but in a thoughtful, individualized way. That means with regard for what's right for you and in your best interest, given the whole of where you are in your life at any given time. And then those tools can be reevaluated and altered or abandoned when necessary. After all, we don't all wear cookie-cutter navy suits with floppy red bows anymore. Fashion has moved beyond that to recognize the strength and individuality of women. Shouldn't health move beyond cookie-cutter approaches, too?

A DOCTOR'S VIEW OF YOUR SOUL

You know why your doctor cares about your body. But why should a physician care about your essence? I'm not your psychologist or your life coach or your guru or your nanny, after all. I care because as a physician, especially one who is actively working to create a better paradigm for practicing medicine in this country, I am committed to health and healing. And if I am to treat a person, I must treat the whole person. As I hope I've illustrated, your body and soul are intimately intertwined. To maintain health, to facilitate healing, and to live the fullest, best life you possibly can require awareness and balance. Therefore, you've got to be conscious of both—and so do I.

Breathing In, Breathing Out

Think for a moment about what happens when you take a deep breath. As you inhale, your lungs fill with oxygen—deeper, deeper, all the way down to your belly. As the in-breath moves air from the outside world to the organs deep within the body, it is transformed. Its very composition changes, from predominantly oxygen and low carbon dioxide to much lower oxygen and greater carbon dioxide. The oxygen is used by the body to nourish itself. And then you exhale—releasing the breath, releasing the carbon dioxide, to feed the external world.

The in-breath and the out-breath are inextricably linked. And they make a good metaphor for what it means to be Consciously Female. The very process of becoming conscious is like taking deep in-breaths, turning inward, toward our souls. As we fill ourselves with insight and self-discovery, we move into those hidden places deep within ourselves that are so often dark and unlit. In so doing, the very essence of who we are shifts. We can then bring forth from deep inside us a new material— not unlike the nourishing oxygen that is transformed into carbon dioxide—to benefit the outer world. That's our out-breath, our engagement in the world beyond the self, the transfer of our energy to our work, our relationships, and our responsibilities.

To be Consciously Female is to live in commitment to the whole of this process. But in today's society, women focus more on the out-breath phase of the cycle. We work like dogs. We manage families. We take on community responsibilities. We nurture relationships. Outward, outward, outward. Pant, pant, pant. Try actually breathing that way for a moment. What happens? You run out of gas. If we do not learn to take full, rich in-breaths to balance the out-breaths, we will not stay healthy. Sure, you can survive on shallow, unconscious in-breaths, but at what quality of life? You tire quickly. You don't feel quite right. You have only enough energy to focus on the present, not on where you're heading. Your inner life and your outer life have little continuity with each other.

The idea that the communication between body and soul is essential to a woman's health should not sound revolutionary. I'm really not saying anything that hasn't been understood by many different cultures for thousands of years. Whole philosophies of health are founded on the notion of balance between inner and outer. The yin and the yang of Chinese medicine is perhaps the most familiar example of this. Health is defined as the state in which the characteristics of yin (such as dark, moon, night, feminine, interior) are in perfect dynamic balance with the characteristics of yang (such as light, sun, day, masculine, exterior). Disease is thought to result when too much yin or yang accumulates in specific organs of the body.

Another example is Ayurveda, the body of Hindu literature regarding medicine, which is guided by the principle that the mind exerts the deepest influence on the body, and awareness is paramount so that you can bring it into balance. Ayurveda requires a state of harmony among the three *doshas* (elements): *vata* (space and air, which includes the functions of movement, respiration, and the nervous system), *pitta* (water and fire, which includes the functions of metabolism, digestion, and perception), and *kapha* (earth and water, which covers the structural and musculoskeletal functions). Similarly, in Tibetan medicine, health is dependent on a state of balance between the three humors: *rLung* (movement or wind), *mKhris-pa* (bile or heat), and *Bad-kan* (phlegm or moisture). Native American practices and beliefs are often based on the four cardinal directions (south, north, west, and east) and the four elements of nature (earth, wind, fire, water), which are thought to provide harmony and balance.

Thinking of your health in terms of balance has a perfectly natural place in mainstream Western medicine, too. By living most of your existence in the exhale mode, not only do you risk your wellness, you miss the amazing opportunity to reconnect your female body with your female soul, to align your outer life with your inner essence. In Part Two of this book I will show you how to take the "in-breaths" that will help you "breathe"—and live—in advantageous equilibrium.

The *Real* Windows to Your Soul

Luckily for women, the nature of being female offers unique access to this "total package," body and soul, that makes up wellness. I've explained what it means to be conscious. Now let's step back and take a brief look at what it means to be female. Obviously a glance at one's genitalia reveals one quick answer. But science is only now beginning to understand the mysteries within that distinguish the sexes. Our genes are one factor, setting the genders apart right from a zygote's very first cell divisions. Our chromosomes are a matched set—until the twenty-third pair. Women have two X sex chromosomes; men get an X and a Y. Call them your personal X files: a world of differences right from the start. Within ten weeks of conception, external genitals in a male visibly differentiate the fetus from a female. By the time she's nineteen weeks old, a female fetus already houses nearly seven million eggs, among them her mother's future grandchildren. (By birth, only two million eggs will remain present, and only about 450 or fewer will wind up being selected for ovulation.)

Hormones further divide the sexes. Both men and women have a complicated, self-remixing cocktail of them circulating within. This includes testosterone, called "male" hormone, and estrogen, "female" hormone, although both occur, in varying amounts, in both genders. Serotonin, a hormone that is used therapeutically to prevent depression, also occurs naturally in both genders, with men having more of it than women. The levels of individual hormones are constantly shifting, particularly in women, because of the cyclical nature of their reproductive system. Even women's daily hormonal fluctuations differ from men's.

Beyond hormones and genes, scientists have discovered a carnival of intriguing differences between men's bodies and women's. We're 10 to 15 percent smaller. Our hearts beat faster. We have twice as much body fat. There are even differences in the way our brains function—

women seem to process language differently and seem more attuned to detail. Blood flow between the brain hemispheres is 20 percent higher in women than in men. What does it all mean? We're not sure yet, but an entire new fascinating field of gender-specific research is exploring questions like this, as well as how men and women experience illnesses and medicines differently. We are learning, for example, that men and women metabolize drugs differently. And women have different symptoms of cardiovascular disease. In 20 percent of heart attack cases, women do not have the classic sensation of chest pressure radiating down the left arm. Instead, they may experience pain in the upper abdomen or back, intense shortness of breath, nausea, and profuse sweating. More women die within a few weeks of a first heart attack than men, and women are more likely to have a second attack within a few years. But until recently almost all the research on cardiovascular disease (and many, many other problems and treatments) has been done with male subjects, so many of these differences are just beginning to be acknowledged.

But the dominant gender difference, because it influences so many dimensions of our lives, always comes back to the X factor. We can reproduce.

Because women are designed to conceive and bear children, our lives are a series of cycles set within a larger circle that is the whole of our reproductive life. (Whether we choose to bear children or not, whether we are physically able to or not, is another story. Either way, we live within this framework of cycles.) *Menses* means "month." Month after month, our bodies release a single egg (or very rarely, two or three) and gear up for conception. If it doesn't happen, the uterus sheds its blood-vessel-rich lining, the nest it had prepared for the fertilized egg, which leaves the body as a menstrual period.

Your menstrual *period,* technically, is the series of days when you bleed as the uterine lining is shed. Your menstrual *cycle,* on the other hand, is the span of days (roughly twenty-eight, or one month) between the start of one menstrual period and the start of the next. (The actual length of an individual woman's cycles can vary tremendously, averaging from about twenty-five days to thirty-five days.) A tremendous cacophony of hormonal activity occurs during the four weeks or so of a menstrual cycle, each day slightly different from the next. Some levels rise; others drop. More than just your uterus is affected by these riotous hormonal undulations. Hormonal action also takes place throughout your body, in your ovaries, adrenal glands, thyroid gland, hypothalamus, and pituitary gland. Every system in the body is influenced, in ways large and small.

In addition to monthly rhythms, a woman's reproductive life follows a certain broader rhythm. Your monthly cycles don't just start up instantaneously one day when you're eleven or twelve and then stop on a dime at fifty. The gearing up and winding down of your reproductive capability works less like a light switch being thrown than like a fire being started, gradually, with the flames first rising and then falling until it eventually extinguishes itself. To use a different metaphor, your reproductive cycle takes you along various pathways of female life. First comes the beginning of menses (menarche) and a pathway of Cycling, in which a female is physically capable of having a baby although she does not choose to exercise that ability just then. Next may come a pathway I call Fertility, during which a woman chooses to try childbearing and may or may not (because of infertility or miscarriage) traverse through pregnancy and postpartum recovery. A woman may travel back and forth between the Cycling and Fertility pathways. Eventually, she enters the pathway of Transition, or the phase consisting of perimenopause (technically, "around menopause") to menopause (technically, the last period), the finale of her reproductive ability. When her periods have been gone for a year she reaches menopause. Its attendant hormonal and soul-level reconfigurations mark the Transformation Pathway, which consumes roughly the second half of life.

Menarche, menstruation, pregnancy, menopause. Once known as the "blood mysteries," there's actually nothing mysterious about them—at least not for women who are living them in a Consciously Female way. Each pathway, like each period, is marked by distinctive physiological changes that affect both body and soul. What's more, the nature of any natural cycle is that there are inward and outward phases. The tides move in and out. The moon waxes and wanes. A caterpillar cocoons and emerges from its chrysalis as a butterfly. The natural rhythms of menstruation and reproduction similarly support periods of external focus and periods of internal focus. It's the way your body is programmed to operate thanks to its hormonal ebb and flow.

I encourage you to engage these natural rhythms as opportunities to tap in to your inward reflections and then take outward actions. There's an old saying that your eyes are the window to your soul, and maybe that's true for somebody else looking at you. But for you, the windows are all those female hallmarks that you've been gliding right past without ever bothering to peek in. Take a look! I think you'll like what you see.

SOME IMPORTANT DISTINCTIONS

Often women think they get the concept of what it means to be Consciously Female, only to reveal in subsequent conversations that they have missed one of three key points. So I want to take a moment to clarify these important distinctions.

Loving Consciousness vs. Critical Consciousness

It's not enough to live with awareness. I also want you to do so *non-judgmentally,* with kindness and compassion for yourself.

If you are your own best listener to the clues of your body and your soul, then you need to have the qualities that make for a good listener. A good listener absorbs before she responds. A good listener is slow to judge. And a good listener is compassionate and forgiving.

The importance of being uncritical can be seen in the story of my patient Audrey, a sixty-two-year-old retired teacher, the hub of her busy family. She'd begun suffering from periodic shortness of breath, which she brushed off as the result of a hard day's work chasing grandchildren, or fatigue from an overlong afternoon running errands. A few months later, she developed chest pains. Still, she put off getting medical help. Audrey was *aware of* what her body was trying to communicate, but she did not heed its message. Why? Because she had been a lifelong smoker and was so filled with guilt over the fact that this might have caused her current problems, she could not bear to make this confession to her doctor. She ignored even those high-decibel shouts of her body and soul because she could not listen impartially. And her judgments worked against her: She had a heart attack.

I see this phenomenon all the time. A woman ignores sporadic unexplained vaginal bleeding, avoids making a doctor appointment because she feels embarrassed that she hasn't had a Pap smear in years. By the time I see her, she's got frank bleeding that she could no longer ignore. Does she think I will lecture her or think less of her because she has not been diligent about her Paps? Of course I won't—I want only for her to be healthy and happy, and that goal is a lot easier to achieve when symptoms are small than when they are full-blown.

Don't worry what anyone else will think. Don't assign baggage to your symptoms. Whether it's your body's symptoms or your soul's sentiments, just meet them and greet them. Let them in the front door, rather than sending them around to the back and hustling them down the cellar stairs, shushing them so they won't make any noise. Deal with them the way they deserve to be dealt with. Remember, they are part of you. Being Consciously Female means meeting yourself where you are. It means accepting yourself *no matter what* so that you can find your own best path to your own best self.

You won't always like the things you discover when you reconnect your body and soul. You might be surprised. You will face some difficult choices. That's all okay. Consciousness requires courage. And the payback will astound you.

Being Aware vs. Being Informed

One of the better developments in medicine over the past generation has been the dawn of the informed patient. We have informed-consent laws, open charts, patient education handouts on every imaginable topic. The average American understands a great deal about sound health practices (even if she doesn't always practice what she knows). More than ever, I find my pregnant patients can toss around terms like *hCG, alpha-fetoprotein,* and *effacement* as deftly as I can. It's been nothing short of a revolution. Having a familiarity with the issue at hand can help you re-lax and better meet it head-on, too. So I'm all for being informed.

I want you to realize, however, that there is a difference between being *informed* about your body and soul and being *aware* of them. A woman can be totally informed—yet totally unconscious. How is this possible? Remember Laurie, the doctor who performed a C-section and three hours later delivered her own baby? As a practicing ob-gyn, she was about as informed as a pregnant woman could possibly be. She knew on a physiological level how the stages of labor proceed and what their signs are. She understood what a protracted process it is, especially for a first-time mom, and how Braxton-Hicks contractions begin days and weeks before the more regular contractions work to thin and dilate the cervix. And I also know that as a caring, attuned physician, she has seen the amazing transformations that childbirth and motherhood have brought to scores of her patients. Yet she chose not to embrace these life-changing events happening right within her.

Knowledge itself is a powerful thing. You can—and should—learn as much as you want about a particular health practice or treatment de-cision. It's also useful to gather perspectives from different people, for example, those who have been through a particular experience before (whether it's pregnancy, miscarriage, ovarian cancer, or menopause). It's valid to seek second opinions and to learn about the full range of op-tions for treating a given problem. Even if you did all of these things, however, you would not meet my definition of a woman who is truly Consciously Female.

All the external information in the world cannot tell you about *your* experience. Only you can know that. And that is the most vital infor-mation of all. In a later chapter I will walk you through the five Centers of Wellness that each woman has—the primary arenas that add up to total well-being—and I'll explain how to evaluate your internal state in each of these domains. And then, beyond that, you need to assess your general body consciousness and soul consciousness. Part Two of this book will teach you specific methods for doing so. If we acknowledge and increase our awareness around the ways that we are in flux every day—if we begin to pay attention and tune in to the ways our bodies, our emotions, and our intellects shift throughout our cycles as well as throughout the phases of our lives—the result will be a prosperous marriage of information and consciousness. We can, very simply, make better choices about our lives. And that makes our existence better and easier.

Making Conscious Decisions vs. Making "Right" Decisions

Surprise! There is rarely a single "right" path to pursue when it comes to health and healing. As much as many patients (and physicians, too) would like it to be this way, wellness is not a matter of diligently following steps A, B, C, D, E. To be sure, there are certain courses of action that we know work better than others. We know daily exercise is one of the kindest things we can do for the body. We know that folic acid helps prevent certain kinds of spinal deformities in a fetus. Yet even when conventional wisdom has been supported by research, many of the particulars can remain fuzzy. How much exercise per day? Twenty minutes? Thirty? Recently the Institute of Medicine recommended sixty minutes daily. What kind of exercise is best? Aerobic? Stretching? Weight resistance? Or a combination of all three?

What's more, truisms we hold dear are constantly being shattered and re-formed. In 2002, two long-term follow-up studies of women who had mastectomy (breast removal), lumpectomy (in which only the tumor and surrounding tissue were excised), or lumpectomy with follow-up radiation to the breast found that there were no significant survival differences among the groups. The studies seemed to prove the validity of lumpectomy as a treatment. Yet twenty years earlier, the procedure was viewed with a great deal of skepticism. At that time, radical mastectomy—the removal of breast, lymph nodes, and muscle—was considered the gold standard of breast cancer treatment, the best hope for a cure. The medical community's general sense of the "right" way to proceed has shifted. Or look at the swirl of contradictory information available about HRT. Each new headline brings calls to my office, as women wonder what they should do in response to the latest finding about hormones and cardiovascular health or Alzheimer's disease or osteoporosis.

Answers aren't easy because there are a thousand variables for every situation, including genetics, individual history, health habits, the severity of a problem, your comfort level about it, and so on. A physician's job is to help the patient make the best decision possible based on the latest, best information available. Ultimately, though (aside from an acute crisis), the decisions are best left in your hands, because only you have access to the information of your soul (yes, that word again). You are steering the ship of your life. So watch where you're going!

I am not asking you to pay careful attention to yourself so that you will never make a misstep. Missteps are a given in life. They are often unavoidable no matter how cautiously we tread. And while we would never plan on a misstep or even wish for one, it is often through them that we learn a great deal. As the Dalai Lama says, "Wherever it is that you stumble—it is there that you find your greatest treasures." I am asking you to listen to the timbre of your body and soul so that you can make decisions about your life that are as fully conscious as possible. If you do so, you are more apt to respect those decisions, feel good about them, and follow through with them. You will know you are moving in the right direction because it feels right to you. And when it no longer feels right or you get new information that tells you it's not right, then you can correct your course.

Knowing that you are making conscious choices about the direction of your life results in a very different experience from just letting your life happen to you, being driven by happenstance and the wishes of others. Susan, for example, is forty-five. Her erratic periods and occasional night sweats and hot flashes indicate that she's clearly peri-menopausal. But when I delivered this information to her, Susan was thunderstruck. She was at the tail end of her fertility and had no children. This turned out to be a fact that Susan neither mourned nor celebrated—yet she felt traumatized by the realization that she had never really paid attention to the idea of becoming a mother and now that opportunity was slipping past her. It always saddens me when I see women who glide unconsciously from the days of "Oh God, I hope I'm not pregnant" to "Oh God, I'm never going to be pregnant!" They have never really asked, "Is this something I want or don't want?" It shifts everything just to ask the question. For someone who never asks, having the answer foisted upon her can be traumatic. Perhaps had Susan had such a dialogue with herself in her thirties, everything might have turned out exactly the same way—she might have consciously decided against having children, for whatever reasons. I suspect if she had, her misgivings (about childlessness as well as about impending menopause) would have been far less severe.

A certain peace of mind results when you know that you're going through your life tuned in. You can't do any better than that.

Chapter 2

Consciousness in Action

Seven good reasons to be Consciously Female

Your vision
will become
clear only
when you look
into your heart. . . .
Who looks outside,
dreams.
Who looks inside,
awakens.

⌒ CARL JUNG

Ignorance is never bliss when it comes to your health. Unconsciousness exacts a price. Some effects are immediately recognizable. Symptoms that are ignored erupt into unavoidable full-blown illnesses. Stress that's unheeded asserts itself in your body as a sore neck, backache, or a pounding headache. The toll of a life lived unconsciously can also be less immediate, although no less painful. Your relationships, your plans, your goals, and the choices you make may all be affected.

A woman who is Consciously Female, on the other hand, reaps a number of health advantages on both an immediately practical level and in ways that can have a ripple effect all through her life. Jon Kabat-Zinn, the founder of the Stress Reduction Clinic at the University of Massachusetts Medical Center, describes mindfulness as a lens, taking the scattered and reactive energies of your mind and focusing them into a coherent source of energy for living, for problem solving, and for healing. I like that description.

This dynamic process is naturally accessible to you every month if you are still menstruating. When women begin to really pay attention to their physical, mental, emotional, and spiritual changes from day to day, most notice the following pattern. In the first half of their cycle (from the first day of menstruation to ovulation), they feel sharper and more productive. They report feeling "on top of things," more "like myself." During the second half of the cycle leading up to their periods, most women notice that they feel increasingly emotional, even moody. PMS-type symptoms, from acne and irritability to weight gain, peak. Women report feeling "less like myself" in body, mind, and soul. (I will describe what's happening behind these shifts in detail in Chapter 9, "The Cycling Pathway.")

Simply becoming conscious that these changes are taking place, owning them rather than dismissing them, can help you improve your everyday functioning. By tuning in rather than tuning out, you can make adjustments in your life that correspond to what's happening within you. These modifications range from changing the supplements you take at different times of your cycle to being more compassionate with yourself and enjoying that longed-for sundae—guilt-free—in the midst of your PMS. You might even rearrange your activities across your cycle. For example, maybe you try to schedule important presentations that require you to feel outgoing and sharp during the first half of your cycle. Or if that's impossible (since many of the realities of everyday life are inflexible), you might recognize that you'll perform better at a big meeting that falls in the days before your period if you allow yourself more time to prepare and get centered, rather than trying to dive in and wing it.

Besides the second half of her cycle, there are other times in a woman's life when she has greater access to her inner reality if she chooses to look. Pregnancy, the postpartum phase, and the peri-menopause years leading up to menopause are marked, like the menstrual cycle, by dramatic hormonal shifts that represent great natural opportunities to get closer to who you really are and what you really need. It's no coincidence that such opportunities are linked with major life transitions, when a woman is filled with reactions, fears, enthusiasms, and ideas as she evolves from one version of herself to another. But even a woman who is postmenopausal can set aside planned time to hear her inner voice. For her, it's simply a matter of being mindful of the need, and of the benefit.

The connections between body and soul, between mindfulness and healthfulness, are amazing and wide-ranging. Every aspect of your well-being will be touched. Let me walk you through seven of the biggest advantages to living Consciously Female.

1. OPTIMIZE YOUR HEALTH AND HEALING ABILITY

Let's start with the broadest, most basic benefit. Consciousness is a tremendously powerful tool for helping your body perform at the peak levels it was designed for. In an oversimplified nutshell: Be aware, be well.

Every human is made up of interrelated systems—circulatory, digestive, nervous, immune, reproductive, and so on. All of these systems interface to create the larger ecosystem that is the human body. It's a perfect example of that old adage that the whole is greater than the sum of its parts. Beyond this, your body (all of these interrelated physical systems, including your brain and mental faculties) also interfaces with your soul (your inner self). Health results from the strength of all these individual systems, both separately and together.

The stronger each system within the body, the better they are able to work together to combat the inevitable adversities that we all face sooner or later, whether that hardship takes the form of a cold or cancer. When the body's systems are depleted, it becomes harder for them to perform. Studies show that the infection rates for cold and herpes viruses increase in a corollary relationship to increased stress, for example. In my own case, I discovered during the stressful days of my medical residency that the severe premenstrual cramps I have always suffered would invariably worsen if that part of my cycle fell during times when I was on call or right after being on call. Why was that? Because being on call would require me to be awake for thirty-six hours at a time, grabbing meals (sometimes from vending machines) on the run. With my systems depleted, my already uncomfortable cramping would morph into the period from hell.

That's not to say that if you do everything "right" and build up superstrong systems that you'll never get sick or die. Sooner or later, everybody does both. In fact, things go awry all the time—we stub toes, get pimples, catch colds, wake up feeling blue. But the body is brilliantly designed to withstand setbacks and to repair itself. You can see this in action the next time you cut yourself. Blood from the broken capillaries beneath the skin immediately begins to flow. Then plasma and fibrin in the blood crowd at the wound's surface to thicken the blood, or clot. A protective scab begins to form from the hardened blood. The scab prevents germs from entering the wound, as do white corpuscles that have gathered beneath the scab. In this well-nurtured microcosm, new skin can then safely form, with the protective scab falling away when the process is complete. *Voilà!* A healed cut. By cleaning the wound and applying a bandage, you're enhancing a natural process of the body trying to regain its equilibrium.

The body is remarkably resilient. It actively seeks to restore itself. No matter how many babies I deliver, I never fail to be impressed how, within minutes of a birth, the uterus shrinks from the size of a watermelon that stretches from the pubic bone to the rib cage down to the size of a large grapefruit. It contracts in order to stop the bleeding; if it didn't, the mother would die of hemorrhage. Other kinds of physical havoc wreaked by childbearing are similarly resolved by the body's cellular and hormonal autopilot. After being stretched flat to accommodate a baby's exit from the womb, the accordion-like pleats lining the vagina, called rugae, gradually reattain their former shape within three weeks of delivery. Perineal tears or wounds from episiotomy repair themselves. By six weeks postpartum, and often earlier, a mother's reproductive system has healed and she's capable (physically at least, even if this isn't the ideal) of starting the process all over again.

My colleague Andrew Weil likes to point out that the word *healing* means "making whole"—restoring integrity and balance. (And the root meaning of *health* is "wholeness.") "Even when treatments are applied with successful outcomes," Andy writes in his book *Spontaneous Healing,* "those outcomes represent activation of intrinsic healing mechanisms, which, under other circumstances, might operate without any outside stimulation." It's impossible to overestimate this extraordinary ability.

We tend to think it's the antibiotics that cure a case of pneumonia, or a cast that fixes a broken bone. But the antibiotics merely facilitate the healing by reducing the bacterial load that your body has to fight. The cast (in a clean break) merely helps the bone stay in a fixed position. These medical interventions don't technically provide the cure; they help your body to do the job it's designed and programmed to do.

So what's your role? How do you optimize the systems that keep you healthy and speed healing when you're sick? How do you make the body's natural healthfulness and healing capabilities work for you? That's where consciousness comes in. *You need to be aware of the needs of your body and soul at any given time and you need to be aware of when they are depleted.* Only then can you modify your actions to best suit your changing circumstances (whether that's a cold, stress, shifting hormonal levels during your period or menopause, or a fetus growing within you).

Let's go back to that ordinary cut. A study of healthy dental students looked at their recovery times from a minor scalpel incision on the palate. Once the experiment was done in the relaxed months of summer; then it was repeated on the same group of volunteers in the middle of exams. When the students were under a great deal of stress during the latter test, their cuts took a full three days longer to heal. Their bodies possessed the same innate healing mechanism as they had in summer, but the presence of untended high stress slowed that mechanism down. The same is true of a woman suffering PMS, recovering from childbirth, trying to conceive, or wishing to avoid preterm labor.

Stress is the body's perception of danger that requires behavioral change. Adrenaline and cortisol levels rise. Blood pressure goes up, as do your respiratory rate and the blood flow to your muscles. It's a no-brainer that circumstances that trigger a stress response—a dizzy work schedule, exams, grief, whatever—are going to compromise the effectiveness of the systems that run your body. If you are conscious of the stress effects and can work to ease them, on the other hand, you clear the way for your body to have a better shot at proceeding the way it was designed.

Karen's Story: Running on Empty

Karen's appointment was for her annual exam. She especially wanted to discuss a specific problem that had dogged her for the better part of the past year. "I always had the usual PMS stuff," began the twenty-nine-year-old mother of two small boys, who worked as an accountant in her father's firm. "But lately it seems to get worse every month. My husband calls me Dr. Jekyll and Ms. Hyde. Some days I feel like such a mess I hardly want to get out of bed. I lose my temper, can't sleep . . . what's wrong with me?"

The exact causes of premenstrual syndrome and its more severe form, PMDD (premenstrual dysphoric disorder, which affects between 5 and 10 percent of PMS sufferers), are unknown. Hormonal changes are almost certainly behind them in large part, but the specific mechanism is still a matter of speculation.

Aside from the debilitating premenstrual symptoms, Karen showed no other signs of illness. What became clear, however, as I updated Karen's history and conducted her exam, was that she was running on empty. She never felt she had enough time. She rushed between work and home and child rearing with little time for herself, much less for her relationship with her husband. Her exercise consisted of walking from her car across parking lots to the office or the store. Her diet was mainly diet Coke, fast food, and leftovers from the kiddie food—pizza, chicken nuggets—she served her finicky sons. In a word, she was depleted.

When I see such a situation, I'm faced with a choice: I can medicate the symptoms, and/or I can show the patient nonmedical steps to alleviate the situation. In Karen's case, we agreed that she would start by making several small but important changes in her life to restore some much-needed balance. It wasn't that anything was clearly "wrong" with her so much as that she needed a bit more to be "right."

Simply pointing out the obvious and having a patient acknowledge it is often a catalyst for change. In fact, making the commitment is the first step in any change program.

Together we created strategies across several different dimensions of Karen's life. She agreed to try consuming fewer prepared foods and more whole foods. She'd try to cut back to one soda a day (and not for breakfast anymore!) and switch to water. I recommended a vitamin supplement with iron, something Karen was lacking. I taught her breathing exercises that she could use for relaxation even at her desk or behind the wheel of her car. She decided to try awakening earlier—especially during the phase of her cycle when she felt great—to exercise to a home video. I also suggested she begin keeping a journal, both as an outlet for venting and as a way to track her symptoms from day to day.

A few months later, I ran into Karen and her husband at the movies. She couldn't help coming over to whisper in my ear. "This sounds crazy, but all the little stuff added up. I feel a lot better. I joined a gym and switched to a flex schedule at work. I still get cramps, but they're manageable now," she said. "And there aren't any more Dr. Jekyll jokes around our house."

2. DETECT PROBLEMS SOONER

Just as paying attention to your needs stokes your overall health, consciousness can help you become aware of the earliest signs of life's inevitable glitches. If you have a good sense of what is normal for you, then you're far more likely to identify when something is amiss. And once you notice the first, slightest evidence of change, you can more quickly take steps to resolve the matter before it advances to a serious problem. In Part Two, I'll give you some tools for making observations about the status of your body and soul.

Being Consciously Female is largely a matter of paying attention—of watching and listening to what your body and soul have to say to you. It's so easy for all of us to disconnect. The buzz of everyday life, fears, prejudices—as I've illustrated, we have no shortage of "good reasons" for ignoring ourselves. Recently a woman came in complaining of vaginal pain. Upon examination, I found a visible cyst the size of a plum. Cysts don't grow to that size overnight. How could she not have noticed it was there? The answer, of course, is that she never looked. And she never noticed the changing sensations until she was in full-blown pain. Like many women, she'd been brought up in a culture that discourages looking at one's own vulva. I've seen women who can't tell me the date of their last menstrual period or how long a typical period lasts. Or who aren't sure how long that discoloration on the areola around their nipple has been there, or haven't noticed that their breasts are always lumpy. We don't know because we haven't taken the time to pay attention. I can slip into this kind of disconnect myself. Consciousness takes discipline.

As you become familiar with yourself, you'll also learn your body's weak spots. We all have them. Although these bellwethers are highly individualized, for women they frequently appear as recurrent UTIs, yeast infections or other vaginal infections, worsening PMS or cramps, easily caught colds, headaches, and backaches. For you, it might be something else—maybe a monthly eruption of acne or a tendency to migraines. For me, one of them is my left shoulder. When I start to notice a tightness there—hopefully before the full-force spasms have begun—I know I need to pay a lot more attention to everything from my overall stress level to what and how I lift. I apply heat, take Motrin, schedule a massage or see an osteopath if I can, do some visualization, and get extra sleep. If I don't respond to those earliest twinges, then the next thing I know, I cannot even turn my head!

The same therapies don't work for everyone. Over time you'll be able to tailor what works best for you. It's a matter of paying attention and experimenting. When my shoulder first began bothering me under stress, someone advised me to work the muscles in order to "work out" the pain. Yet when I tried weight lifting, the muscles became even more prone to spasm. Eventually I discovered what worked better. Over time I have fine-tuned the plan described above, adding B_6 in the second half of my cycle and taking time to journal. Someone with similar symptoms might benefit more from exercising through the tight muscle. You have to find out what works for you.

Often, noticing the early signs and symptoms allows you to self-treat or to take preventative steps so that you never get to the point where you need to see a doctor. When you consider that 60 to 90 percent of physician visits are related to stress, a condition that is very much within your power to address, the financial savings alone make it worth paying attention. Here's an example of appropriate self-care responses in action: Relaxation training has been found to produce a 38 percent improvement for people with migraine headaches and a 45 percent improvement for those with tension headaches. When combined with additional therapies such as biofeedback (a relaxation technique that uses electronic equipment to amplify body responses) or cognitive restructuring (a way of revising how you think about a problem by rewriting your internal "script"), up to three-fourths of chronic headache sufferers find relief.

However, if you can't resolve the problem on your own and feel it's right to see a doctor, of course you should. Even if you're very good at picking up on early symptoms, you might not know what the information points to—not in the direct way that, say, chest pains are solid clues to cardiovascular problems or a breast lump needs to be biopsied for cancer. If you have symptoms that concern you, present them. And be persistent about making sure your doctor hears you instead of dismissing you. At the Duke Center for Integrative Medicine, I see a lot of women who have been to other doctors already. Over and over I hear, "You're the first person who has taken me seriously!" If a complaint doesn't fit into an obvious diagnosis, doctors may dismiss it—causing the patient to leave the office even more stressed. That's counterproductive. I'm not trying to encourage you to be a hypochondriac scurrying to the doctor to report every unusual event. Rather, I want to encourage you to value and honor your experiences and observations—and to find a physician who does the same.

Moira's Story: Sending Up Flares ⌒

Moira, forty-four, had begun spotting between her periods. This is not especially unusual in perimenopause, which Moira plausibly qualified to be in considering that this prelude to menopause can run several years before the final period. Still, the spotting did not seem natural to her at all. She had no other symptoms of perimenopause. What's more, her Paps had always been normal and she had no history of abnormal bleeding and no other gynecological problems. Indeed, nothing else seemed wrong except the breakthrough bleeding and a nagging sense of discord.

"This just feels wrong," Moira insisted.

Since I had recently sampled her endometrial tissue for something else and it was normal, I might have said, "Don't worry, we'll just keep an eye on it." I could have planned to repeat the sample at a later date and meanwhile watched for more symptoms of menopause. But I didn't, because I knew that Moira typifies what it means to be Consciously Female. She knows her body well and is aware of what's normal for her. Therefore her concern about her symptom was a bit of data I could not ignore.

I did an endometrial biopsy in the office that day. The tissue from her uterus showed a precancerous pathology. Uterine cancer is not an aggressive disease, but her uterine lining was abnormal enough that, if left untreated, it would eventually have progressed to cancer. It's possible that her previous sample had not picked up the precancer (although a later one probably would), but more likely the tissue had changed across time. We scheduled a simple hysterectomy.

Would Moira have died of cancer within six months if we hadn't done the biopsy that day? Almost certainly not. Had we monitored the situation, we'd have caught it later in plenty of time. But she's undoubtedly in a better position for having been persistent about her doubts; not only has she resolved the problem early, but she has the peace of mind of not having cancer or worrying about the possibility. And she can feel good about having listened to and respected her body's and soul's messages.

3. BOOST YOUR HEALTH GOALS

Trying to get pregnant? Maybe you'll get lucky within the first few times you try to conceive. On the other hand, your body furnishes many clues to fertility that you can read to aid the pursuit of your goal. For example, knowing precisely where you are in your cycle, which is indicated by the quality of your cervical mucus and your basal body temperature, can help you pinpoint your most fertile times. So can more subtle clues, such as a dip in your mood or a bump in your libido. Alice Domar, director of the Mind/Body Center for Women's Health at Boston IVF, a fertility and in vitro fertilization center, has demonstrated that using relaxation tools and having support can improve fertility outcomes. And of course such information is also useful if you're trying *not* to conceive.

Want to lose weight? You'll need to understand the health habits that have packed on the pounds in the first place before you can effectively (and permanently) shed them by altering those habits.

Determined to remain fit in your fifties and beyond? Postmenopausal fitness involves more than making a commitment to exercise every day and taking vitamins and possibly hormones. You will want to be alert to the shifts in every part of your makeup so you can make the adjustments that will most benefit you individually. You'll want to avoid writing off every change as "just age" until it's too late to do anything about them. For example, glucosamine sulfate supplements can help prevent the rapid advance of osteoarthritis if begun as soon as symptoms of joint pain appear. Vision changes need to be monitored closely, since the outcomes for treatment of macular degeneration and glaucoma, two common sight thieves, are better when caught early. A sudden tendency to constipation can be a surprising presenting symptom of colon cancer. To meet the goal of health requires a multidimensional awareness.

Many of my new patients are dubious that keeping journals, doing body checks, monitoring the experience of their periods, and other Consciously Female tools can impact their presenting problem. But all of these practices are ways to collect information. And the more data you have to work with, the better equipped to achieve your health goals you will be. This point is fairly obvious but worth highlighting because I consider it one of the most positive benefits of a Consciously Female life. There is no downside.

Tamara's Story: Seeing the Bigger Picture ⌒⌐

By the time I met her, Tamara weighed 250 pounds and had been fighting fat for thirty years—more than three-fourths of her life. "I can't remember a time when food wasn't both my comfort and my enemy," she told me. In school, Tamara took refuge in being the smart, caustic one in her crowd and eventually channeled these characteristics into a career as a newspaper reporter. "It was a perfect choice for someone used to being on the outside looking in," she explains. "And instead of being judged by my looks, I am judged by my words."

But life-threatening high blood pressure was increasingly putting her at risk for stroke and heart attack, and she was borderline diabetic. "I didn't want to go from one medication to another, until taking prescription pills became as much a part of my life as eating Oreos," she confessed. Although Tamara understood very well about nutrition and how to lose weight, she was unable to make it happen.

I introduced Tamara to my Consciously Female approach with the idea of getting her in touch with her whole self—not just the morbidly obese outer package. Through guided imagery (see Chapter 8), she found insights into the dynamics behind the disconnect between her mind and her body. Her head knew what and how much she should eat, yet her body was unable to comply.

Once the imagery exercise was under way, I asked Tamara to think of an image that represented her weight—whatever popped into her head. "A straitjacket," she said, "with only my hands, feet, and head able to wiggle." I then asked her what she might want to say to that image. This kind of imaginary conversation, which later I will show you how to do, can be a constructive way to tap in to one's inner feelings—feelings that you may not even be aware that you have.

"Why are you here?" she asked the image of the straitjacket. She reported imagining that it replied, "Because I define you. You need me. Without me, you wouldn't know who you are."

I asked Tamara to begin a journal to write down her dreams, observations, and thoughts. I also asked her to take one step that would demonstrate a behavioral commitment to controlling her weight. (She gathered information on joining Weight Watchers.)

In the next guided imagery session, the image that came to Tamara's mind was a box, the kind that a stove or refrigerator could come in. She could move around in it but not get out. The box image conceded that she could cut a hole in the top to stick her head out, but she had to come back inside if it wanted her to. She continued Journaling and in her next behavioral step joined Weight Watchers and signed up for a gym. A third session conjured up the box again. This time, Tamara found herself telling this image that she needed to be able to stand outside it. It was fearful and resentful. "I care for you deeply, but I am ready for more independence," she found herself saying.

By our fourth session, the image that came to mind for Tamara— now able to put in a half hour on a treadmill and work with free weights—was a ladder, with endless rungs stretching to the sky. "I was stunned that my conversations with the box—my own unconscious metaphor for my fat self—were so power-packed with uncomfortable truths," she told me later. "I felt almost a physical rush, a feeling of joy and weightlessness."

What Tamara experienced was not a simple matter of "mind over matter." Rather, the exercises allowed her to realize that a part of her felt very much at home in her obesity, and that part of her would sabotage her at every turn until she became conscious of it and could work through it. Over the next six months, she lost fifty pounds, was able to decrease her blood pressure medications, ran a seven-kilometer charity race, and applied for a promotion at work.

4. SPARE YOURSELF THE "RICOCHET EFFECT"

There's a very common phenomenon I see: putting it off. There are a million reasons for ignoring a problem, none of them particularly good.

Maybe you're afraid, or preoccupied, or busy, or in denial. (Or all of the above!) So you put off dealing with it, until tomorrow, or next week, or maybe (you hope) never. Or you repress it, so that the worry immediately gets buried in your unconscious, never to see the light of day. The problem is that ignoring a health problem is only your *wish* that it will disappear. It almost never does. Unless you actively process a problem—for instance, by having a symptom checked out, by self-treating, or by venting an emotion—you will wind up having to deal with it later, because it will eventually express itself again (or continue to express itself), and very likely in a more intense and significant way than it did at first. Often this later expression appears in an unexpected way not obviously linked to the first instance.

I call this "paying now, or paying later with interest." And it's why it's best to be attuned to the here-and-now of your body and soul, and to respond promptly and accordingly. During a postpartum checkup recently, Sarah, a twenty-seven-year-old first-time mom, mentioned that her dad had just died. She hastily added that her instinct was not to let herself express too much grief. "Even though I really wish my dad could see his granddaughter, I figure I have a lot to be happy about with the baby and he wouldn't want Gracie to see her mom crying all the time," she told me. I cautioned Sarah that by ignoring her very real feelings of grief, by not honoring them and allowing herself to express them, she was in fact putting herself at risk for physical problems. Humans are uncannily good at repressing psychological pain and unpleasantness. But these same strong emotions will find a way to express themselves somehow. Often they translate into stress—muscles tense, tempers flare, and so on. I didn't want Sarah to wind up with a bad back or postpartum depression because of very real emotions that she had brushed aside. Better to "pay now" (grieve openly) than to "pay later, with interest" (get sick, and still have the grief to confront on top of it).

Sometimes cultural pressure leads us to avoid an issue. Miscarriage is a perfect example. To suffer one can be devastating. The physical recovery can be quick, but coming to terms with the loss (whether the pregnancy had been planned or not) can take longer. Yet a woman who suffers a miscarriage is not typically encouraged to grieve or even dwell on the experience. "At least it happened early," she is often told. Or "At least you're still young." Or "At least you have other children to enjoy." After a day or two's rest, she is expected to go on about her business. But without an opportunity to reconcile what this loss means for her, she's placing herself at risk for later problems. These might include depression or difficulty conceiving later.

This concept of an ignored issue turning up again later is often surprising to women. Sometimes it's hard to connect the dots, because an emotional issue can manifest itself later as a physical one, or vice versa. But manifest themselves they will.

Gloria's Story: What's the Worst That Could Happen?

During her annual exam, Gloria, a fifty-five-year-old marathon runner, told me she was in great health except for a sore ankle she was nursing. When I found a small lump in her breast, however, she burst into tears and confessed she'd been ignoring the lump for several months, hoping it would just "go away." "What's the worst thing that could happen?" I asked her.

"It could be cancer," Gloria whispered.

"Yes, that's scary," I agreed. But I told her that when such a worry is left to the unconscious, it freezes us, rendering us unable to act. Becoming conscious of it—saying "Okay, this could be cancer and that's scary, but now I can find out" helps take you out of "frozen mode." I continued, "You're scared, that's very real. And now you can take steps to find out for sure. And even if it *is* cancerous, you'll be better able to deal with it physically, because you will have intervened early, and you'll be better able to deal with it emotionally, because you're no longer living with a pack of hidden fears that will rear their ugly heads later."

Fear is one of the strongest motivations women have for ignoring problems. I see it every single day in patients with breast concerns. Finding a lump during a self-exam is a terrifying experience for most women. Nine times out of ten, everything is fine. But the possibility that it might not be fine is so overwhelming as to freeze her ability to act. When a woman in such a situation doesn't "pay now" by seeing a doctor about the lump, she "pays later, with interest"—gnawing anxiety and a potentially worsening medical condition. Plus she still has to have the initial problem investigated. This was Gloria's situation. She had lost sleep and even injured her ankle in the intervening months. Maybe she would have injured the ankle anyway. But might her concentration have been wandering when she was running because she was thinking about the lump? Might stress have left her muscles more vulnerable to damage? It's impossible to say. Owning the fact of having found a lump can be hard, but not as hard as trying to hide it in a mental trash can. Women with breast lumps often simply avoid looking at or touching their breast. By going into the experience head-on, as I encouraged Gloria to do, through tools ranging from Journaling to body monitoring (which encourages touching the breast with the lump), they put themselves in a far better position to cope with treatment options and make healing progress. As it happened, Gloria *did* have breast cancer. Acknowledging this reality enabled her to be a more proactive patient, with her full self behind the problem. Her recovery was smooth—and, having recently celebrated her fifth cancer-free year since the lump was discovered, Gloria not only is back to marathoning, but helps organize her local Race for the Cure breast cancer fund-raiser.

It's always better to take the direct route with health problems. Go right into it. Ask yourself, "What's the worst that could happen?" Then take a breath and dive in.

5. ENRICH AND EASE YOUR FEMALE LIFE TRANSITIONS

Having been born female, you were automatically signed up for certain linchpin events in life: getting your first period and going through menopause. In between those markers, you're likely to also experience other touchstones unique to our gender: becoming pregnant, becoming a mother, suffering a miscarriage, being unable to conceive, or choosing not to bear children. A woman's transitions are very rich invitations, if you can see them as that, to align your physical state with your deeper sense of who you are in your soul. Transitions are by definition all about changes. And change brings great opportunities to learn new things about yourself.

As you travel the pathways of your female life, from your cycling years (before you want to have children), through your fertility and pregnancy phase (when you do), through motherhood and menopause and beyond, you basically have two options. You can go through each stage unconsciously, or you can go through it consciously. The good part is, it's entirely within our power to choose. As I wrote about Laurie, the ob-gyn who gave birth just three hours after delivering a patient's baby by C-section, do you want to have just the event—or the experience and all the blessings that come with it?

Living unconsciously means living through things as though they are not really happening to you. You disconnect from the experience physically and emotionally. You pretend there's no *there* there. An example of a woman denying a transition to both the outer world and herself is the woman who hides her pregnancy at work, even though she's well into her second trimester, telling no one even though she is running to the toilet every fifteen minutes or is long past the stage where she can fasten the top button on her skirt. Concealing your hot flashes from your partner because you don't like the idea of being menopausal is another common kind of denial.

Being Consciously Female means being mindfully involved in all the changes taking place in your own body. You don't necessarily go out and trumpet them to the world, but you do approach them matter-of-factly as part of the package of who you are. Women who understand the intricacies of their menstrual cycles stop viewing them as a monthly drag and instead gain a new respect for them as an opportunity for self-awareness worth anticipating. *That's* a dramatic change. Over and again I've seen women who have had troubled relationships with their physical selves in the past—who were unathletic or held a poor body image, for example—come out of childbirth absolutely agog at what their bodies were capable of, and developing a new self-respect as a result. I've seen women shift from fearing menopause to using it as an opportunity for transformation.

As an added benefit, being mindful of the dramatic changes associated with these passages is likely to give you a better outcome. For example, Alice Domar's research has shown that women in menopause who learn the relaxation response (a technique to counter the body's stress response) can decrease the intensity of their hot flashes. Anecdotally, I've seen that women who allow themselves more downtime and, often, more time for creative pursuits at this stage of their life, experience a decrease in the characteristic fuzzy thinking of this transition.

If you're navigating a new passage consciously, it's like trying to do so in the daytime with a compass and a map. That's so much easier and more rewarding than trying to sail without any navigation aids in the fog at night.

Zoe's Story: Moving Past Clichés

Zoe, twenty-five and married barely a year, is pregnant for the first time. During our initial visit, our conversation begins easily, although I notice that she shifts constantly in her chair. Finally she blurts, "You haven't congratulated me on being pregnant yet."

I smile. "So tell me, how do you feel about this pregnancy?"

With that, Zoe bursts into tears. "I know I'm supposed to be thrilled, but I don't feel wonderful at all. I'm constantly sick. And I'm terrified about what having a baby will do to my life." I hand her a fistful of tissues.

Zoe and her husband want a family; that's why they finally married after five years of dating. But the reality of impending motherhood is nevertheless a shock. Zoe has severe nausea. It's so disruptive that she dreads what other physical changes are in store. She wonders how pregnancy will affect her relationship with her new husband, their sex life, and her career. People are already asking her about the array of childbirth options, and she's panicky about how soon she has to decide about the kind of birth experience she wants. She finds it hard to honor these uncertainties while friends and family exude their joy.

Our culture leans on many clichés about the transitions of female life. The dewy virgin. The blushing bride. The radiant mother-to-be smiling serenely in her rocker knitting baby booties. The scatterbrained menopausal matron. Since new transitions are uncharted territory, women who are living them unconsciously are often unsure how they really feel about the changes rattling them inside and out. Often they fall back on the stereotypical images that they think are expected of them: *Okay, I'm pregnant. So I'm supposed to be happy and calm and walk around acting like I know just what to do while everybody's patting my belly and my head, right?* Actually, wrong! The trouble is, life's transitions aren't one-size-fits-all propositions. There are many, many different reactions and responses to each, colored by your individual personality, history, and other factors. Every response is legitimate, because it is *your* response.

The way to get past the clichés and to get at your own true experience is to become Consciously Female—conscious of the fact that you are ambivalent, nervous, and afraid about becoming a mother, for example. These "side effects" of pregnancy are just as normal and common as overwhelming fatigue or constant visits to the bathroom. And just as those physical symptoms indicate great changes afoot, so do your emotional reactions to them. They are not something to dread, dislike, or feel ashamed of. Rather, they are brilliant opportunities to more fully embrace the experience of pregnancy, the primal transition that is becoming a mother.

I explained this to Zoe, and we spent time working through many of the tools in this book. Understanding the reasons for her nausea and learning coping methods and new treatments helped her to resent the disruption less. Through imagery, asking open-ended questions, and other methods, she explored her conflicting reactions to impending motherhood. "I realized that I wasn't scared of having a baby so much as scared of change," she said. "When I learned to take things one day at a time, it gave me a sense of peace. I began to see being pregnant more like an exciting adventure ride instead of like a terrifying roller coaster in the dark."

After her rocky, tentative start, Zoe grew more confident and excited as her pregnancy progressed. Better yet, she was able to carry her Consciously Female mind-set through delivery, the topsy-turvy postpartum weeks, and on into motherhood.

6. OWN YOUR FEMALENESS, ON YOUR OWN TERMS

Being Consciously Female does not mean obsessing about being female all the time. Nor does it mean accepting any one particular notion of what *female* is supposed to mean. *Female* is a gender. It's defined by your anatomy and your biology. It's not to be confused with *feminine*. That's a different word, which according to the dictionary means "the quality or nature of the female sex." But qualities and nature are culturally shaded terms. To be "feminine" in today's world implies a certain set of ever-shifting interests, tendencies, and appearances. Apply the word *feminine* to other eras in history and you'll conjure up a museumful of different images, from nineteenth-century crinolines and parasols to the 1960s California girl cliché to the especially broad range of feminine icons we have today. It's the same with masculinity. All humans contain varying degrees of both masculinity and femininity within them. You can be a woman (or a man) who likes needlepoint, playing the flute, and wearing silk. Or you can be a woman (or a man) who's drawn to motorcycles, electric guitars, and denim. None of those preferences makes a woman more or less female.

Neither the noun *female* nor the adjective *feminine* should be confused with a third term *the Feminine*, which (like *the Masculine*) refers to archetypes with which we are all familiar. The Feminine is more about partnership, collaboration, communication, intuition, emotion. Associated adjectives are *soft, spatial, opening, creative*. Other frameworks for the same distinctions include right brain (as opposed to left brain), yin (as opposed to yang), and heart (as opposed to the mind or head). Compare this to the Masculine, which is more about hierarchy, authority, intellect. Associated adjectives include *hard, linear, closed, logical*. The Feminine is about the internal, the Masculine the external.

Neither is good or bad, right or wrong. And though women have certainly not cornered the market on the Feminine, nor men on the Masculine, as you become more Consciously Female, you may find that you have slightly easier access to, or greater familiarity with, the Feminine. That's what happened to April as a result of a situation that demanded she pay attention to what being a woman meant to her.

April's Story: Feeling Something "Click" ⌒⌐

April, thirty-three, is a successful engineer in a manufacturing firm. Single and very career-focused, she was stunned to find herself pregnant. April wasn't sure whether she was ready for motherhood, and the baby's father was definitely leery about settling down to be a dad. She didn't have to mull her situation very long, however. Two weeks after the twin blue lines showed up on her home pregnancy test, April miscarried.

This stressful event wound up having an unexpected benefit in her life. Through the process of recovering from the miscarriage and working through the constellation of feelings the event inspired, April changed in ways that were subtle but profound.

"I'm a very driven person. But working with all men in a very male-oriented environment, I always felt I had to play by their rules," she tried to explain to me at a checkup some weeks after a D&C. "I was very careful to be unemotional and logical, and cautious about what I said. You always have to have your facts in order. That's just smart business. But somehow being pregnant and then not being pregnant made something click—that I'm a smart engineer but I am also a woman."

April, who had always worn a uniform of dark pantsuits, began to loosen up her look, allowing her clothes and jewelry to be more an expression of herself and her moods. She lost her former reluctance to use collaborative approaches to engineering problems. She engaged colleagues in personal conversation, a useful bonding skill she enjoyed but had once dismissed as a waste of time. She found herself working less overtime.

These changes were gentle and gradual; it's not like April suddenly began wearing flowing gowns to job sites and strewing rose petals behind her. No doubt many of her colleagues didn't notice a thing. But because I know her well, and knew of her experience, the shift was clear. Actually, April seemed to exude a new calm confidence that I attribute to the realignment that had taken place between her internal life and her external one. April's new attention to her reproductive life, as it moved from subtext to forefront, had left her freer to express the female side of her personality. Interestingly, she began to be more careful about taking care of herself as well. She had come into greater balance. Her story reminds me that we all tilt from the Masculine to the Feminine at various times in life—and that balance really is what life is all about.

7. FEEL MORE ALIVE (AND LIVE LONGER)

One of the best benefits of becoming Consciously Female is that you will gain a deeper sense of fulfillment that comes from having your internal world mesh with your external world. You will feel more whole within your own skin. That's a confidence-inspiring, health-enhancing, peaceful feeling that can't be matched by any pill or medical procedure.

I've known many women for whom this kind of consciousness has clicked on only at menopause. Alice had raised a family, gone to med school in midlife, started a practice, and was in the middle of a very full life when one day she realized that the life she was living bore little resemblance to who she felt she really was. Every minute was full, yet she was not fulfilled. Alice wound up quitting her practice and turning to teaching and writing. Today she says she feels absolutely more alive than ever. And you can see in her face and her eyes that this is true.

Study after study has established that people who have a sense of purpose and meaning in their lives, who feel that their outer lives have some connection to their inner lives, live longer in comparisons controlled for other risk factors. A positive attitude toward aging has been shown to increase the average life span by 7.3 years. Optimism has repeatedly been shown to be a reliable predictor of good health twenty years down the road. Never underestimate the power of the mind-body interface.

The evidence of that connection is abundant. And the surest way to harness it, and to reap the full benefits of having your body and mind functioning in unity with your soul, is *through consciousness*.

Natalie's Story: "Who I Really Am"

Natalie is sixty-one. When I met her she had just earned a black belt in karate and finished teaching a seminar on sexuality at a local college. She's a master gardener and is writing her first book. Natalie exudes an enthusiastic outlook, walks with confidence, looks great, and seems really interested and engaged with the world. She's one of the coolest women I know.

Five years ago, when her husband, Mac, retired, he and Natalie began a long-planned, yearlong voyage on their sailboat. Three months into the trip, Mac died. The couple had been very connected, and Natalie went through a very long mourning period. This coincided with a time when she was still wrestling with the physical and emotional changes of being postmenopausal.

Despite these potentially grim events, Natalie today says she feels "breathtakingly alive." She certainly projects that exuberance to all who meet her. What accounted for the change? Natalie used those transitional years to grow reacquainted with herself. "My life had changed with Mac gone, my body was changing—it all made me wonder who the 'real' me was," Natalie says. Simply asking that question is a great first step that women experiencing big life changes are often too disconnected or afraid to ask. Foremost, Natalie gave herself the gift of time to process her grief. She sought therapeutic support and also joined a church bereavement group. Tools ranging from meditation to writing letters to Mac also helped bring her feelings to the fore.

Because she was aware of her physical needs—and her changing postmenopausal body—Natalie also gave herself a great deal of compassion in these arenas. She might have just shut down; instead, she realized that she needed to give herself extra nurturing. She experimented with adding supplements and more soy to her diet, for example—needs she had been aware of but previously ignored. She joined a walking group in her town, as much to make friends as to get weight-bearing exercise. Keeping a written record of her emotional and physical progress was a tool that she found especially useful.

"Some people told me I was grieving too intensely," she says.

"Some family members were just surprised I was making so many changes instead of just hunkering down and clinging to the past." But Natalie rediscovered who she is now, both within her body and within her soul. "I no longer do all the things I think I 'should' be doing," she explains. "It's clear I won't live forever. So I am determined to take care of myself as I am, to live each day I have from the core of my being."

That philosophy just shows on her face, in her form, and especially when you hear her talk. Whenever I see Natalie, I always think, *I want to be just like her!*

Chapter 3

Health Care a Woman Can Love

What being a Consciously Female patient looks like

> This is the great error of our day in the treatment of the human being, that the physicians separate the soul from the body.
>
> ⁓ PLATO

Let's take a sneak peek at the future. It's time for your annual exam with a new ob-gyn. Two weeks before your appointment, you are sent a long questionnaire. It asks some familiar questions about your health history: Chronic illnesses? Allergies? Previous surgeries? Date of last menstrual period? But there are also dozens of other questions. The form asks about your relationship with food, your relationship with your parents, whether you have a routine around exercise, who and what the stressors in your life are. Do you like your job? What is your typical sleep pattern? What brings you joy? What are your greatest sorrows? You're instructed to answer as many of these as strike a chord, and mail the questionnaire back.

On the appointed date and time, you take a seat in the cozy waiting room. You check to make sure you have everything you were asked to bring: a bag containing all of your prescriptions and supplements in their original bottles, notes about your records, and questions and symptoms you've jotted down. Your visit will take a full but efficient hour, not forty-five long minutes leafing through old copies of *Lifestyle and Travel for Physicians* followed by ten hurried minutes perched on the exam table.

First you are escorted to an exam room that's decorated much like the waiting area. Relaxing music fills the air. You take a seat in a comfortable chair next to a vase of fresh flowers and examine the painting hung on the opposite wall. The floors are warm polished wood and all of the lighting is indirect. Soon the doctor arrives and takes a seat opposite you. No awkward handshakes while you're already half undressed and wondering whether or not to place your freezing feet in the stirrups that are already set up. Your doctor exchanges greetings and makes eye contact as she speaks. "I read your medical history in your chart. But I'd like to hear more about what brings you here today."

You explain that you're here for a regular checkup, although a couple of things have been bothering you. So a conversation follows in which you sketch your current concerns. Your doctor asks you a number of open-ended questions. Do your symptoms seem to vary in response to other aspects of your life? To your stressors, maybe, or the ups and downs of your relationships, the changes in your diet? What do you notice? How do you feel about your irregular periods (or being pregnant, or being perimenopausal, or being postmenopausal)? She inquires about your long-range health goals and your attitudes toward different types of treatments. Together, you review details about your current medications and the kinds of therapies you've pursued. She also asks about your typical diet, your exercise habits, your stress level, the role of spirituality and social connectedness in your life, and your sexuality—topics you recognize from the questionnaire you filled out previously.

Then it's time for your physical exam. The doctor leaves the room while you change into a comfortable gown and sit on the comfortable wooden exam table. When a nurse comes in to raise the stirrups, you notice they're covered with the same pretty fabric as the curtain behind which you changed.

After a conventional physical exam, during which you and the doctor talk throughout about what she's looking for and observing, it's time to talk again. Your doctor summarizes the follow-up lab tests she'd like to order and gives you a few handouts on subjects that have come up during your visit. Finally, she helps you create a health plan that focuses both on your general health and on your current concerns. (Today there is plenty of time for this step; if not, the doctor sometimes asks patients to return a week later to finish this part of the visit and review any lab work.) The plan is broken down into specific steps that you can take each day. At each step, the doctor asks if you think it is reasonable and doable. If not, she suggests an alternative. Once you agree, she writes it down. You will get a copy of your health plan before you leave, and another copy will go into your record. Finally, your doctor makes referrals to a stress-reduction clinic and a massage therapist she thinks can supplement your plan. You're asked to check back with her in six weeks so you both can evaluate how your plan is working and tweak any areas that need to be changed.

Does all that sound idyllic? Far-fetched? Actually, this picture is not too far off from the way I practice medicine now. As the director of the Duke Center for Integrative Medicine at Duke University, I am privileged to be on the forefront of exciting initiatives that are helping to change the way that medicine is being taught and practiced. As an ob-gyn, I get to see firsthand how these changes are of particular benefit to women.

I want to share them with you because they are intimately tied up with the idea of being Consciously Female. In fact, you might say that being Consciously Female and practicing integrative medicine are two sides of the same coin. One side is the patient's perspective, and the other is the physician's. The Consciously Female approach is a way of living your life, and integrative medicine is a way of practicing medicine. Both stem from the same set of values. Both redefine the role of "patient" from passive recipient of medicine to dynamic participant in the processes of health and healing. Each side informs the other. I'm fond of the symbiotic nature of cycles, as you've probably guessed. Well, this is another great example of one.

WHAT IS INTEGRATIVE MEDICINE?

Integrative medicine (IM) is relatively new, yet grounded in concepts that are as old as anything being practiced on the planet today. IM is a multidimensional approach to health care that's firmly rooted in the best of the scientific approach to medicine, while refocusing in several key areas.

Integrative medicine:

- Pursues a "best of" approach to medicine (combining state-of-the-art conventional Western treatments with careful selections from a range of other, less mainstream therapies)
- Is healing-oriented rather than disease-oriented
- Emphasizes the whole person—body, mind, and soul
- Is proactive rather than reactive
- Is self-directed rather than physician-directed
- Uses low-tech, low-cost methods wherever appropriate

To integrate means "to form, coordinate, or blend into a unified whole." Integrative medicine views the individual patient not as a set of isolated body parts and symptoms, but as an integrated whole, body and soul. IM integrates conventional Western medicine with traditions from around the globe. It integrates the actions of physician and patient toward a shared goal of health and healing.

There's little that's radical about integrative medicine. It's simultaneously commonsensical and cutting edge. In many ways, IM revives the best of the era of old-time docs who thrived in a landscape of house calls, home remedies, first-name friendliness, and cradle-to-grave care. Certainly many good doctors still have practices that combine a warm bedside manner with practical, prevention-oriented care. But such values have grown harder and harder to sustain in the face of managed care, liability concerns, and rapidly advancing technologies.

Integrative medicine is piquing interest because it fills a growing gap in the health care marketplace. People are beginning to reject the impersonal world of PPOs, HMOs, preauthorizations, gatekeepers, and insurance company domination of medical choices. Everyone's alarmed by spiraling costs, especially for the care of chronic conditions, which eats up a full 70 percent of medical costs today yet is not always well addressed by conventional medicine.

IM is also a response to the fragmentation of medical care. A woman might see an internist for high cholesterol, an ob-gyn for Pap smears and mammograms, a massage therapist for stress reduction, an acupuncturist for a bad back, and an herbalist for help with hot flashes—and none of these professionals might have any knowledge of the others. Indeed, in one study 72 percent of patients who used unconventional therapies did not inform their physicians. That's a lot of missing information. And therefore very often there's no one health professional piecing together the clues in order to see the big picture. Perhaps the most poignant victim of our divided health care system is the cancer patient. Here is someone whose life is literally on the line. She receives one set of recommendations from her oncology care team. Or perhaps she has a surgeon, a radiation oncologist, a pain management specialist, and a variety of other specialists issuing *conflicting* recommendations. Then she's inundated with still other information— from friends and family members, from fellow cancer patients, from the Web, from the media—regarding an array of alternative options. Yet she has no way of assessing what is safe, effective, or dangerous, and she lacks the medical expertise to know how these alternative therapies interface with mainstream treatments. She's left to negotiate this confusing, frightening path virtually alone.

Patients and physicians alike are beginning to say, "Wait a minute. Is this the best we can do? What's missing here?"

Chances are good that some elements of integrative medicine are more present in your life than you might first have thought upon hearing the term. Nearly half of adults used alternative and complementary medicine in 1997, spending more than $27 billion in out-of-pocket costs, according to a study by David Eisenberg of Beth Israel Deaconess Medical Center and Harvard Medical School. That's a 25 percent increase from an earlier study he conducted in 1990. In fact, there are now more visits annually to nonconventional healers (six hundred million a year) than to primary care providers. This includes such services as support groups, massage therapy, relaxation/meditation, and acupuncture. The percentage of Americans taking botanicals quadrupled between 1990 and 1997. More than half of all gynecological cancer patients (ovarian, uterine, cervical) use alternative approaches as part of their healing plan. Eighty percent of menopausal women use nonprescription therapies either instead of or in conjunction with conventional prescription therapies. In the Eisenberg report, 74 percent of patients used alternative medicine with conventional medicine; 15 percent used it as a replacement.

The conventional medical community, too, is looking more broadly at forms of healing. A study by the Maryland Commission on Complementary Medical Methods found that almost half of physicians sampled had made a referral to or had discussed complementary therapies. Fully 96 percent of the two hundred physicians affiliated with the Duke Health System said they would refer to an integrative medicine center, half said that they were willing to collaborate with complementary or alternative therapists, and 30 percent expressed interest in integrative training for themselves. The budget for the National Center for Complementary and Alternative Medicine (NCCAM), which is a branch of the National Institutes of Health, has grown from $2 million in 1992 (when it was a small office and not a center) to $100 million in 2002. Formal programs in integrative medicine or mind-body medicine now exist in more than twenty American universities. With coursework in complementary and alternative medicine (CAM) now available at two-thirds of medical colleges, we are beginning to train a new generation of physicians in a different—and I say vastly better—model of health care. Even insurance companies are increasingly covering alternative therapies, although this is only beginning to change.

Let's examine more closely the core values of integrative medicine. Notice how they echo the themes of what it means to live Consciously Female. Being more conscious is as empowering to your life as a patient as it is to every other facet of your life.

TAKE A "BEST OF" APPROACH TO MEDICINE

There's plenty to be said for the miracles of modern Western medicine. I wouldn't hesitate to perform an emergency C-section under general anesthesia, prescribe antibiotics for a sexually transmitted disease, or recommend a mammogram as a screening test for breast cancer. So many advances are nothing short of fabulous. These deserve to be embraced.

Integrative medicine is *not* about turning your back on modern medicine. Integrative medicine is about incorporating a different kind of care into the current model.

As things are now, the degree to which conventional medical care is an ideal fit with an individual's health needs varies considerably. It's a good fit for dealing with acute problems such as infection or trauma (as from an accident). Make that a *great* fit. If something goes drastically wrong with me—I collapse from bacterial pneumonia, my appendix is about to burst, or I'm in a car wreck—take me to the closest hospital emergency room, stat! (Of course, it'd be even better if there was a hypnotherapist in the ER to help me slow my heart rate and my hemorrhaging, too!)

The remedies of conventional medicine are a less good match, however, with most chronic conditions. There is no magic fix for diabetes, for coronary artery disease, or for chronic pain. Conventional medicine unleashes a battery of medications, tests, therapies, and surgeries to help remedy or control the problem. Often these interventions are of enormous help. But they are not as surefire as removing an appendix or repairing a wound. They don't generally eradicate the problem in a few simple steps. The underlying factors that led to the disease often go unaddressed. The ongoing life impact of these chronic conditions may never be assessed or even acknowledged.

And finally, conventional medicine is the least good fit when it comes to life transitions. Think for a moment about what drives you to seek a physician's help. An injury? Management of your high blood pressure? Sure. But women also tend to enter the health care system for reasons that have little to do with illness or injury. The onset of menses often brings a young girl and her mother in for the girl's first gynecological exam. A young woman becomes sexually active and seeks advice about birth control. In neither case do these patients have anything "wrong" with them. So it continues throughout a woman's life cycle. Pregnant? One of the first things you do is make a prenatal appointment. Thinking about becoming pregnant? Even better that you would check in with your doctor ahead of time. Unable to conceive? There may or may not be a disease at root, but again, it is the life issue, rather than physical symptoms, that precipitate a call to an ob-gyn. Experiencing irregular cycles or want to change your birth control? The pattern continues right through menopause.

Integrative medicine recognizes that different health situations require different responses. IM seeks to match the best practices to a given situation. Very often these may be state-of-the-art conventional treatments. But sometimes the best treatment may be a careful, scientifically supported, but less mainstream therapy. Such therapies can variously be used to supplement, augment, or replace conventional practices.

Because of this open-mindedness toward finding the tools that are the best fit, some people confuse integrative medicine with alternative medicine. The two terms are not interchangeable. Integrative medicine neither rejects conventional medicine nor uncritically accepts alternative practices. It recognizes that good medicine must always be based in good science that is inquiry-driven and open to new paradigms.

Complementary and alternative medicine is generally considered to consist of those medical interventions not taught widely at U.S. medical schools or generally available at U.S. hospitals. This is NCCAM's definition of what CAM encompasses:

- Alternative systems of medicine built on complete systems of theory and practice, such as Oriental medicine (including acupuncture), Ayurvedic medicine, homeopathy, and naturopathy
- Mind-body interventions such as meditation, prayer, biofeedback, hypnosis, art and music therapy, hatha yoga, and other mindfulness-based stress reduction techniques

- Manipulative and body-based methods, such as osteopathic manipulation, massage therapy, and chiropractic care
- Biologically based therapies such as botanicals, supplements, and vitamins
- Energy therapies, based on the idea that energy fields (biofields) originate within the body or come from other electromagnetic fields, such as reiki, qi gong, and therapeutic touch (acupuncture and shiatsu massage can also be included here, as they are considered ways to move or unblock the body's natural energy pathways)

As you see, it's a huge list. The challenge in understanding and embracing CAM is that alternative therapies fall along a massive spectrum, from the very useful and widely accepted to outright quackery. Most physicians today have not been trained to understand most CAM therapies. Research on them is often scanty. No single process can evaluate them all. To be sure, more and more mainstream physicians are becoming certified in acupuncture, for example, and use it as a treatment for pain, migraines, menstrual cramps, or nausea and vomiting. Many physicians regularly include mind-body techniques, nutritional therapies, botanical supplements, and physical manipulation in their treatment plans, and willingly refer patients to CAM practitioners. But resistance is also common, and lack of knowledge more common still. When you factor in the current time-pressured environment in which most physicians are forced to practice, it's easy to see how, from a physician's perspective, sometimes the simplest (and safest) response is to steer clear of it all, and advise patients to do the same.

A doctor may not recommend a single alternative treatment to a given patient, yet if he or she embraces all the other principles of IM, that physician would still be practicing integrative medicine. Conversely, a doctor who exclusively embraces alternative techniques but employs none of the other key elements of an integrative approach is not really an integrative practitioner. That's because IM is about more than which kind of tools are in your black bag. When you limit your idea of medicine to simply fixing problems, which is the way students predominantly have been trained in medical schools, everything is boiled down to the problem/solution paradigm. Problem: pain. Solution: acetaminophen. Problem: PMS. Solution: a triphasic oral contraceptive. It doesn't matter if your solution is coming from conventional medicine or alternative medicine. The paradigm is the same. Problem: pain. Solution: acupuncture. Problem: PMS. Solution: chasteberry. A great deal of current research into alternative medicine is at a this-vs.-that level. St. John's wort vs. Prozac. That is important research, but I think it misses the boat in terms of better patient care.

IM isn't merely about trading one set of tools for another. IM is about finding the best ways to promote optimal health and healing. That means being open to the best tactics and therapies available, conventional or alternative—and more, as the following sections will show.

What You Can Do

- Make sure all of the parts of your care team subscribe to the value of integration. They don't all necessarily need to confer with one another, but they should be open-minded about the benefit of a broad approach to health and healing. They should be willing to entertain your questions and comments about a range of modalities, even if the answer is a frank "I don't know much about that." Alternative providers and conventional providers alike can stubbornly believe that they have all the answers, shunning the concept that the best approach in a specific situation may be one different from what they practice. Open-mindedness is healthy.

- Take the initiative in reporting your use of alternate and complementary therapies to your conventional physician (and vice versa). If you're using homeopathy or massage therapy, for example, don't keep that experience isolated from your mainstream care. Fuller knowledge always yields better results.

- Dig a little. Before you blindly plunge into any kind of therapy, find out what kind of scientific studies have been done on its safety and effectiveness. Evaluate the potential for benefit as well as the potential for harm. (Harm can come directly or indirectly, as from delaying more proven techniques while pursuing one that is unproven.) Know your sources, too. Don't believe everything you read on every Web site. Medical libraries and federal databases can be good places to start, such as CAM on PubMed, which was developed by the National Center for Complementary and Alternative Medicine and the National Library of Medicine (NLM).

- Network for recommendations. If you're choosing a CAM practitioner, ask around for recommendations, including asking your doctor—just the same way you would network to find a conventional practitioner. You might also want to ask a nearby hospital or medical school if they maintain lists of CAM practitioners. NCCAM recommends contacting a professional organization for the type of practitioner you're seeking. In addition to offering referrals, it can explain the standards of practice for that specialty, provide information that explains the therapy, and describe the training and licensure requirements of its members. (See "Readings and Resources.")

- Evaluate the cost. Most CAM therapies are not covered by health insurance. As a result, the charges may not be regulated or may be open to negotiation. Many are pay-as-you-go and can require frequent visits initially. Know what you are willing to spend. Stop at various points in therapy to evaluate how you feel about your progress.

- Trust your instincts. If a therapy doesn't sound right to you, maybe it's not the way to go, or maybe it's not the right therapist or practitioner for you. Make your decisions based on the information you collect and how it ultimately squares with your gut reaction. Have reasonable expectations, not miracles, in mind for any therapy, conventional or CAM. Know which problems a given therapy is most successful in treating, and how long you should wait before reasonably evaluating the results. Make sure you and your provider share the same perspective on the treatment.

THINK HEALING, NOT DISEASE

The health care system that healthy, normal women frequent when they begin to menstruate, need birth control advice, become pregnant, or face menopause was not designed to partner with people through the life cycle. It's a disease care system. The entire process has been conceived to ferret out problems and cure them, from the initial visit (focused on the "presenting complaint," in the medical parlance) through treatment. And for women, especially, that's its number one shortcoming.

When a woman's life-cycle concerns are overlaid into a disease-based system, you wind up with the medicalization of those perfectly natural life stages. A pregnant woman may see her obstetrician for endless monitoring and tests but receive relatively little information about her changing nutritional needs, safe exercise during pregnancy, or where to find emotional and practical support about the transition to motherhood. Menopause has often been viewed as a disease of hypoestrogenism, to be treated with supplemental estrogen. There's no room in that efficient problem-solution equation for acknowledging menopause as a broad life transition—the end of fertility—that also warrants self-assessment and a fine-tuning of one's lifestyle, habits, and life course. And when the problem seems to defy an X, Y, Z diagnosis and treatment, it receives a medical label—premenstrual syndrome, fibromyalgia, depression—that implies a single disease without offering much of a probe into the myriad root factors (including physical, emotional, and lifestyle-related) that may be intertwined.

Now let's shift mental gears. Let's imagine health care as a prevention- and healing-oriented system rather than a disease-oriented one. Suddenly everything shifts. The entire *orientation* for how you think about health and how you act on it is by necessity different.

Remember our present disease-based model of care: You break it, we fix it, you go on your merry way. Health, of course, isn't like that. It has no end point. You don't ever reach a place where you say, "Okay, I am well. Now I can stop exercising and eating vegetables and all that."

If you stop doing what's keeping you well, somewhere along the line your system will break down and you'll be ill.

We cannot ignore the fact that the body has its own awesome capacity for healing. If you strengthen your system—fuel it, not drain it—you can help to maintain its healing capacity at its greatest. When you are conscious (yes, that word again) of this ability, then you can make choices that support and optimize the body's natural healing. Ideally, your health care provider works with you to develop that consciousness and to make those choices. What a tremendous difference from the customary system, in which you aren't encouraged to pay attention too closely until something goes wrong, and then you see your doctor to get it fixed.

People innately seem to prefer the hands-on, work-together, healing-over-disease mode of health care. According to a major 1998 study by John Astin at Stanford University, people aren't turning to CAM because of a dissatisfaction with conventional medicine. Rather, they find CAM "more congruent with their own values, beliefs, and philosophical orientations toward health and life." This is key. In other words, people aren't saying, "I'd rather have an acupuncture needle than a pill, thank you." They are responding to the values inherent in many of the CAM therapies. For example, an acupuncturist doesn't merely stick you with needles; he or she also spends a lot of time talking with you and touching you. And patients are responding to that. They are saying, "These are my philosophies about life and wellness: to be treated as a whole person, to work in partnership with my practitioner, to go low-tech if that works, to learn how to facilitate the healing process, rather than to be patched up and sent out until I break down again."

Health and healing result from a continuous cycle of reflecting inward, evaluating the needs of your body and soul, and then taking an outward step in response to those needs, with a goal of restoring balance. Even when a cure is not possible, you can continue the process represented by the metaphorical in-breath and out-breath, of reflecting inwardly and then taking action, of seeking to achieve the optimum within a given situation. So often in conventional health care, a dying patient is viewed by a physician as the ultimate "failure." When a doctor thinks he or she can't help a patient any longer, it's often seen as time to refer the patient to hospice and remove him- or herself emotionally. Move on to the next problem to cure. But if helping a patient is viewed as healing, not "fixing," there is no failure, only a continuum of care. A tremendous amount of healing can happen within dying.

As Hippocrates himself put it, physicians and health care professionals should seek to "cure sometimes, heal often, and comfort always."

What You Can Do

- Develop an appreciation for the fact that you have a healing system. The best way to do this is to observe it in action. Pay close attention the next time you get a cut or a cold. How does your body react? What happens? Notice how healing is more than a matter of applying a Band-Aid or taking an antihistamine. Most medicines don't "fix" the problem; they support the innate healing that your body has triggered on its own.

- Ask your physician what you can do to promote healing when something's wrong. Don't assume he or she will just tell you if there's anything you can do on your own. Sometimes physicians are so lost in the "my job is to fix it" mind-set that they overlook the fact that the patient can help! I'll never forget how a woman I once met while accompanying a resident on rounds brought this message home. Admitted to the hospital for a heart arrhythmia, she was found also to have chronic anemia. "Really?" she asked the resident. "What can I do?" He was dumbstruck. No one had ever asked him that before. "Well, there's nothing you can do. We'll take care of it for you," he assured her. It was now the patient's turn to be dumbfounded. "I'd really like to do something to help the process along," she persisted. "Isn't there anything I can do about my nutrition, for example?" The resident again insisted there was nothing that she could do, and left the room. By then both doctor and patient were feeling uncomfortable, perplexed, and disempowered.

EMPHASIZE THE WHOLE PERSON

As an IM physician, I never look on a patient as a uterus, or as a cancer case, or as an estrogen-depleted reproductive system. I see each person as a complete, complex package, a human being made up of an intermingled body and soul. I know that disease can manifest itself on either plane, and that imbalances within either can cause problems. So seemingly disparate events are often linked. Your nutritional status can affect your mental health, for example (and vice versa). Events from your past can cause problems today. It's as important for me to know if your husband is being treated for leukemia and it's no longer in remission or if you've just lost your job as it is for me to hear your physical complaints. What's more, an individual has the potential for healing at the soul level even when physical healing cannot take place.

I use a handy framework in order to evaluate a patient's health and healing status and to assess the changes she wants and needs to make. It consists of five Centers of Wellness, five different (albeit overlapping) domains of your well-being that, when strong and balanced, help add up to optimum health.

These five Centers of Wellness are:

1. *Movement:* exercise for fitness as well as movement that brings you joy
2. *Nutrition:* food, drink, and supplements, and your relationships with them
3. *Mind:* the state of your mind, including your stressors and your perceptions
4. *Spirit:* connectedness, whether via spirituality, community, religion, or other vehicles that take you beyond your self
5. *Sensation:* sensuality (e.g., tactile, oral, visual, aural) and sexuality

It's through these five centers that you nourish your body and soul. Conventional medicine tends to value the first two and acknowledge the third. The last two are rarely even considered in a medical setting.

Maybe you've had the importance of daily exercise and the food pyramid, for example, drummed into your head since childhood, and as an adult you've been hearing more about stress reduction. Researchers are just beginning to demonstrate the importance of the fourth center, which I call Spirit, with evidence underscoring the effect of community and faith on physical health. And most health experts completely ignore the fifth category, Sensation. Maybe this is because it tends to influence the soul more than the body. But I think an awareness of sensuality and sexuality in one's life is absolutely necessary, especially for a woman, in order to achieve a real sense of balance, and because it impacts our health in a very real way.

The needs you feel in each of these centers are not something static that you figure out once in your life and can then forget about. They are incredibly dynamic, especially for women, constantly shifting, depending on where you are in life or in any given day or week. To use an obvious example, think about how a woman's needs change in all five centers during pregnancy. She's encouraged to consume more folic acid, to watch out for fish from polluted waters. Her body moves differently, and she may give up unsafe sports such as scuba diving. Her thoughts and emotional needs change; she begins to focus on becoming a mother. She seeks advice from other pregnant women and needs different kinds of support from her partner. The sensations (from scents to sex) that give her pleasure tend to shift. But these same kinds of fluctuations occur throughout every woman's menstrual cycle as well. They can happen from month to month in a woman no longer cycling. Everyone experiences subtle shifts from day to day, as well as profound shifts throughout the life cycle.

Being Consciously Female means fine-tuning your awareness of your needs within each of these centers as they fluctuate in order to constantly best maintain balanced, optimal health.

Let's take a brief tour of these centers. (They're in no particular order of importance, because *all five are important!*)

Center 1: Movement

Notice I didn't call this section "Exercise." The word *exercise* has become a loaded one, implying activity undertaken specifically to burn calories or build muscle or trim a waistline. Movement is any kind of activity, both the sweat-it-out kind and the joyful, fully engaged kind, such as gardening, dancing, or walking the dog. Being in motion requires an active decision for many of us. The modern lifestyle is sedentary by nature; we mainly move from car to elevator to desk to sofa to bed.

I won't bore you with the vital statistics here about how important physical exercise is and how the average American woman does not get enough. But I want to point out that movement is also important to a woman's soul. You can choose kinds of movement that align to what's going on in your body and in your soul on a given day. For example, estrogen levels in the first half of your cycle support more vigorous, hard-charging exercise; after ovulation, when estrogen drops and other hormones shift, you might find high-impact aerobic routines less appealing and more difficult. Rather than fighting through such reactions, you might drop back the pace for a few days, substituting stretching or low-impact movement. In doing so, you're responding not just to a physical need but to an inner calling as well. I'll show you more examples in Part Three.

Center 2: Nutrition

It's generally easy for women to grasp the idea that food nourishes not only our bodies, but also our souls. Many of us actually use food to soothe our souls. (That's why we call it "comfort food.") And yet food is also something we often consume unconsciously. (That's why we call it "fast food.") Our relationship to food and our nutritional needs shift across the pathways of our life, across our menstrual cycles, even across the hours of a given day. Tuning in to these relationships, as well as to our shifting nutritional needs, allows us to make conscious decisions about the foods that best stoke our total health.

Center 3: Mind

Your mind is the interface between reality and your body's response. I strongly believe we have not begun to fully understand the power of the mind. I hope that fifty years from now the use of mind-body techniques will be an integral part of health care. The bottom line: Your *perception* of reality becomes the reality to which your body responds. You can be lying on a beach, but if you are ruminating over your work to-do list, problems in your marriage, or financial stressors, then your body will respond as if you are home and in the thick of those messes: Your adrenaline will jump, your blood pressure will increase, you'll experience the whole stress response. Conversely, you can be in the middle of a hectic, stress-filled situation but realign your thoughts and breathing pattern to a calmer, relaxed mode, and your body will respond accordingly. An interesting study that drives home the power of the mind over the body concerned Japanese students with lacquer tree allergy (like poison ivy). The students were blindfolded and stroked on one arm with either a lacquer tree leaf or a (nonallergenic) chestnut tree leaf. Rashes developed only on the arms of the students who *thought* they were being exposed to lacquer tree. They had no rash if they thought it was the nonallergenic leaf. Learning to use this mind-body connection consciously is a central spoke of wellness.

Center 4: Spirit

If tending to movement and nutrition can be a challenge for a busy woman, Spirit needs tend to get particularly overlooked. Taking time to reflect on what makes us feel more connected to the world beyond our immediate concerns, and to what helps us to feel a part of something bigger than ourselves, is essential to wellness. Numerous studies have established the benefits of relationships—married men live longer than single men, for example, and women with pets live longer than women without pets. Cancer patients with social connections have longer overall survival rates. Infertile women who participate in support groups have slightly higher pregnancy rates. Tending to the needs of one's spirit can also involve as small an effort as spending a few moments gazing up at the stars or reading poetry. All of these things lay down direct connections between our bodies and our souls. You wouldn't go for a week without feeding your body. Neither can you afford to go for weeks on end without feeding your spirit.

Center 5: Sensation

While sensuality and sexuality are rarely thought of as part of any wellness plan, they should be. Becoming aware of the richness of your senses, including your sexual nature (regardless of whether you are sexually active or not), and then nourishing those sensations are essential components of achieving balance between body and soul. These needs can be nourished in a multitude of ways, from things as small as wearing clothing that is pleasing to the touch to things as broad as being comfortable with your sexuality. To not be at peace in this area is to invite discord into your life. And to have your Sensation realm well tended is to be constantly replenished and more complete.

Just being aware of your five centers is an important first step in making you healthier. Simply by paying attention, by making these things conscious, a shift begins to occur in your overall health. And further, the five centers give you a practical mechanism through which you can bring about real change in your life. Once you understand how these five dimensions work in your life, you can make conscious choices about them that optimize your general well-being.

When I am evaluating a patient for the first time, my medical health history canvasses all five Centers of Wellness. (I'll show you a way to do this yourself in Chapter 5: "Explore.") I probe for how each center is being nurtured both at the physical body level and at the deeper soul level. I will also use the centers framework when I am helping a patient devise a daily wellness plan to improve her health and healing. Together, we come up with goals in each center that the woman can then take steps toward every day. The specific steps she takes each day are based on her awareness of her body and soul during that phase of her cycle and that phase of her life.

I use the five centers every day to check in with myself. Conveniently, there are five fingers on each hand! At the start of each day, I check in to gain an awareness of how each center stands. Then as each day winds down I run through them again, reviewing whether I attended to each center, and how.

What You Can Do

- Grow familiar with the Centers of Wellness concept. Think about how each dimension plays out in your daily life now. Are your body and soul being satisfied by each, or is something out of whack? I will return to this concept throughout the book to show you how to embrace and find consciousness about your "whole self."
- Take time during the day to reflect on the centers. Which ones feel fueled? Which ones feel depleted? How does each vary across your cycle or your week?
- Think about whether your doctor views you as a whole or as a bunch of disconnected parts. If the latter, he or she may be doing so unconsciously. Because most physicians' training is so problem-based, it's easy not to see the person who is having the problems. Present your situation in terms of both your body and soul. For example, if you've developed pounding headaches since taking on a new assignment at work, don't just describe the headaches; mention the work situation as well.

BE PROACTIVE, NOT REACTIVE

Once you see the value of optimizing both body and soul for healing, it should not be much of a stretch to recognize that your health habits (i.e., lifestyle choices) are a key factor in the development of disease. In fact, lifestyle—nutrition, exercise, habits such as smoking and drinking—is responsible for 60 to 70 percent of the illness that doctors see. Taking control of these lifestyle factors is what being Consciously Female is about.

From a simple dollars-and-cents viewpoint, one of the single biggest problems dragging down our current health care system is chronic illness. Cardiovascular disease, for example, is the leading cause of death for women, followed by cancer, stroke, chronic lower respiratory disease, and diabetes. Most cases of these problems are either preventable or could be delayed for decades. Some 125 million Americans have a chronic condition. The cost of treating them tops $1 trillion, of the $1.5 trillion total spent on health care every year. In other words, of the tremendous amount of money poured into the health care system in the United States, two-thirds of it is going to treat people who are sick with diseases that might have been prevented in the first place!

The cost to an individual woman's life can be just as staggering. Through a series of simple steps that you take responsibility for at home, you can spare yourself thousands of dollars in health care costs and untold hours, days, weeks, months, and years of suffering. You can literally add years to your life and raise the quality of your life—the most priceless savings of all.

Although we don't understand the mysteries of what causes every disease, we have learned plenty about how to prevent them. Look at one common example, hypertension. Recent government guidelines state that lifestyle changes alone—at least a half hour of daily exercise plus a diet high in fruits and vegetables, high in potassium, and low in fats and alcohol—can be enough to prevent hypertension for the twenty-three million Americans with "high normal" blood pressure (120 to 139 over 80 to 89).

As a Consciously Female patient, you want to learn everything you can about preventing illness. As an integrative medicine physician, I am committed to showing you what those things are. The Consciously Female approach that I present in Part Three represents a new level of proactive care. Because it's a health plan that women tailor to their individual changing needs throughout their reproductive cycles, it is proactive in a day-to-day sense as well as in a general sense.

What You Can Do

- Set goals for your health. What's your ideal vision of well-being? How do you envision yourself a year from now? Or you may have a very specific goal in mind: to walk a 10K race, to stop smoking, to have painless periods.

- Devise a plan to get there. Use the Consciously Female tools and approaches to map out a personal strategic health plan.

SEE HEALTH CARE AS SELF-DIRECTED, NOT PHYSICIAN-DIRECTED

So many patients say that they have never had a physician listen to their story. It's sad but true. On my first day of clinic as an intern, a senior resident pulled me aside. "Okay, let me tell you truly and honestly the key to success in clinic," he confided. "*Never* ask a patient an open-ended question. Because the second you do, you're screwed. You will hear the whole story of their life and you will never stay on track. Only ask yes-or-no questions." Unfortunately, the human connection is drilled out of doctors right from the start.

Doctors are also trained that it is their job to know everything, even when they don't. There is a joke that goes like this: A team is making postoperative rounds. The attending physician says to the chief resident, "What is the patient's postop hematocrit?" The chief doesn't know, so he asks the resident, who doesn't know, who asks the intern, who doesn't know, who asks the med student. None of them know. So the student says to the intern, "I forgot to look." The intern says to the resident, "It is stable." The resident says to the chief resident, "It is mid-thirties." And the chief resident says to the attending physician with full confidence, "It is thirty-seven." Now, that little exaggeration might sound horrifying to you, but every time I tell this joke in front of a medical audience, it gets a big chuckle. Anyone who has been through conventional training knows that not only is it your job to know everything, but if you don't, you'd better pretend you do. And this mind-set, unfortunately, can't help but pervade the relationship the physician has with his patient.

I don't think the doctor-on-a-pedestal model serves either party well. What's the matter with saying, "Gee, I don't know. Let's see what we can find out"? Or with giving a patient a welcoming hug? Or sitting on the edge of her hospital bed? The knee-jerk reaction for a newly minted MD is "Oh no, I mustn't do that!" And as recently as ten years ago, most physicians rarely did. Fortunately, medicine is far more informal—more human-faced—than it once was. Respectful informality helps both sides remember that behind the white coat is a person, and behind the flimsy exam room gown is another person. And both are working together toward a goal of improved health.

It's also important to feel your practitioner takes your observations seriously. A survey done for the National Consumers League in 2003 found that about one-third of women facing menopause don't talk to their doctors about it because they find their symptoms are trivialized. The more severe the symptoms, the survey found, the less satisfied the patients felt with their doctor-patient relationship. How unfortunate that at a juncture where a woman would so benefit from a dialogue, there is no conversation.

A partnership dynamic works in both directions. Each learns from the other. Not only are doctors better doctors, but patients become better patients. I believe that magic happens when you give patients the right and the opportunity to be their own healers.

What You Can Do

- Take the initiative. Think about whether you automatically fall into a passive mode regarding your medical care—it's easy to do. Don't wait for your doctor's office to remind you when it's time for an annual exam; mark it down yourself in your date book. When you get there, don't just sit there passively hoping that your doctor doesn't find anything wrong. Jot down questions or symptoms of patterns and bring your notes to your appointment. Ask yourself what you want to get out of the meeting.
- Follow through. Don't wait to hear about test results and assume everything is okay if you don't hear back; follow through yourself so that you're sure.
- Be honest with your physician. If I say, "Okay, you need to do X, Y, and Z for optimal nutrition," but those suggestions are

an awkward fit with your life, you are not likely to follow them. And if that's so, then what has been accomplished? Be as candid as you can about your reactions, your symptoms, and your worries.

- Make sure that your concerns are addressed. There's a very common phenomenon in which a patient comes in with a particular concern, the doctor finds something wrong and fixes it, and the patient goes home—with her original complaint unaddressed! For example, a woman might complain of fatigue. The doctor does a complete evaluation. The workup reveals that the patient has high blood pressure, which is then treated. The doctor feels satisfied that he's done his job. Meanwhile the patient still has fatigue. Her high blood pressure was real, and it's great that it was caught, but that wasn't causing her tiredness. Unless she articulates her needs and concerns, she'll never have the fatigue responded to.

CHOOSE LOW-TECH, LOW-COST, HIGH-TOUCH WHERE POSSIBLE

Women's health is full of examples where expensive, fancy techniques are trumping those that are plainer but equally effective (or more so). Often this latter group is high-touch rather than high-tech. For example, doulas, women trained to serve as lay support for moms during childbirth, have been demonstrated to significantly lower the rate of cesarean sections, of forceps use, of maternal infections, and of length of labor—yet their use remains rare. Studies have documented the benefit of exercise and herbal approaches in the treatment of depression, yet pharmaceuticals remain the dominant route of treatment. Among the many other examples are the use of acupuncture to treat nausea and vomiting (which was supported by a prestigious 1992 National Institutes of Health consensus panel) and glucosamine for arthritis of the knee. Guided imagery, hypnosis, and other mind-body techniques before surgery have been proved to reduce blood loss, decrease the amount of pain medication needed, speed the return of bowel function, and shorten the length of hospital stays, all at very little cost or risk. Relief bands, simple bands that deliver pressure or mild electrical stimulation to acupressure points, significantly decrease nausea and vomiting after surgery. I could go on and on.

So many of these examples provide such amazing benefits, it's almost dumbfounding that they have not gained universal acceptance. It's not that I automatically prefer low-tech to high-tech. If there is clearly a best way to proceed, I'll recommend it. But with so many aspects of medicine, especially within women's health, there is often no one right way. So much is dependent on the individual. And many women—particularly those who are really in tune with a given situation—would rather start with the prudent, low-risk, low-cost steps, and escalate if and when necessary. Many of the courses of action just cited not only save money, but give the patient a greater sense of control over the situation—for example, using doulas in childbirth.

Yet as a culture, we've grown so enamored with, and in many cases so dependent upon, the high-tech route that it's become the road of first choice. This tendency is illustrated perfectly in an advertisement for the antidepressant Paxil that runs in women's magazines. The ad's headline asks, "What's standing between you and your life?" It then offers a checklist: "Depressed mood, loss of interest, sleep problems, difficulty concentrating, agitation, restlessness." Under a photo of a vacant-looking woman in her forties being looked at with concern from across the page by her husband and young son, the copy continues: "Life is too precious to let another day go by feeling not quite 'yourself.' If you've experienced some of these symptoms of depression nearly every day, for at least two weeks, a chemical imbalance could be to blame.... Feeling balanced, more like 'yourself,' is within reach." Certainly depression is a very real health condition. And certainly the symptoms listed in this ad can add up to depression. But those very general symptoms might describe problems that stem from a number of situations: high stress, severe premenstrual tension, grief, perimenopause, infertility. Rather than jumping right to Paxil, as the ad implies, there are a number of low-tech steps a woman (and her doctor) can take to assess what's behind her problem, and what she might do about it besides (or in addition to) a prescription medicine.

What's one of the simplest, lowest-risk, lowest-cost, highest-touch ways to improve your health? Learning to live in a Consciously Female way, of course!

What You Can Do

- Keep an open mind. A treatment does not have to cost a lot of money, be covered by an insurance company, or come in a manufacturer's package to be effective. Sometimes less really is more. When discussing treatment options, ask your physician if there are any other low-tech alternatives.
- Keep reading to start learning to live more consciously!

Part Two

The Consciously Female Tool Kit:

How to Tune In to
Yourself Every Day

Chapter 4

Commit: Tools 1–5

Creating the space to begin

A journey of a thousand miles begins with a single step.

⌒ LAO TZU

A woman must have…a room of her own.

⌒ VIRGINIA WOOLF

Articulating a desire to be more conscious about your health is a terrific, commendable, and brave first step. You have decided your own well-being is a high priority in your life. Now what?

In the back of your head you might already be thinking, "Sounds good, but I don't have time!" Now is the time to remind yourself that self-care is not really an optional thing. It's not selfish, a matter of indulging yourself to wake up feeling nicer tomorrow. It's not a transient pleasure. Becoming conscious of what's transpiring within your body and your soul concerns all of your tomorrows. We're talking about your health, your healing ability, your very being. *Your life!*

Your journey to living more Consciously Female begins with the concept of space. You can't begin to be more conscious or create greater health by adding one more thing into your life, by declaring with all the verve of a New Year's resolution, "I will be more conscious!" We all know what happens to those resolutions. No, instead of forcing a new bunch of edicts into your day, you need to first do the opposite: clear the decks. You know the saying, Don't just stand there, do something! It's important to change the words around sometimes: Don't do anything, just stand there. In order to hear what your body and soul have to tell you, you need to create a quiet space for listening.

I call space a "container for change." *Container* is a good word for this metaphor because it implies any empty form ready to be filled—a room, a blank canvas, an empty sheet of paper, an abstract shape, a thought bubble. You can create the following different kinds of containers for change:

- Space in time
- Physical space
- Inner space (through relaxation)
- Space on paper (through journaling)
- Space through talking (one-to-one or in a group)

All of these are essentially ways to gain readiness, or openness, for the Consciously Female process. I'll walk you through each one. Some may appeal to you more than others. But I'd encourage you to at least try all of them.

Sherry, 26:
— *"Sitting in traffic yesterday, I watched all the people walking down the street talking on their cell phones. It was a perfect autumn-in-New-England day, all the leaves aflame. But nobody seemed to notice. Now that we can always be in conversation with somebody else, we no longer have time to enter into a dialogue with ourselves. Who has time to smell the roses when the phone in their pocket is ringing?"*

Debra, 41:
— *"I'm drowning in chaos. I feel empty, lost. How can I find out what my health needs are when I can't even find myself?"*

Lucy, 32:

～ *"I have twin toddler boys, a house with a yard and a swing set, and a sweet and wonderful husband. I also have a full-time job, a mother, a mother-in-law, and a bunch of friends who haven't had kids yet. I've seen enough to count my blessings, and I do. But I wake up almost every morning—five seconds before the boys—with my heart pounding. I just start running. It's lunches and what's for dinner. Mascara and stockings. Their backpacks. My briefcase. When I'm home, I hate to go to work. When I'm at work, I hate to come home. In my car, I curse every stoplight. When my friends call, I feel annoyed about the time it takes to be social. My focus seems very narrow these days—if you can call being the mother of twins narrow. But I feel like I have no sense of myself anymore, other than as a mom, a wife, a daughter, an employee. Is there any of me still left? Where would I look? When would I find the time to look? I want to protect a private piece of me before there isn't any 'me' left."*

TOOL 1: SPACE IN TIME

Time is a form of space. Of course, you only have a finite amount of time in any given day: twenty-four hours, to be exact. Cramming more things into an already jam-packed day is setting yourself up for failure. You'll collapse from exhaustion or feel nagged by guilt over not being able to keep up. The solution to creating more time so that you can begin developing your female consciousness, therefore, is to subtract a few of the existing time suckers from your life.

The time is there, somewhere, in your day. To find it, ask yourself what you can subtract from your current lifestyle. These might be big things: cutting back on your work hours, saying no to one more volunteer committee, hiring a baby-sitter or joining a baby-sitting co-op to give you more support with your kids. Most women find it easier to start with the smaller things that are draining time and energy. Give some conscious thought to how you spend your time. What would your life be like if you changed some of these habitual activities? Imagine it, and then try it. Isolate the activities that most drain you. See what happens if you take them away. Obviously it's not possible to erase every time-gobbler in your day. Kids need to be fed, responsibilities still need to be met. But as you break down the hours and minutes, you may find different ways to meet those needs. What can you jettison, ignore, pass off, or hire out?

Taking time for yourself is a commitment, as worthy as anything else on your agenda right now, and probably far worthier than a good many of the to-do items in your life. But know that you may disappoint—even anger—some of the people you care about most. Or you might just feel guilty. When I married a few years ago, I went through a period of adjustment in which I felt that the time I spent on meditation and journaling was taking time away from Rich, when it seemed we had so little time together as it was. Eventually I realized that although my self-focused periods seemed to take time away, they actually add to our life because they allow me to be more fully present with him when we are together. Now he takes time for himself, too.

Reconnecting with yourself allows you to give a precious gift to those you love: a fuller, more balanced you. A healthier and therefore better wife, lover, mother, daughter. A better—*truer*—version of yourself. Sure, you benefit more than anyone. But there's nothing selfish about this equation. You'll be able to give more to others, too. It's not a you-vs.-them proposition.

Especially at the outset of this process, it can be useful to figure out when coming-to-consciousness time works best for you. Is it the first hour when you come home from work? First thing in the morning? Last thing before you climb into bed? After exercising? It doesn't necessarily require a lot of time. I'm not asking that you dedicate ninety minutes a day to self-focus. (Though more power to you if you can!) The Consciously Female process might require as little as thirty minutes, or twenty, or fifteen, or ten—whatever is comfortable for you. In fact, the amount of time you spend may fluctuate according to your cycle or your life pathway, and probably should.

However much you set aside, make it your sacred time, and let the others in your life know about this commitment. Ask not to be disturbed. And don't disturb this time yourself, habitually shunting it aside on hectic days or allowing yourself to be distracted by other tasks. If you're all alone but you're balancing your checkbook or skimming a paperback, then you're not engaging with your inner voice!

All that is easier said than done. I know. I keep mile-long lists of things to do myself, and my assistant keeps adding to them when I'm not looking. I have days (though luckily not all of them) that begin with 7:30 A.M. staff meetings and end thirty-four hours later after a night on call delivering babies. But I have trained myself to make spending time on myself a priority. I block in time for myself on my day planner, just as I schedule appointments and meetings. I can't afford to leave it to chance. Please know that it's still tough to keep this commitment, even for me. The instinct is that *this* can be sacrificed when push comes to shove on a busy day. I try to remind myself that they are all busy days, and if I let it slide, I will feel worse for it.

One way to start is to practice being unavailable for fifteen minutes a day. Ask others not to disturb you unless there is truly an all-out, life-threatening emergency. Turn off the phone, the beeper, the radio, the TV, the pager. Don't choose a crazy part of the day when everybody's coming home and you're fixing dinner or the kids are in the bath. Try to find a time when there's usually a lull. If fifteen minutes is too daunting, start with ten, or five. Then work your way up to an amount that feels right to you. Remember, this time not just for relaxing and unwinding, but for active listening, thinking, and observing. Focusing on your body and soul requires as much structure as anything we hope to build into our lives on a regular basis.

Gold Mines of Found Time

To get you started, consider these common places to find time:

- *Housework.* Can you lower your standards of excellence? Can you skip some of the things you're in the habit of doing every day or every week, or space them out further? Divide the work with your partner or your children? Be less critical about allowing someone else to help in his or her own way?

Can you organize your shopping in a different way (such as buying in bulk) so that you're not running to the store several times a week?

- *Personal care.* Are all the elements of your morning routine really necessary? How many different products are you using on your face and body? What would happen if you skipped a few? (I'm not suggesting that it is unimportant to spend time on yourself; I want you to think about *how* that time is spent.)

- *Clutter.* Is your house full of mystery mounds you don't have time to tend to? They're sucking up your time anyway, because you use energy feeling vaguely bad every time you catch a glimpse of that paper-piled dining room table or over-stuffed closet. Toss unopened mail. Free those file cabinets you never look at. Donate the outgrown toys and clothes to Goodwill. The time you spend tackling and clearing is nothing compared to how much more you'll reap by not having to deal with the stuff anymore.

- *Work.* Are you driven by some unconscious work ethic that's neither healthy nor productive? What would really happen if you worked thirty minutes less each day? You have to draw a boundary somewhere, so why not choose to draw it in a slightly different place?

- *Your calendar.* Is your "free" time overscheduled with things you don't really feel you have a choice about? (You always have a choice.) Can you contribute your time in flexible ways (bringing refreshments, making calls) rather than in fixed ones (being present at meetings)? Do you know how to say no? What if your default was maybe, rather than yes? Really re-examine your choices. Others' expectations are often created by your own behaviors. Have the courage to make conscious choices and put things on your day planner based on your wants, not shoulds.

- *Children.* No doubt about it, raising kids takes time, and for the most part it's time well spent. But are your kids involved in more extracurricular activities than you (or they) can comfortably manage? Are their schedules so full of doing that they grow up not knowing how to be with themselves? Do they pitch in with chores? (Even preschoolers can be put to work.)

- *Shortcuts.* Can you shop online or sign up for home delivery services instead of running to the mall? What if you picked up ready-made meals at the grocer or a restaurant once or twice a week? Are there elements of your life you can outsource? Everybody needs a wife. Can you hire one for a few hours a week—for example, in the form of a cleaning service or a yard-care company? Recognizing that I don't want to do it all, and that the time I gain is more than worth the added cost, has made all the difference in my life!

Try It:

Take a week in your life and question or examine everything you spend time doing. Imagine what it would be like, what the consequences would be, if you made different choices about how to spend time. Pay attention to what knee-jerk responses come up: "But I have to." "I have no choice." "I could never drop that." Why do you have no choice? What would happen if you dropped it? Ask yourself, "And then what?" Follow the consequences in your imagination, carrying the fantasy to the absurd.

Next, try over the following week to initiate some of those cutbacks. Often women start by finding just a small block of time once a week–then they find the experience so rewarding that they find ways to find such a block every day, and gradually lengthen it as they realize how much they get out of it.

Second-guessing everything you do can be an eye-opening exercise. I have seen women drop whole relationships, activities, and commitments after truly examining what they were putting into them, what they were getting out, and whether this was truly a way they wished to invest their time. One woman, a mother of four children ages three to fourteen, told me she was "sure" she could not enlist her family in help with the housework. "What about laundry?" I suggested. "Oh, they'd ruin it!" she replied. So I persisted with, "But what if you did the sorting and the kids handled the drying and folding and distributing? Or what if they washed and dried the sheets, towels, and underwear?" She conceded that this might just work. Where there's a will there's a way.

If your knee-jerk reaction is to say, "Oh no, I can't let go of *anything!*" I would submit that you're not being fully conscious of your needs. Your stress is trying to tell you something. Try one of the other mechanisms in this chapter to begin creating your space for change.

Tricia, 33:
⌒ *"I joined a gym that has child care. Since I was already covered with baby-sitting, I decided to use the time right after I work out to check in with myself. It might just be a sweaty locker room, but for me it represents a kind of freedom to just think about myself for a few more minutes, so it works for me."*

Nia, 28:
⌒ *"It makes my girlfriends so mad when I can't do this or that in the hour right after work. But I need to unwind from my hectic job and everything else that's going on, so I devote an hour all to myself. Working my Consciously Female process into that time has worked out just perfectly. I wish I could make others understand how I actually look forward to that time."*

Carey, 56:
⌒ *"Even though in theory it should be easier to have more time now that my kids are grown, somehow that hasn't worked out. I seem to work all the time, and I prize my relationships more and want to spend time on them, too. I don't know—I can't account for the days. But the other day I went on a mad-tear cleanup. Tossed out piles of unread old magazines and newspapers, gave away a bunch of junk; I even got rid of worn old sheets and towels I'd been hanging on to just because. I have a real sense of found energy from all that letting go."*

General Guidelines About Sacred Space

We all need to carve out space to discover greater self-awareness. Whether the format you use is written or verbal, physical, mental, or some combination of these, there are certain characteristics needed for such a sacred space (sacred to the purpose of building consciousness):

- It should be safe. You should feel totally comfortable.
- It should be private. You should not have to worry about intrusion.
- Anything goes there. You should not feel constraints, whether self-imposed or externally imposed.

If you choose to let others in your sacred space (for example, a group of women exploring their consciousness together), they should enter with respect for its sanctity. All must agree that confidentiality reigns. Ordinary social constraints can't apply within such a space, where the purpose is self-discovery, not pleasing others.

TOOL 2: PHYSICAL SPACE

Though coming to consciousness is an internal process, some women find it useful to set aside an actual physical space in which the process can unfold. The space can be something as modest as a corner of a room or even a piece of furniture. Maybe it's a chaise longue in your bedroom. Maybe it's your bed, covered with your childhood quilt. Maybe it's your yoga mat or your favorite chair at the kitchen table at dawn. It's simply a place where you can be.

I keep a sacred corner in our bedroom. All that it consists of is a comfortable place to sit, facing a shelf with symbols of people who are important to me and a candle from our wedding. When I travel, I bring a kind of portable space with me, in the form of a favorite pillow I use for meditation. Candles, incense, and chimes can also transform any foreign space into a familiar and intimate spot.

Your physical surroundings can definitely influence your soul. Remember the soothingly decorated exam room I described at the beginning of Chapter 3, with its fresh flowers, artwork, wood exam tables, and relaxing background music? When I was directing the Program in Integrative Medicine in Arizona, we happened to have four exam rooms; for a while, half had been remodeled to look much like that cozy space, and half still looked like conventional fluorescent-lights-and-beige-linoleum exam rooms. Before long, the fellows were reporting that the environment of the rooms was transforming the experience of the interaction. Patients seen in the remodeled rooms seemed more comfortable, at ease, and open to intimacy. The conventional rooms made patients seem more tentative, formal, and nervous. This made perfect sense—they looked like places where you were supposed to be sick, scared, or both! Even some cutting-edge hospitals are beginning to redesign in the belief that a calming, healing environment helps foster a more conducive environment for healing. After a Detroit cancer center overhauled itself for a more soothing look, for example, it discovered that sickle-cell anemia patients used 45 percent less self-administered pain medication than before the redo. My take-away message: Your surroundings do matter!

Think about what you can do to evoke a sense of sacred space. Light scented candles if you enjoy them. Play some music (although ideally it should be very soft and in the background, because you don't want this time to be about the music; rather, it's about the space that the music helps create). Fill your space with objects that symbolize or connect with your authentic self: family photographs, a painting of a scene you love, crafts made by a child in your life, objects that you collect. It's wonderful if you have an object that reminds you of a place or experience in which you were really in tune with yourself—a postcard from a spa visit, a seashell you picked up during a long, contemplative walk on the beach. Or perhaps you have a piece of clothing, such as a favorite silk robe, comfy sweats, or a cozy pair of wool slippers, that invariably soothes and calms you.

Especially at the start of this process, your inner voice is like a small, unformed part of yourself. It needs a quiet, protective environment in order to develop and thrive, a womb to nurture your developing consciousness.

Try It

Identify a physical space that would help you to be receptive to the process of tuning in.

Helen, 66:

— *"When I am sitting in my armchair by the fireplace after supper, Hank knows not to disturb me. I started doing this back when my kids were younger, just taking time for myself with a cup of tea in the evening. Back then I think I did it just to catch my breath. Now I find myself using this time to try to focus on who I am, where I'm heading, what kind of old lady I want to be!"*

Alexandria, 26:

— *"I decided I was going to do this right. I cleaned up a corner of my bedroom and turned it into my own sacred space. I put down my favorite Oriental carpet and reupholstered a chair to match it. I filled the bookshelf with inspirational books I'd collected, and a tiny old framed photo of my grandmother when she was a girl. She's so inspiring to me. I don't do anything else in this space except write in my diary and spend introspective time. A place for everything, you know? If I didn't have a specific place for this, it might get lost."*

Mandy, 39:

— *"I keep a crystal bowl on my desk filled with smooth rocks that I picked up on the shore of Lake Superior, at my favorite place in the world. When I need a little restorative break, I finger a few of the rocks and let my mind wander back to the last time I was there. I purposely put the rocks in a fancy lead-crystal bowl that I had received years ago as a wedding present because it signals that they are important to me. I don't care much about the bowl, but those rocks really take me away."*

TOOL 3: INNER SPACE

Another way to make yourself ready for consciousness is to create space in your mind. Some people refer to this practice as "centering" or "meditation," but basically it's a way to transition out of a busy, preoccupied consciousness and into an inner-focused one. The following breathing and relaxation techniques allow you to shift to a different place, to quiet the external noise around you, the better to hear those all-important inner whispers.

You can practice these techniques as a way to mark the beginning of a period of consciously focusing on your inner voice, such as before you begin writing in your journal. Or you can use them throughout the day whenever you need a brief time-out. They're portable and discreet. And they make you feel instantly calmer and more refreshed.

Tool 3A: 4/7/8 Breathing

Have you ever thought, *I just need a few moments of privacy* (or sanity, or relaxation)? As Andy Weil, who taught me the following technique, is fond of saying, "It's right under your nose!" Conscious breathing is a powerful mental space-maker. If you were to sit next to me on an airplane or pull alongside my car at a stoplight, you might see me doing my favorite mental space-maker, the 4/7/8 breathing pattern. (Actually, there's not much to see. You might just think I look very relaxed.)

When we panic, we tend to take shallow, panting breaths. They're part of the body's stress response. But you can reduce the tempo of this escalation simply by changing your breathing pattern. The 4/7/8 pattern, based on an ancient yoga tradition, most likely works by sending the opposite of a crisis signal to the nervous system, thus triggering a relaxation response to counteract the stress response.

Here's how it works:

• Breathe in through the nose for a count of four.
• Hold for a count of seven.

- Exhale through the mouth for a count of eight.
- Repeat these steps four times.

As you breathe, rest the tip of your tongue on the ridge behind your front teeth. When you exhale with your tongue in this position, it should create a *shoosh* sound. In the yoga tradition, this position is believed to close an energy channel. Be sure to breathe in through your nose and out through your mouth.

The exercise is traditionally done in multiples of four. You should notice calm descending after you finish the fourth exhalation. Because this technique is fast and portable (and not particularly apparent), you can repeat it as often as you need.

Try It:

Take a break and do a series of 4/7/8 breathing right now. Try it out periodically through the next day. Notice if some of the edge softens for you afterward.

Tool 3B: Mental Muscle Relaxation

Have you ever awakened in the morning to find your fingers curled into a fist? Or suddenly rubbed your temples and realized that your entire scalp feels tight on your head? Do you find yourself grinding your teeth, or have you ever been told by a dentist that you do? Often we hold tension in our bodies without even being aware of it. This exercise for relaxing your major muscle groups is a handy way to both relax your body and calm your mind.

Here's how to do it:

- Sit or lie in a comfortable and quiet place with your body fully supported by a chair or the floor. Close your eyes. Take a few deep breaths: deep inhale, deep exhale.
- Begin at the top of your head, with your scalp and your forehead, noticing whether there is any tension there. Give it permission to just let go.

- Progress down your body, from head to toe, assessing the muscles along the way and then mentally releasing any tension that you find. Move from your head to your neck, your shoulders, your upper arms and lower arms, your fingers, your back all down your spinal column, around to your belly, your hips, your buttocks, your thighs, your knees, your calves, the arches of your feet, your toes. The idea is simply to let the tension go in your mind.
- Take all the time you need. If there are places that still seem to be holding tension after you finish, return there. Give that place permission to let go. Only when you feel completely relaxed should you slowly bring your attention back to the present.

Try It:

This exercise is a great one to practice at night before you fall asleep. When you are comfortable with it, you can use it to begin other Consciously Female tools.

Tool 3C: Progressive Muscle Relaxation

This technique is a slightly more active variation of the previous one. You basically do it the same methodical, stem-to-stern way, but instead of patrolling for tension and then mentally letting it go, you physically tense the muscle and then release it. This exercise helps make you more aware of when your muscles are tense or relaxed, and can help invite the relaxation response in your body.

It works like this:

- Lie on your back with your arms at your sides, on a firm but soft surface, such as a soft carpet or a workout mat. (A bed, though, is too soft.) Alternatively, you can sit in a chair that supports your head and neck. Loosen any tight clothing and remove your shoes.
- Ideally, you should have someone slowly read the instructions below to you, or make a tape of them for yourself.

- First tense the muscles throughout your body, from head to toe. Tighten your feet and your legs, tense your arms, and clench your jaw. Pull in your stomach. Hold the tension while you sense the feelings of strain and tightness. Notice the difference between how this feels and how the muscle feels when it is relaxed. Then take a deep breath, hold it, and exhale long and slowly as you relax all your muscles, letting the tension go. Notice the sense of relief as you relax.
- Now you will tense and relax each individual major muscle group. Keep the rest of your body as relaxed as you can as you tense for a few seconds, getting a clear sense of what the tension feels like. Then inhale deeply, hold the breath, and release the tension as you exhale.
- Start by making your hands into tight fists. Feel the tension through your hands and arms. Relax and release the tension. Now press your arms against the surface they're resting on. Feel the tension. Hold it... and let it go. Let your arms and hands go limp.
- Hunch your shoulders up tight, toward your head, feeling the tension through your neck and shoulders. Hold... and release. Drop your shoulders down, free of tension.
- Now wrinkle your forehead, sensing the tightness. Hold... and let it go, so your forehead is smooth and relaxed. Shut your eyes as tightly as you can. Hold... and release them. Now open your mouth as wide as you can. Hold... and let it go, letting your lips gently touch. Then clench your jaw, teeth tight together. Hold... and relax. Let the muscles of your face be soft and at ease.
- Take a few moments to sense the relaxation through your arms and shoulders, up through your face. Now take a deep breath, filling your lungs down through your abdomen. Hold your breath while you feel the tension through your chest. Then exhale and let your chest relax, your breath natural and easy. Suck in your stomach, holding the muscles tight... and relax. Arch your back. Hold... and ease your back down gently, letting it relax. Feel the relaxation spreading through your whole upper body.

- Now tense your hips and buttocks, pressing your legs and heels against the surface beneath you. Hold...and relax. Curl your toes down so that they point away from your knees. Hold...and relax, letting the tension go from your legs and feet. Then bend your toes back up toward your knees. Hold...and relax.

- Now feel your whole body at rest, letting go of more tension with each breath. Your face is relaxed and soft...your arms and shoulders are easy...your stomach, chest, and back are relaxed...your legs and feet are resting at ease...your whole body is soft and relaxed.

- Take time to enjoy this state of relaxation for several minutes, feeling the deep calm and peace. When you're ready to get up, move slowly, first sitting, and then standing up gradually.

Try It:

The first time you try progressive muscle relaxation, you might want to have someone read the directions to you so that you can focus on relaxing. Or record yourself slowly reading the instructions and play the tape whenever you want to use the technique.

Whichever of these tools you choose to use, don't underestimate the value of creating mental space where your consciousness can come out and play.

Lorelei, 25:
"I am absolutely hooked on progressive muscle relaxation! I used to have my roommate read the directions to me, but now I know it by heart and kind of go in a trance state, silently saying it to myself."

Del, 55:
"It's like my little secret, that although there is chaos all around me, I can close my door and, just by the way I breathe, get centered and calm. Although I started doing this as a way of centering myself before writing in my journal

and focusing on the state of my body and soul, now I sneak in relaxation at all sorts of times."

Karin, 32:
— "I have practiced meditation for years, and for me this is a good way to lead in to my Consciously Female explorations."

TOOL 4: JOURNALING: THE PAPER SPACE

Even if you have never kept a diary, hate taking notes, and rarely make lists, I suggest you use a journal as a companion for your journey. A journal is a very useful way to create space. The space that a journal offers is symbolized by its blank pages. Gradually, words will flow onto the page, your consciousness taking form.

A journal can be whatever you need it to be at the moment you choose to write in it. Sometimes it may be a confidant, recording your most intimate thoughts; other times it will be a lab assistant, recording physical data about your body. How you use it, and in what form, is completely up to you. It doesn't matter whether you use complete sentences, write in shorthand or cursive, use profanity, or even choose to illustrate your thoughts as drawings rather than express them as words. Some women like to organize their books into daily entries. Others dedicate different sections to specific purposes. For example, you might have sections on My Menstrual Cycle, My Dreams, My Body, Diet and Exercise, My Moods, General Thoughts, and so on. Still others like a totally free-form approach. All up to you.

Nor does it matter what your volume looks like, whether it is lined or unlined, large or small. I do think it's useful to have a book that you enjoy holding and using because it makes the whole experience more pleasurable, more a reflection of you. Depending on where you use it, you might prefer a small, portable book, or a weighty desktop one. Maybe you're drawn to a cover that is beautiful to look at or you appreciate the tactile appeal of suede or embossed leather. Or maybe a dime-store notebook works just as well for you. Maybe you don't want a notebook at all, preferring to write on your computer. There's nothing magical about writing in longhand versus writing digitally, although the process *is* different. Try experimenting and see what you notice.

Here are some ways you can use your journal:

• Write down basic observations about your menstrual cycle and physical symptoms.
• Describe your daily experiences.
• Assess your five Centers of Wellness and describe the ways you are nurturing them.
• Explore your unspoken feelings surrounding a specific issue.
• Begin to find your inner voice.
• Let your mind wander; express whatever happens to be in your mind or heart at the moment.

You might be interested to know that keeping a diary carries built-in health benefits. Two separate impressive studies showed that people with asthma and rheumatoid arthritis who journaled for several months had marked improvement in their functional status, compared with those who didn't journal. And both kinds of Journaling patients were able to reduce their medications as a result. James Pennebaker, the University of Texas psychologist who has conducted many studies on Journaling, believes that repressing difficult emotions leads to stress; journals provide a venue for feelings and defuse their ability to harm. Other studies have shown that Journaling improved outcomes for insomniacs, depressed people, cancer patients, and those wishing to lose weight. A study of students found that writing about painful events for just twenty minutes on four consecutive days boosted immune function. The process of writing down insights is a way of tapping one's consciousness. That's why it works, whether you're suffering from a chronic problem or trying to maintain good health.

The main thing about keeping a journal is to make it personal and private, a place where you can truly explore your inner self, free from worry about how it will sound to someone else or how it might affect someone else. The act of voicing thoughts on paper can't truly be help-ful unless you feel confident enough to make no-holds-barred entries in your journal.

You might take to the process like a duck to water. You may, in fact, already keep a diary that performs many of these functions. On the other hand, you might find writing in a journal burdensome. Like any new habit, it can be difficult to start. Allow yourself to stop and start; don't beat yourself up or throw it away altogether if you can't manage to write in it daily. As you begin to fold Journaling into your Consciously Female process, its value is likely to grow more apparent, and you may find that you are more inclined to persist—and even look forward to this way of dialoguing with your inner self.

Try It:

Have some fun picking out a book to use as a journal, if you don't have one already. How to use the book will be-come clearer to you over time, so experiment a little. You could start by finishing some open-ended sentences: "Today I feel _____." Or "What I like most (or least) about being a woman is _____."

Tammy, 42:
⮑ *"I have kept a diary forever, since I was eight years old. When I was a kid it was all about what books I was reading and how I hated my sister that day because she ripped my Barbie's dress. But through sheer force of habit, I guess, my inner thoughts began to seep onto the page. I now can't help writing things down—what happened each day, how I'm feeling, my dreams, random ideas."*

Concetta, 52:
⮑ *"I use it to get down all my greatest fears and the stressors in my life—I really unload. And then after I write it, I feed the pages to a paper shredder and shred them. I can't tell you how much I have learned about myself through this process, and I don't have to worry about who might find it someday. There's also something very therapeutic about seeing all those fears shredded away to an inconsequential pile of scraps!"*

Bethany, 33:

☞ *"Sometimes I write pages and pages; sometimes I doodle and only write three words. But when I read it over at the end of the month, I am always surprised by the kinds of insights I shared with it."*

Sally, 27:

☞ *"For the first three weeks, I wrote in my journal religiously. I focused most of my observational energy on my femaleness. I tracked the details of my cycle—when my breasts started to feel tender, when I started to have a little discharge, when I found myself getting kind of withdrawn or edgy. I pinpointed the day I started to bleed and how I felt about it. I was so detailed in my observations that I felt I wasn't in my life so much as watching my life. It was making me a little crazy, so I had to take a step back and stop writing for a week or so. Then I began to journal again, but not as compulsively. It's been an excellent exercise for me—but I didn't get it right on day one."*

TOOL 5: THE WIDE SPOKEN SPACES

Another way to create space for your inner voice is to let it be heard—literally. Saying what you are feeling out loud helps make it real. Bringing your feelings into the world brings them more fully into your consciousness.

Sharing is something that comes naturally to many women. We confide. We commiserate. We give counsel. We cry together. In twos or threes, or in larger groups sitting together in trust and intimacy, women tend to like to come together to hear each other and to be heard. Sadly, this natural, healthy process seems less and less available in our culture. What do you think was part of the attraction of women gathering together for quilting bees or coffee klatches, or, to take an example from further back, going to the menstrual huts described in Anita Diamant's novel *The Red Tent*? Today, busy women often don't even have enough time for their best friends. Time for talking with other women is something that I think is sorely missed by women today! Of course, the person you share with doesn't have to be a woman, but truly listening (as opposed to fixing) is generally a more natural process for women than for men. Whomever you find to talk to, know that there is tremendous healing power in speaking and in being heard.

The process of speaking your truths aloud forces you to honor your demons and your dreams. In so doing, you acknowledge and respect their influence over the woman you are becoming.

Tool 5A: One-to-One Talk

To find someone to share this process with, choose a woman you know and explain to her that you are working on a project in which you have to find someone to listen as you share your story. Sometimes it's best if the person is not a close friend or relative who already has her own version of your history. On the other hand, you may prefer to build on an existing level of comfort and intimacy by exchanging stories with someone you already trust. Whoever you choose should be an openhearted, kind witness who will honor what you have to say mainly just by listening.

(Some women may choose to explore these issues with a therapist, someone who is trained to listen, which is another form of making space for one's consciousness.)

Being a witness is not necessarily easy. Many of us have a hard time with the art of active listening. We're all so used to interrupting a narrative with suggestions, reactions, and questions. Clarify your expectations before you begin. Here's a brief sketch of the job of a witness:

- You don't have to solve my problem.
- You don't have to commiserate or feel sorry for me.
- You don't have to share the stories that my story brings up for you. In fact, as a witness, you *can't* share your story just now. If you choose, you may share when I'm finished.
- You simply need to give me your full and undivided attention, to be present and listen.

After you have shared your story, invite the other woman to share hers. When you are the witness, of course, you follow the same rules that she did. Use this process on an ongoing basis, as a way of regularly checking in with each other. Work out a structure together, deciding how often you will set time aside, whether you both will speak at the same gathering or whether you'll alternate, and so on. Ideally, you will continue this sharing throughout your Consciously Female process.

Try It:

If you have a friend you trust, ask her if she'd like to try this exercise with you. It doesn't hurt to ask, and it doesn't hurt to try.

Cara, 26:

⌐ *"It is such a relief to have Dawn to talk to. We meet once a week for lunch, religiously. I'll just go and go for twenty minutes straight, and then she talks for the next twenty. Maybe it's just getting it off our chests, but I always feel lighter afterward."*

Dominique, 40:

⌐ *"I had been having a very rough time coping with infertility when I met Sara, my new neighbor. I didn't really know her well but one day mustered the courage to ask if she would let me tell my story, to be a witness, as you say. I had been hiding all this from people at work and from our families. Sam and I basically avoided the whole subject for two-week chunks, unless it was time to make love or time to run another pregnancy test. Until I began talking to Sara, I didn't realize what a toll my stiff upper lip was taking on me. Once it was out there—'it' being the reality of my not being able to get pregnant—it seemed like a more manageable situation, somehow."*

Val, 33:

⌐ *"My friend Cheryl helped me tremendously when I was working through a decision about whether or not to have an abortion. She listened more than she gave advice. But allowing me to say, 'Well, maybe I feel like this,' and the next day, 'Now I feel like such-and-such,' let me walk through the different scenarios and try them on. All she would do is prompt me with things like, 'You sound scared.' Or 'What do you think of that?' I was so bombarded with people telling me what I should do, but the most useful thing was having* someone just listen as I figured out what deep down inside I wanted to do. That was priceless."

Angel, 45:

⁓ *"Lynne, who is my neighbor, and I decided to go through the Consciously Female process together. Even though on the one hand it's so personal and individualized, we found that it helped to have another person to report to. I'll say stuff like, 'Guess what I learned?' or she will ask me how I'm doing on a particular goal. We'd be talking about stuff anyway, but it worked out for us to have a framework for our conversations."*

Tool 5B: Group Talk

When a group of women is gathered, the process works best if it becomes a bit more formal in terms of ground rules, but even when it doesn't I've found it to work very well. Again, there's plenty of precedent for the idea of women sharing and witnessing in circles. Think about sewing circles, bridge clubs, book clubs, recreational sports teams, and friendship groups. Think about consciousness-raising groups during the women's movement in the 1960s. Then, too, women gathered to explore what it meant to be female, although their idea of consciousness tended to tilt to the political ramifications of personal experience.

One interesting dimension to a group is that while the details of our lives are all unique, it quickly becomes apparent how many life-cycle experiences we have in common. Our first brushes with puberty, getting our periods, being pregnant, and/or experiencing menopause serve to link us to one another and, in so doing, help smooth our own transitions.

I've facilitated many of these groups, and here are some guidelines I've found useful for organizing one:

- *Make the intention of the group clear when you invite participants.* It's not for everyone, and no one should feel goaded into joining or caught by surprise.
- *Pay attention to the physical space.* Lighting, music, and food can

all add to a comfortable mood if they are unobtrusive and soothing.

- *Agree on a process.* I suggest beginning each meeting with a ritual such as a few quiet moments of reflection to make space for the conversation to come. Sit in a circle so that everyone can be seen and heard. You can choose to focus on specific topics (such as those described in different parts of this book) or have no agenda other than to share whatever comes up for each woman. Decide whether there will be a leader or not, whether that leader will rotate, and how long you will meet.

- *Agree on the ground rules.* The woman who requests the floor speaks without interruption. Remember that it's a forum for giving voice to inner thoughts. It's not a forum for group-think problem solving. One way to reinforce this is to have a "talking object" (a stone, a pillow, anything) that is held by the speaker. You may speak only when you're holding the talking object. If you want to make sharing advice a part of your group, set careful boundaries. Advice time should be distinct from storytelling time, perhaps taking place during a social period afterward. Knowing that we can/should/will give advice totally changes the listening mode, making us more preoccupied with what we will say than with truly and fully listening.

- *Periodically reassess your group.* Groups are as dynamic as people. You may want to change the format based on changing needs in your group.

Try It:

Consider starting your own Consciously Female group. This format doesn't work for everyone, but when it does fall into place it can be a powerful and enjoyable experience. Having a mix of women from different stages of life can be especially inspiring and informative as you learn from one another's stories.

Lana, 51:

⟳ *"I can't tell you how much this group has meant to me, how much it has helped me heal my wounds. I have been thinking about things that I must have just squashed down deep, like a trash compactor does. For instance, I never really thought about how wounded I was by having a hysterectomy. I was so focused on healing physically that I would not allow myself to think about emotional issues. I was in my forties, in what turned out to be a dying marriage, with my family almost grown. It was a shock when the doctor said I was pregnant. And another shock when, since I wasn't ready to start over again and had other gynecological worries, he suggested a hysterectomy and an abortion in one swoop. I recovered physically and never thought about it again—until this group. It's allowed my wounds to open up, and that's been painful, but it's also allowed them to finally heal. That's felt like fresh air and sunlight for me."*

Tool 5C: Solo Talk

Not all of us are comfortable confiding in another person. You could decide not to have another person witness your story but still say it out loud to yourself. Or talk to your pet. You might even choose an inanimate object to address—say, a stuffed animal, a plant, or a doll. One great advantage is that these witnesses never interrupt! This method of voicing your story works just like the other ways. Having thoughts transformed into sounds that are projected into the world seems to make them more real, less scary, less intimidating, more matter-of-fact. This, too, can deepen your self-discovery. If you're a person who talks to yourself a lot and always thought this was crazy, maybe it's time to view the habit in a new light!

Try It:

Talk to yourself in the mirror or in the car on the way to work. At first it can seem strange, saying words you don't intend for anyone else to hear. But *you* will hear them; that's the important thing. See if this exercise helps you illuminate thoughts or problems.

What all of the activities in this chapter have in common is that they create a place to start. Whether you find space within your schedule, your home, your mind, your journal, or your friendships—and ideally, you will craft your space from most of these things—you need this space before you can continue on your journey. All are ways to create the container for change, the space within which the Consciously Female process unfolds.

Chapter 5

Explore: Tool 6

Taking inventory of your health

This being human is a guest house
Every morning a new arrival.

A joy, a depression, a meanness,
Some momentary awareness comes
As an unexpected visitor.

Welcome and entertain them all!
Even if they're a crowd of sorrows,
Who violently sweep your house
Empty of its furniture.

Still, treat each guest honorably.
He may be clearing you
Out for some new delight.

The dark thought, the shame,
the malice;
Meet them at the door laughing,
And invite them in.

Be grateful for whoever comes,
Because each has been sent
As a guide from beyond.

— RUMI, "THE GUEST HOUSE"

Now that you've made a commitment to change and created the space for it, you're ready to move forward. Except that the first thing I am going to ask you to do is to look backward.

What is your health story? What is your story as a woman? Taking inventory of the history of your body and your soul is an important way to uncover information about who you are now, which can influence the choices you make in the future. It's your "her-story," so to speak.

The tool that you will use to get at this information, the Consciously Female Inventory, is a cousin of the conventional health history, with a few twists. Before I explain its use, let me tell you what inspired me to work with my colleagues—first at the Program in Integrative Medicine at the University of Arizona, then at the Duke Center for Integrative Medicine—to create versions of the document I've included below.

I had been so excited when I began med school. Then the hours and hours spent in class, in lab, and at the library began to make me feel like I'd signed on for a dry doctorate in biochemistry instead of a dynamic one in medicine. But once we began our clinical rotations, I was finally able to remember what had drawn me to a career in medicine in the first place: helping real people.

Clinical rotations were the first time I was allowed to wear a white jacket and talk to patients. The first task I was given was to take a medical history. I sat down next to a patient's bed and began this slightly intimidating (for both of us) encounter. I had a clipboard filled with pages of questions, and because as a student I had no real clinical duties, I had hours to listen if I needed them, and if the patient wanted to talk. And she did. A seventy-four-year-old woman with acute abdominal pain, at first she seemed grateful simply to have one-on-one attention and a personal connection in the bustling, sterile hospital. I learned through taking that first history how involved and complex people's stories are. Clues to a patient's presenting abdominal pain may turn up in the woman's surgical history, her diet, her car accident last fall, or any number of things. By asking the right questions you can learn new information found nowhere in the medical charts.

I soon became the patients' primary relationship in the hospital, their key listener. By the end of the hour (or sometimes two, or even three), a close bond had formed between us, the lowly but all-ears medical student and "my" patient. I was learning that these interviews shouldn't be perfunctory exchanges; they could be a wellspring of real data. A dialogue with a patient is more than a shortcut to problem solving. Yes, it highlights the medical background, points out clues to the possible causes of complaints, and lets you know what treatments have been previously attempted. But if the doctor is willing to try to go beyond these basics, it can also be a collaborative effort that uncovers deeper, back-of-the-mind information offering insights into the state of the patient's body and soul that can serve as a starting point for action.

Unfortunately, the gift of being able to conduct as-long-as-it-takes medical interviews was not long-lived. Although a medical resident is supposed to take detailed and complete health histories, once I began working on the wards full time with a full patient load, I (like all of my colleagues) rarely had the time. There wasn't enough time to sleep or eat hot meals, let alone spend hours listening to every patient's life story. I had only a few minutes. We were trained to get right to the "chief complaint," in order to make a quick diagnosis and set a workup and cure in motion.

I was frustrated. I knew I was missing the big picture. Technically I was becoming a better doctor as I learned to treat a myriad of diseases and disorders, but I didn't feel I was becoming a better healer.

Once I finished my residency and the intense years of hospital-based training, I made it a point to return to that big picture. As an integrative physician, I know that the time I invest in understanding a patient's life helps me better understand the interconnected factors behind her current medical issues and guide her through the lifestyle decisions that will keep her healthier in the future. What good is it to tell a single mother working full time that her headaches are caused by tension if I don't also talk her through choices within her control to reduce the stress in her life? How can I tell a frantic woman that her "fuzzy thinking" is related to menopause without getting a sense of how this is affecting her life and what she can do about it?

You're probably familiar with the conventionally conducted health history. You give your name and insurance card to the receptionist in the doctor's office; she hands back a clipboard with a page or two of questions and check boxes. You struggle to remember when you had your last tetanus booster, the date of your last period, and whether your maternal grandmother had diabetes or not. That's all useful information, but it only scratches the surface. To get a truer picture of the state of your health, you need lots of detail. The questionnaire that my colleagues and I developed is lengthy. Comparing a conventional health history and the Consciously Female Inventory is like putting a quick pencil sketch next to a meticulous oil portrait. In the hands of a competent artist, both should conjure up an accurate picture of the subject. But the oil portrait is much more likely to reveal subtleties and textures, and to supply a background and a context. And it's in those intricacies, I submit, that we can really begin to see the big picture.

The health inventory process is time-consuming. I typically send a questionnaire to a new patient in advance of our meeting, and then spend as much as forty-five minutes at the intake appointment going over the highlights. Most physicians are under such time pressure that they cannot afford to do this; the managed care system simply doesn't permit it. But this time that I spend up front is extremely worthwhile to me, because it establishes the framework for a healing relationship.

WHAT'S YOUR STORY?

The benefits of a detailed, open-ended health history are not limited to physicians working with patients in exam rooms. You can access this knowledge yourself, at home. It can help you to get at what's working and not working in your life, where your trouble spots are. It enables you to reflect on your history—the events that were pivotal, that helped make you who you are. You can then act on that information on your own as well as share key parts of it with your physician as needed.

The Consciously Female Inventory is not just a fact-gathering process but a series of questions meant to encourage exploration of the inner workings of your body and soul. It's a tool for connecting with your inner wisdom.

You might think, "Well, I already know all these answers, so how is this going to help me?" You may indeed have top-of-mind responses readily available for many of these questions. But I daresay that your answers aren't really informed by *consciousness*. And some of the questions raise issues that you may never have entertained before in your life. I like to call the inventory a "soul magnet," because it's meant to exercise a pull on your inner self. As you run through the lengthy list of questions, some will nag at you or upset you and some will intrigue you, while others will evoke no response at all. The emotional quality of your immediate reaction can be as informative as the actual answers that you provide.

Guiding Principles

Here are some suggestions for getting the most out of the Consciously Female Inventory:

- Don't feel overwhelmed by the sheer size of this questionnaire. There are more questions than you can reasonably be expected to answer at one comfortable sitting. You won't win any brownie points by diligently responding to each and every one. If that's what you choose to do, great. But ideally, I want you to skim through the list and reflect on the questions that resonate with you. When I do this exercise with groups, I call it a "monologue of questions"—I deliberately ask away faster than they can be answered, just to ignite sparks in the listeners' heads.
- Don't feel that you need to write out answers to every question—or any of them. Many women find it useful to jot notes when a question strikes a chord or elicits an intriguing answer. You can do this in your journal or right in this book.
- Don't feel compelled to answer each question at first glance. Initially you might draw a blank. If you do, that's fine; move on. But do jot down any responses that come instantly. You can then return to those immediate responses and see whether you wish to refine them upon further reflection.

- Ask yourself if the question has ever come to mind before. When, if ever, did you last think about it? Has your response changed over time, and if so, how?
- Be open-minded. Entertain everything. Realize that there are no right or wrong answers. In fact, usually the answers you give are less important than the simple fact of introducing the question to your consciousness. You might find that these questions spur a process that continues long after you think you've finished. You might find yourself returning to a certain question in the shower, in your dreams, or in conversations with friends, for example.
- Come back to the questionnaire as often as you feel you need to. It's not a one-time-only exercise. Your life changes, and so do your perspectives. Comparing your responses from one run-through to another can also be illuminating.

TOOL 6: THE CONSCIOUSLY FEMALE INVENTORY

General Questions

- **What does health mean to you?** Reflect on your general wellness.

_____

_____

- **Think of a time when you felt most healthy.** What were the circumstances? Were you conscious of how you felt at the time? What's different now?

_____

_____

- What are your overall goals in terms of your health and lifestyle? Where do you want to be five years from now?

Your Periods

- When did you get your first period? What's your story around your first period? Who else knew—your mother, father, siblings, friends, relatives? How did they deal with it? How did their response make you feel? When was your first pelvic exam? How was that for you? Were you embarrassed? Scared? Calm?

- What's your relationship with your periods? Are they a normal rhythm in your life now? What are your concerns regarding your period? Your fears? Your hopes? How have your feelings about your period changed over time?

- What is your period like? Do your periods come and go almost unnoticed? Are they painful? Do they seem long or short to you? Do your moods change when you are premenstrual or menstruating? Does your energy change? Your libido? Your relationships? How is your mental health affected? Your physical health?

- If you no longer have periods, how do you feel about that? Is it a blessing? A curse? Something of both?

_____

_____

Your Fertility

- What are your thoughts around having children? What are/were your wishes surrounding fertility? Are there times when you tried *not* to become pregnant? Are there times when you tried hard to become pregnant? If you are just now heading into this time in your life, what are your hopes and concerns? If you are past this time, do you regret choices you made during it? Or did you make decisions you are comfortable with now?

_____

_____

- Do you use contraception now? What form? Do you have any fears or concerns about its effectiveness?

_____

_____

- What form(s) of contraception have you used in the past? How did they work for you? How do you feel about each of them?

_____

_____

- How does your current form of contraception make you feel physically? Emotionally? Does contraception change your enjoyment or the sensuality of your sex life?

- If you have no need for contraception, does that make you happy? Sad? Something of both?

Pregnancy

- If you have ever been pregnant, what was the experience like? Was your pregnancy difficult, energizing, or both? What did you like most about being pregnant? What did you like least? What was the hardest part? What was the easiest?

- What was the range of your feelings about being pregnant? In what ways did your feelings shift over the course of the pregnancy? From one pregnancy to another? Did you want to have a baby at that moment in your life?

- How did pregnancy affect your body? Did you feel at home in your body? How did your body change from trimester to trimester?

- Who and what were your supports?

- If you have been pregnant more than once, how did each pregnancy differ?

- Reflect on giving birth and on how you gave birth. Did you labor or not? What was labor like? Did you have a vaginal delivery or a C-section? How do you feel about the birthing experience you had? How did it match with your expectations? How did it surprise you?

If Never Pregnant
- If you haven't had a baby, how is that for you? Are you eager? Afraid? Ambivalent? Frustrated? Relieved?

- If you know that you will never have a baby, are you glad? Regretful? Something of both?

Miscarriage and Loss

- Have you had a miscarriage? More than one?

_____

_____

- How did it make you feel? Did you grieve? Are you still grieving?

_____

_____

- Who and what were your supports?

_____

_____

- Did miscarriage affect your relationship with your body? Your sexuality? Your partner? Your femaleness?

_____

_____

- What other losses have you experienced in your life as a woman? The death of a child? The surgical removal of parts of your reproductive system? Losing the possibilities of motherhood? An abortion? How did, or do, any of these losses affect who you are?

_____

_____

Menopause

- Do you remember your mother or other important women in your life going through menopause? What did you observe or learn from their experience?

_____

_____

- What thoughts or feelings does menopause conjure up for you? What images does the word _menopausal_ bring to mind? What does it mean, or what do you think it will mean in your life, to reach menopause? Does the idea upset or frighten you? Make you feel relieved? Not bother you much at all?

_____

_____

- What physical changes have you experienced during menopause? Are they scary? Uncomfortable? Alarming? Surprising? More or less upsetting than you imagined?

_____

_____

- What are your hopes and desires about menopause? What are your concerns?

_____

_____

Your Daily Life

- How do you spend your days? What does a typical day look like? How much of the way you spend your days is a reflection of who you are? Do your work and other primary activities bring you joy and a sense of connection, or do you feel disconnected, as if you are just doing what you have to do? Do you look forward to Monday mornings?

_____

_____

• What are your main sources of stress?

_____

_____

• How do you typically cope with stress? Do you sleep more or less? Eat more or less? Exercise more or less? Do you feel that you have enough coping strategies?

_____

_____

• How do you relax in the course of a normal day? What gives you the greatest sense of letting go and feeling at ease (whether you've done it recently or not)?

_____

_____

• What do you worry about?

_____

_____

• What are your greatest challenges?

_____

_____

• What makes you feel happy and fulfilled?

_____

_____

• What kind of role does your femaleness play in your life? What are the ways that being female gets in your way? What are the ways it helps?

_____

_____

Your Relationships
• Who is your community?

_____

_____

• Who do you define as your family? Your biological family? A chosen family? Who do you think of when you think of family? Who in your family gives you the most support and in what ways?

_____

_____

• What is your relationship with your parents like? If they are still alive, how involved are they in your life? How is that for you? Does the state of your relationship feel right and comfortable, or something else? If they have passed away, do you miss them? Do you have regrets about things said or not said, done or not done?

_____

_____

• What is your relationship with your siblings or stepsiblings like? How involved are they in your life? Do they add to your enjoyment of life or take away from it?

_____

_____

• Are you married or do you have a significant other? What are the qualities of that relationship? What is it about it that feeds you or drains you? Do you feel that there is mutual love and support?

_____

_____

• If you're not in a couple relationship, how does that make you feel?

_____

_____

• Do you have children? Stepchildren? What is your relationship with them like? In what ways do they enrich you? Drain you?

_____

_____

• Do you have friends? How many are those rare friends to whom you can say anything no matter what? Do you have friends who drain you? If you have a close woman friend, how often do you get together?

_____

_____

General Health

- **How is your energy level?** Overall, do you wake up with lots of energy? Or do you wake up tired? Is there a specific pattern of rising and falling energy throughout the day?

  _____

  _____

- **Reflect on your tendency toward illness.** Do you catch a lot of colds? Or do you seem pretty resilient? Has that changed over your lifetime?

  _____

  _____

- **What's your typical sleep pattern?** Do you fall asleep easily? Do you have difficulty falling asleep and staying asleep? What feels like an ideal amount of sleep for you? Do you dream? Do you remember your dreams?

  _____

  _____

- **Do you know what medications, vitamins, and supplements you are taking and why?** What's your comfort level about your medications—does it feel right to you or do you have any concerns?

  _____

  _____

- **Do you use tobacco, caffeine, or alcohol?** Why? In what quantities and how often? How does the use of these substances affect your life and the lives of those around you?

  _____

  _____

Nutrition

- **What kind of eater are you?** Do you eat three meals a day? Or are you a grazer? A binger? When do you eat?

  _____

  _____

- **What's your relationship with food and how has it changed over time?** Are you conscious of why you eat as well as what you choose to eat? Is mealtime a special time or done on the run?

  _____

  _____

- **Are you happy with your weight?** Is your weight fairly consistent, or are you always gaining and losing?

  _____

  _____

Movement

- **What movement brings you joy, whether it's something you've done recently or not?** When was the last time you experienced that kind of movement in your life?

  _____

  _____

- **What about exercise?** Does the very word make you cringe, or is it something you look forward to? Do you have a routine around exercise that is built into your day? How often do you usually exercise? What kind of exercise do you usually do? Aerobic? Strength training? Stretching and flexibility-oriented?

  _____

  _____

Spirituality

- What in your life connects you to things bigger than yourself? What gives you a sense of strength? When was the last time you did something that made you feel connected?

  _____

  _____

- What brings you joy and a sense of fullness? When was the last time that you experienced that feeling?

  _____

  _____

- What do you do well? What are you proud of? What are your gifts (everybody has them)? How do you express your gifts?

  _____

  _____

- What gives you a sense of meaning and purpose in your life? How palpable is it for you, and how has that shifted over your life?

  _____

  _____

Sensation (Includes Sex and Sensuality)

- Can you recall your first sexual experience? Was it what you had imagined? How did it affect your subsequent sexual encounters?

  _____

  _____

- **Are you sexually active now?** Is your frequency of sexual activity what you want it to be? Do you want more? Less? Or just something different?

_____

_____

- **Are you comfortable in your sexuality?** Do you feel free about expressing yourself sexually? Are your needs met? How has this shifted over time? What role does body image play in your sexual life? Do you feel you know who and what you want sexually?

_____

_____

- **To what degree are your sexual encounters driven by your partner?** How much are they driven by you? How much is a merging of the two of you?

_____

_____

- **What do _you_ bring to the sexual encounter?** Just your body? Or the whole of your being?

_____

_____

- **What are your hopes around sexuality?** What are your fears? Your concerns?

_____

_____

- **What about sensuality in your life?** How do you define your sensuality? What kinds of experiences do you consider sensual? Are there enough of these experiences in your life? How does your sensuality relate to your sexuality?

Remember, the exact content of each and every answer is less important than the fact that asking the questions brings them into your consciousness. Focus on those that you are particularly drawn to. The questions that catch your attention or interest will undoubtedly change as your journey does. Noticing that is part of the exercise. This is not a one-time exercise. I hope you will return to these questions again and again and reflect on the ways in which your story changes.

Now you have made a solid beginning on your road to a more Consciously Female life.

Try It:

Every woman should do this questionnaire. But save this exercise for when you're able to make space for it. Allow yourself time and privacy as you read through the questions. Try using the space-making techniques in the previous chapter—relaxation exercises, moving to a special private space—to help you shift your consciousness. Nondistracting background music can help to get you out of your buzzing everyday head and into a quiet place, where you can bring intention and focus.

Alternatively, some women may choose to do this with another woman as a framework for the story-sharing technique I described in the previous chapter. One person reads the questions aloud while the other reflects on them (not necessarily aloud) and writes down her responses, and then considers her experience; then they reverse the roles. These questions can also be used to frame group discussions. It's great fun to share responses within a group of women—so many commonalities and so much uniqueness all at once!

PERIODS

Stella, 30:
—"I remember my first period, I threw myself on my bed and cried for hours, I was eleven and wasn't ready to be a grown-up."

Marion, 45:
—"I was with my mom in the kitchen putting away dishes. I went to the bathroom and noticed a spot of blood. I felt as though I had finally reached a landmark as a woman (even though I was only eleven years old), and when I went back to school in the fall I was anxious to see which of my friends had started theirs. I recall feeling as though I had joined a club of sisters who had reached a level of maturity that our friends who had not started yet could not possibly understand."

FERTILITY

Kate, 30:
—"When I decide I want to get pregnant, I want it to happen after one month of trying, and have no problems."

Dee, 35:
—"I'm anxious about being infertile or having a baby with birth defects because of the drugs I took when I was younger."

Sudie, 25:
—"After years of trying not to get pregnant, I freaked when I did get pregnant for the first time. I had to remind myself it was okay. I was married."

Pregnancy

Bethann, 32:

⌒ "I didn't love being pregnant at all. I didn't like feeling nauseous or ungainly. I felt like a joke."

Marta, 26:

⌒ "Life before and after pregnancy are totally different. Not even connected."

Miscarriage and Loss

Nancy, 39:

⌒ "I couldn't talk about it to anyone. And many of my friends were pregnant at the time and I didn't want to spook them."

Menopause

Mary-Elizabeth, 50:

⌒ "I am terrified. I don't want it—life as I know it—to end."

Augusta, 48:

⌒ "I hope that I will use this next part of my life to think about what mark I want to leave on the world, beyond children."

Chapter 6

Observe: Tools 7–10

Learning to pay closer attention to your body and your soul

We don't see things as they are, we see things as we are.

⌒ANAÏS NIN

Now that you've begun to explore the big picture of your life, we're going to focus more narrowly. Quite narrowly, in fact—on each individual day.

This chapter is about the art of paying attention to the "now." After all, if you don't learn to slow down and be present in the moment—or at least in *some* of the moments that make up your day—you can't be fully aware of what your body and soul are up to. You won't know your individual baselines—what's normal for *you*—day to day and over time. Nor will you be able to identify changes as they occur, whether they're positive, negative, or neutral.

Becoming actively engaged in observation is a skill that takes time to cultivate, and it is an ongoing process. You can't merely plug in one day and learn what you need to know. A woman's nutritional needs, her exercise patterns, her moods, and indeed her physical self and her inner sense of herself all fluctuate throughout a given cycle and across the span of her life.

THE ART OF OBSERVATION

Once in Arizona at the end of a long morning meeting of professionals and therapists from both alternative and conventional medicine, my friend John Tarrant spoke. A Zen Roshi master and Jungian analyst, John has a soft yet charismatic manner. "Before we all leave," he suggested in his Tasmanian accent, "why don't we all pause a moment? Take a breath, maybe close your eyes, and just check in with your body."

There we all were, itching to exit, shuffling our papers and reaching for our white jackets to move on to the next meeting. In all my years of medicine, I had never thought about checking in with my body. My body was something that was simply *there;* it did what I needed it to do. And unless I was in really bad shape with a flu or PMS or exhaustion, I wasn't in the habit of giving any special consideration to what it needed from me. But, dutifully closing my eyes to turn my full attention to my body for a rare moment, I discovered that it had a lot to say—starting with a sense of amazement that I was actually noticing it. The ache in my stomach was complaining about the two cups of coffee that I'd had that morning. The crick in my neck wanted relief from the stress of an unusually hectic pace. Overall, I felt depleted.

This short exercise made me realize that I normally went through the entire day—in fact, through many, many days—without being aware of my body. I lived so much in my head, thinking about the next meeting, the next item on my to-do list, that *not* focusing on my body had become my normal path.

Once I was willing to begin to listen to my body, to give it my full attention, even if only periodically, I learned what it wanted from me. Although it wasn't too happy, my body did seem honored that I'd taken the trouble to notice. It had long since given up hope that I would.

Slowing down to pay attention to my body equipped me to pay closer attention to my soul, too. I quickly realized that what I was feeling on any given day wasn't limited to cricks in the neck and a queasy stomach. On a deeper level, I realized that on some days I felt more confident and secure—"in the zone" of who I was and what I wanted out of life—while on other days I felt depleted. Over time I began to read the barometer of my inner self as avidly as I explored my outer physical self.

With rare exceptions, I haven't stopped paying attention since. Now I habitually check in with my body before I get out of bed each morning. I conduct a quick review of my muscles, my head, and my internal organs. Am I getting a cold? My period? Does my back feel stiff? How about my neck, a particularly tender spot with me? Where once I believed that my neck pain pounced on me out of nowhere, over time I discovered that if I paid careful attention, I could sense the buildup of tension and then intervene to do something about it before getting to the stage of being immobilized with pain.

Each morning while still in bed I also assess the state of my soul. Am I feeling sharp and raring to go? Drifty and dull? Do I feel a sense of purpose? Do I feel loved? Connected to others? The answers I uncover can help shape my day, in terms of which tasks I approach or how much time I allow myself to do them. Tarrant's simple suggestion—"check in with your body"—became a turning point for me.

I find that most women are not very practiced at observing. We're all much more skilled at doing than we are at being or tuning in. But that's only because we've had more practice in the "do" mode than in the "be" mode. Luckily, the more you observe, the better you get at it.

You can develop keener attention in many ways. Mindfulness, the subject of this chapter, is one way. The art of being mindful can be practiced formally (by learning to meditate) or informally (by learning to apply purposeful, nonjudgmental observation to life). But where meditation involves setting aside time for the formal practice, informal mindfulness involves simply learning to pay attention to the moment.

Becoming observant in this way is challenging. It's a different way of going through your life. Half the challenge is basically a matter of developing the habit, of having it become the lens through which you see the world. I'm not exaggerating when I say that cultivating an awareness of yourself is the linchpin of better health, and that's why the mindfulness-based tools described in this chapter are among the most essential ones on the journey to becoming Consciously Female.

Watching vs. Observing

I've chosen the word *observe* deliberately. Watching is passive; observing is active. It is watching with engagement, noticing all. When something is watched, the image merely presents itself. It's not necessarily absorbed in any particular way. When something is observed, it means you have trained yourself to use all of your senses to pay attention.

By making focused observations over a period of time, you learn to detect patterns, which enable you to understand what's normal for you. One woman's breast lump may be another woman's characteristically fibrocystic tissue, depending on whether what she's observing is new for her or not. A grouchy "fat" day becomes not just some random day when you're in a bad mood with the munchies, but part of a familiar constellation of changes that you notice occurring every month at a particular point in your cycle. A midafternoon diet breakdown is perhaps not a weak moment but something that occurs regularly when you skip breakfast and lunch. The only way you can assess these subtle (and not-so-subtle) changes within you is through continual awareness.

Paying attention to yourself is a form of love. Ever notice how when we fall in love with someone, we focus our attention on the object of our interest like a laser beam? All that the loved one does is interesting, every word or gesture memorable. This is the kind of love I'm asking you to lavish on yourself. Observe yourself, and watch your world unfold.

Observing vs. Obsessing

Don't worry. I'm not going to suggest that you spend every waking moment scrutinizing yourself and scribbling down what you discover in a handy-dandy notebook. You won't need a measuring tape or a Polaroid camera. There's no need to record every snippet of your life. I'd call those behaviors obsessing, rather than observing. Obsessing is a common pitfall of women who feel more comfortable in or more accustomed to the realm of black-and-white facts. Time and again patients will come in with long, detailed charts about what kind of discharge they had on day X and day Y, or what they felt like on each day of their cycle. But when I ask such a patient about the changes she has noticed over time or what kinds of patterns are usual for her, she can't say. It's easy to get bogged down by minutiae, to be unable to see the forest for the trees.

To be sure, looking at and recording factoids about our physical selves can be an important tool for observation, but too often it becomes an end in itself, yielding data that don't tell us what we need to know.

The kind of observing that I'm describing takes place not solely in the head, but in the heart and head together. It's not about scientific analysis. It's about taking it all in, being totally present with all of your senses and seeing what comes in. I tell patients, "Just observe what you observe." That Dadaist saying means just what it appears to: It's interesting simply to notice what captures your attention.

Observing vs. Interpreting

At this point you shouldn't be concerned about the meanings behind your discoveries. It's not necessary to analyze, critique, or judge what you are noticing. In fact, those activities get in the way of observing. All that matters is to make note. Cumulatively these observations will allow you to understand what's normal for you. Try to just notice what you notice, without judgment. Wondering about the meaning of every twinge and cramp can actually distract you from the important task of observing; it's possible to overintellectualize. You don't have to understand what's going on the moment it's happening.

When you are beginning the process of cultivating awareness, I think it's usually most helpful to write down all your observations. Later you may feel that you are familiar enough with the process to do a quick body-and-soul check in your head, or you might be selective and write down only certain kinds of observations. For example, a woman trying to conceive might carefully chart her basal body temperature and cervical mucus, along with her periods. A pregnant woman would want to monitor fetal movement with special focus. Or a woman wishing to lose postpartum pounds might rely on a nutrition diary in which she writes down everything she eats and what she was feeling at the time. But for now, when you are just beginning the process of becoming mindful, make a practice of writing down a broad spectrum of information—from both the body and the soul.

Some of my patients have a particularly hard time getting what I mean by observations of the soul. When you focus on feelings rather than facts, you assess your personal experience of the events. Ask, "How does this make me *feel*?" "What is my gut reaction?" Although this sounds more abstract than the relatively straightforward messages sent by the body, it's really not. We've all heard the nagging voice in our heads urging us to check out a problem, slow down, or be alone. We've all experienced sudden blues, bursts of energy, or other emotional data. Accessing this information requires making systematic observations of your soul, just as you make systematic observations of your body.

As the Persian poet Rumi said about prayer and piety, "There are a thousand ways to kneel and kiss the ground." So are there many paths to greater mindfulness. The following tools will all help sharpen your self-observational skills. Although they overlap somewhat, I'd encourage you to practice all of them at first in order to gain the fullest picture of where your body and soul are each day. Later you may do some, such as the all-important Five-Center Review, daily, but the others less often. It depends on what seems to work for you.

TOOL 7: THE FIVE-CENTER REVIEW

This is a tool that you can use every day. Your Centers of Wellness are the five main components of a well-stoked, balanced system: Movement, Nutrition, Mind, Spirit, Sensation.

The Five-Center Review is very simple. You only need to pay attention. But pay attention to each center on two levels—the body level and the soul level—because there is a two-way flow of information within each center, even though you may tend to think of some of them as being more body than soul, or vice versa. Your emotions on a given day will affect your appetite, just as your physical state may affect your ability to connect with the world beyond yourself. This tool is best used at the start of the day so that you can get information to inform your choices throughout the rest of the day. I like to do it in the morning to assess my needs, and again at day's end to check whether I fulfilled those needs. Sometimes I do it once or twice more as the day progresses. It doesn't need to take very long. Go right down the list:

- *Movement.* What is my body feeling today? Am I in a place that feels revved up, full of energy, or more lethargic and slow? How am I going to enhance its well-being today?
- *Nutrition.* Am I hungry? What for? How am I feeling toward food—do I have the munchies, a nervous stomach, cravings? Am I or do I feel depleted in any nutritional arena?
- *Mind.* Am I centered, calm, and focused? Or anxious or distracted? What's my stress level? Is anything on my mind manifesting itself in my body—a tension headache, sore back? How am I feeling in general: Confident? Sad? Nervous? Happy? Upset? Worried? Excited about the day?
- *Spirit.* Do I have a strong sense of purpose and connectedness? Is the meaning in my life palpable and real, or disjointed and vague?
- *Sensation.* Am I aware of all of my senses? Do they all feel well nourished? Do I feel sensual? Sexual? Very much so, slightly, not at all?

Some women like to keep systematic charts on this information, even after they've been doing it for years. Others prefer to do the Five-Center Review as a mental exercise, keeping tabs on how things change throughout the day. You can also jot key elements in your journal. As suggested above, when you're just starting out on your journey to mindfulness, writing it down is a good idea. You'll use this running account to inform your decisions about how to nurture each of these centers during the day.

Resist the temptation to judge this information or to make critical evaluations in any way. If, for example, you notice that you are craving sweets or wishing you could skip the exercise class you signed up for, don't criticize yourself for those thoughts and feelings. That's not the point of this tool. The point is simply to notice what you notice. Gather the facts of yourself. (Later, as with all of these tools, I will show you how to utilize the information you collect.)

Try It:

Track your five Centers of Wellness on paper every day for at least a month. Use the categories in the sample chart below to help you get started; later you might improvise your own system. By staying true to this process for several weeks running, you'll be best able to develop the habit of paying attention. The process itself is easy, but the ongoing practice of it requires discipline. Without consistent awareness, you risk falling back into watching, not observing.

Sue, 52:
⌒ *"At first I said, 'I don't have time to hear myself think, and you want me to evaluate five different aspects of my life?' But it hardly took any time at all, and before long I started to look forward to checking in."*

Martha, 26:
⌒ *"You'd think you just know when you're low on community and friend interaction, or haven't exercised in ages. I mean, I sort of do, but when I started to check in with the five centers every day it made me far more aware of where I was depleted. It's like a safety net before things get too out of control."*

TOOL 8: THE BODY SCAN

The Body Scan is a quick method for assessing yourself. Do it first thing in the morning. Ideally, you should repeat it several times throughout the day, but at least once a day. A good way to develop the habit of doing it daily is to incorporate the Body Scan into your normal routine. For example, you might do a quick scan before you step into the shower, or just before you leave for work.

SAMPLE CHART

Here's what I recorded on a recent morning using the Five-Center Review. Notice that it's not overly detailed, but rather more of a top-line view of what's happening within each center. Realize that "body" and "soul" are somewhat artificial distinctions, different points on the spectrum of who you are. One doesn't stop *here* and the other begin *there*. But noting distinctions between the two is a useful tool for making you a better observer.

CENTER	BODY	SOUL
Movement	Sluggish, hard to get going, leg muscles feel tight.	Want to crawl back under the covers; feel in retreat and in need of TLC.
Nutrition	Crave salty foods; don't really feel hungry but want to snack and graze.	Turning to food absentmindedly, as if for company or to provide myself with that TLC I'm craving.
Mind	Busy day ahead; already feeling scattered and having a hard time concentrating.	Feel a little fragile today, anxious, and worried about how I will get everything done when I don't feel like doing anything.
Spirit	Want to be alone as much as possible today.	Feel disconnected from everyone around me—my family and my friends.

CENTER	BODY	SOUL
Sensation	Have no libido; old sweats feel comfortable.	Don't feel like a sensual or sexual being—don't even want to be touched unless it's a big comforting hug.

The Body Scan should take only a few minutes. Your goal is to pay attention to what your body is saying to you, right now. You basically scan yourself with your internal eye. The exercise will provide you with an intuitive picture of how you're feeling. Here's how to do it:

- Sit down and close your eyes. Take a few deep breaths to get yourself centered.
- Turn your attention to the top of your head. Do you feel any tension? Any pain? Check your posture. What do you notice?
- Now continue to mentally scan your whole body, muscle by muscle, all the way down to your toes. As you go along, just notice what you notice.

This tool helps you make a snapshot of what's happening, providing a tip-off to what you might want to pay more attention to as the day progresses.

Try It:

Perform a Body Scan right now. What do you notice? What does it tell you about your stress level? What behavioral changes does this exercise inspire you to make? Next think about a point or points in your day when you could most easily incorporate a few minutes for a Body Scan.

TOOL 9: THE BODY-AND-SOUL QUICK CHECK

Even though the Body Scan tool is fast, here's an even quicker way to run an immediate assessment of your body as well as your soul. You can do it when you have a few minutes before meetings or in the car between errands. The Quick Check is essentially what John Tarrant asked my group of colleagues to try. I tell patients who are mothers that it's like stopping to look in on your kids while they're playing—a nurturing act that's done almost reflexively to reassure yourself and to keep in touch with them even in the midst of a busy time for you both.

Here's how it works:

- Pause and close your eyes. (You can even leave them open if you prefer.)
- Take a moment to tune in to your body. How is it doing today? What is its state right now? Is there anything it needs?
- And then turn your attention to your soul. How is it doing today? What is its state right now? Is there anything it needs?

That's it! The mere act of connecting with your body and soul, of paying attention—even for a few moments—brings them to the fore of your consciousness. It's like saying, "Hey there—how are you doing?" I hope the Quick Check will demonstrate to you that mindfulness is not a far-out, complicated thing that you have to study up on. It can easily be a habit that is an automatic part of your daily life.

Try It:

Do a Quick Check now. Be patient while the responses register. Until you become accustomed to zeroing in on yourself this way, it can take a little time to observe the state of your body and soul. Alternatively, you might be surprised to discover how quickly and clearly the observations come, now that you've created the space for them.

TOOL 10: BODY MONITORING

Here's a tool to help you become more conscious of your physical baselines—your personal norms. A baseline is not an ideal or a goal; it's simply where you are right now. If you weigh 160 pounds, your baseline weight is 160, even though you may have a goal of weighing 140. By tuning in to yourself, you'll become intimately familiar with what your baselines are. And then you can more effectively monitor changes (positive ones and potentially negative ones, as well as changes that are neither positive nor negative, but simply normal effects of aging, childbirth, etc.) and plan action steps in response to them.

It's important to mindfully monitor your whole body. But for women, that can be more easily said than done, since your vulva, your cervix, your vagina, and your breasts—those parts that make you quintessentially female—are out of sight. This exercise asks you to pay special attention to those places, since they are where things most often go wrong and where things change a lot. You don't have to rigorously monitor your thigh, because unlike your breasts or vulva, it's not a very dynamic part of your body.

You also want to pay special attention to those aspects of your physical being that can yield information of particular interest to you now—for example, your menstrual cycle if you are having PMS, or your cervical mucus if you are trying to avoid pregnancy or conceive.

The easiest way to learn how to monitor yourself is within a structure. Follow these steps until the Body Monitoring idea becomes second nature. You may choose to use this tool every day after you step out of the shower, or once a week on a leisurely weekend morning. Know that different parts of this tool will become more or less important to you at various stages of your life, but you should maintain some degree of consciousness about all of them. There may also be additional things to monitor during your various life pathways (e.g., during pregnancy).

- *Stand naked in front of a full-length mirror.* That request alarms many of my patients who are unaccustomed to their own nudity or have body image issues. Start with what makes you comfortable. Wear as minimal an amount of clothing as you're okay with, but with the intention of becoming increasingly aware of your body and working up toward full nudity.

- *Assess your general appearance.* What do you notice? How is your coloring, your energy level, your posture? My mother used to be the first to notice when I wasn't feeling well, even before I knew it myself. She was used to observing me. Therefore she was well positioned to discern subtle changes—whether I was pale or my eyes looked glassy, for example. I think we generally observe others, especially our loved ones, more than ourselves. When I see my husband, Rich, with his shoulders up to his ears, one side higher than the other, and wrinkles across his forehead, I know he's feeling tense, often before he realizes it! Learn to focus the same kind of attention on yourself that you might be used to giving to others.

- *Inspect your skin.* Become familiar with its markings, freckles, moles, scars. Use a mirror to see your back. Over time, look for changes in the shape and size of these markings. Report anything out of the ordinary to your doctor.

- *Check your breasts.* What do you see in the mirror? How is the color and tone of each breast and the areola? Touch them all over, from the nipple up to your armpit, as well as any part of the breast that may rest against your rib cage. How do they feel? Any rough, bumpy areas on the surface? Lumpiness or thickening underneath? Is there any discharge? Even if you have had a mastectomy, you want to continue to monitor what's normal around your breast area.

- *Do a vulvar self-exam.* Many women have never even heard of this, but it's based on the same idea as examining your own breasts. The vulva is an incredibly dynamic part of your body and therefore is vulnerable to changes you'll want to keep track of. It's hard to see anything without a mirror and bright light. First, wash your hands. Then, in order to keep your hands free to perform the exam, try straddling a mirror placed on a closed toilet seat or sitting on a towel on the floor facing a mirror. What do you notice about your pubic hair? The color and surface of your labia? What does the skin feel like? Do you notice any lumps or bumps?

• *Examine your vagina and cervix.* Insert your finger into your vagina and notice how it feels. Are the tissues smooth or rough? Moist or dry? Try to tighten the muscles around your fingers; these are the muscles of the pelvic floor. Now slide your middle finger as far back as it will go. As you feel around, you'll come to an area that feels firmer than the surrounding tissue. This is your cervix. It feels just like the tip of your nose, rubbery yet firm. And just like your nose, it can angle in different directions, to the left or right, or up or down, for example. (The position of your cervix doesn't influence your fertility; all of these variations are normal.) Mucus is usually all over the cervix, but gathers in the center. Some days you may notice no mucus, but other days there may be a lot. When you pull your finger out, look at it. What does the discharge look like and smell like? For some women this step involves mustering some courage, but remember why you're doing it: because it's *your body* and it's great to know what's happening inside it. And as vulvovaginal specialist Elizabeth Stewart says, "If in the process of touching you become sexually aroused, fine. That means you're properly wired, which should be reassuring." You should not experience any pain, however; if you do, figure out exactly where the pain trigger is and ask your doctor about it.

Try It:

Do the Body Monitor every week for a month. Write down what you find. This will help you become familiar with your baselines, what's normal for you.

Dee, 34:

"At some point in the year after my baby was born, I noticed all these bumps in my vulva and freaked out. I thought it was a sign of some kind of weird infection. It was pretty embarrassing to learn that they were just the torn bits of my hymen, which was shredded during childbirth. I guess if I had been paying closer attention, I would have noticed earlier that something was different down there!"

Jinny, 40:
⌐ *"I have never liked looking at my naked body. I always thought of it as the enemy—something that needs to be thinner or more pert and is never good enough. But forcing myself to really look at it all the time has changed my vision. It just is what it is. And it isn't so bad."*

The BSE Debate

Several recent studies have shown that breast self-exam (BSE) does not reduce morbidity and mortality rates of women from breast cancer, or catch breast cancers early. Instead, some research has shown that doing breast self-exam increases fear and anxiety more often than it helps detect cancer. Women tend to be immobilized by the very idea of a lump being found. So instead they commonly convince themselves that "it's nothing," and *do* nothing so as not to counteract that wish. I see this in my clinical practice all the time. Women say, "You check them. I'm not sure what I'm feeling" or "I'm not a doctor! I don't know what to look for!"

The medical establishment has made manual self-exam a woman's responsibility. Even though we doctors also perform it as part of the annual exam and may recommend mammogram screenings, the overwhelming message has been for women to follow up every month at home. And I think women have internalized this to mean, "Finding breast cancer is up to me."

The U.S. Task Force on Preventive Services says there currently are not enough data to recommend for or against BSE. I think self-exam is a good idea, just not in the way it's been framed and presented. We've done women a disservice by suggesting that they should move their fingers in a just-so formation every month in order to look for breast cancer. That's frightening and off-putting, not empowering.

A better way to discover whether there is anything wrong is simply to know what is normal for you. Be familiar with your breasts. Look at them. Touch them. Be alert for changes in their coloration or feel. Look at the nipple and notice if there is discharge or anything else unusual. Spend time handling them. Notice whether they feel different at different points in your cycle. Do they feel different to the touch? A great and caring way to do this is to pay particular attention to them when you are applying lotion or soap. Be systematic about it.

Your intention is to know what is normal for *you,* rather than to find anything abnormal. If you do this on a regular basis, year after year, and something different does show up, believe me, you will notice it.

Chapter 7

Imagine: Tools 11–12

Using dialogues and imagery to discover and focus

> Problems cannot be solved at the same level of awareness that created them.
>
> — ALBERT EINSTEIN

The previous chapter provided tools for identifying patterns, symptoms, and behaviors that are readily recognized once you've stopped and paid attention to them. That symptom might be painful intercourse, a tension headache, bloating, loneliness, a rash, lethargy, or a sweet tooth, all noted through checking in with your Centers of Wellness and using other observation tools. But what about the sources of those symptoms, their root causes?

Many of the root causes consist of experiences, feelings, sentiments, and impressions that have been pushed into the subconscious, beyond our everyday access, often with good reason. Some have been tamped down by fear, ambivalence, or horror. Others we ignore, avoid, or forget simply because we have packed schedules, complex relationships, tough choices, and too much going on in our lives.

This chapter shows you how you can access and observe some of what is held in your subconscious. Bringing this material into consciousness is a hugely useful tool for becoming Consciously Female.

Until you make a concerted effort to access this buried wisdom, you'll be making your health and life decisions based on only a partial picture. For example, a woman who has no conscious desire to become pregnant keeps forgetting to use her diaphragm. Although she may have noticed this pattern, that data would not necessarily yield any insight into the meaning of the behavior. Asking herself what feelings might be causing her to act that way could reveal that she is madly in love with her partner and conflicted about whether to make the relationship serious; becoming pregnant would be a test of the relationship, not a fulfillment of the wish for a child. Or she might be ready for a baby even though she hasn't yet articulated this idea to herself. Once she becomes aware of the real reasons for her forgetfulness, she can consciously address her unspoken longings, rather than simply acting them out in an unconscious and possibly harmful way.

Earlier I described the concept of "paying now or paying later, with interest." That is, it's always better to consciously process things as they evolve, rather than ignore or bury them, because if you do the latter, you're bound to be ambushed later, perhaps in an unexpected and physical way, by those feelings or symptoms that went unprocessed.

Ultimately, you want to get as full a picture as possible of what both your body and your soul have to report. One way of doing this is through imagery. Imagery is the language of the subconscious, providing us with a way of translating the messages from our subconscious. It's an incredibly useful tool, giving voice to what is otherwise amorphous and hidden, which is why I love it so much. Think of the dreams you have while you sleep, or midafternoon daydreams. While your conscious mind sleeps, some of what normally remains in the shadows comes out to play. That's why many therapists do dream analysis—to help people access this rich lode of information about themselves. Imagery can be similarly revealing.

Using imagery is a bit like dreaming while you are still awake. It's a way to bring the unconscious parts of your female soul closer to the surface. When you are comfortable with these tools, you will be able to use them at your convenience to check in with your subconscious and hear messages that might otherwise go unnoticed in the din of everyday life. The net result will be to bring you closer to a well-balanced state of health. (This work, of course, doesn't replace dreams, which are unplanned gifts of potential insight, and entertaining to boot!)

Sometimes my patients are surprised that a physician puts so much stock in the world of imagery. Aren't doctors supposed to be governed by precisely measurable data? But as I pointed out in the previous chapter, health information comes from two sources, the body and the soul. The techniques in this chapter focus on the soul. I certainly wouldn't diagnose a problem or outline a course of treatment based solely on what kind of imagery a patient experienced. But imagery is a powerful tool for gathering information that can influence a woman's course of treatment, choices in life, or state of wellness. I've often treated a symptom in a patient (say, pelvic pain), seen it go away, and then had the patient tell me she developed a different problem, such as a ruptured disk in her back. Coincidence? Sometimes. But just as often, there is an underlying issue that was not addressed the first time (for example, severe stress), which has found a new way to call attention to itself. The more clarity a woman has about an issue she faces, the better equipped she is to get to the real root of a problem and deal with it appropriately. Her life is also enriched by these insights and by her greater overall level of awareness.

TAPPING THE ACTIVE IMAGINATION

There are a thousand different ways to access one's subconscious. But I like the following two tools because they give the biggest bang for the buck, so to speak. They can be learned quickly and easily, without formal training. They can be done over and over, anywhere and on your own. Yet for all their simplicity, they can be potent windows to the hidden corners of your subconscious. Both are rooted in a long tradition in psychotherapy, formalized by Carl Jung as the "active imagination."

The first tool, Dialoguing, relies on imagination and is a kind of bridge between consciousness and imagery. It's an interactive conversation between your conscious mind and your subconscious.

The second tool, Dreamagery, relies more directly on imagery. It's a somewhat deeper and more visual kind of conversation with your subconscious.

When most of my patients hear the word *imagery,* they tend to think of visualization, or imagery that's used to alter. That's where you visualize an outcome you desire, whether it's being calm and well spoken at a meeting, crossing the finish line as you beat your best time in a 10K, or healthy cells in your body gobbling up cancerous ones. As a physician, I have used that kind of imagery to help ease patients through labor and delivery, recover from chemotherapy, and accelerate postsurgical healing. Used in this way, imagery is a wonderful, low-risk, high-reward therapeutic tool that empowers patients to participate in their own healing in a very significant way.

The kind of imagery I am going to suggest to deepen your journey of becoming more Consciously Female, however, is rather different. The tools in this chapter use imagery to reveal personal insights, to gain understanding, to glean information that might otherwise not be appreciated by your crowded conscious mind. You might observe that you are avoiding intimacy or are afraid of labor, for example. You can use the active imagination to help understand why.

You will not be in a trance as you do these imagery exercises. No one can make you say or do anything you don't want to. Nor is imagery hypnosis. You will be conscious and aware at all times, able to hear the phone ringing and the dog barking. You'll simply be in a relaxed and receptive state of being.

Suggestion: Read through each technique in its entirety before you begin. Since the best way to understand a technique is through example, I've included many within the instructions. Then follow along step by step. Eventually, as they become more familiar, you'll be able to do them on your own without having the steps written down in front of you. You might also want to perform one or both techniques with a friend.

TOOL 11: DIALOGUING WITH YOUR REPRODUCTIVE SYSTEM

I like to use this tool to help focus the big picture: What is your relationship with your reproductive system? By "relationship" I simply mean that we each have a unique partnership with our reproductive system—that dimension of us that makes us biologically female—whether we're aware of it as a partnership or not. And by "reproductive system," I mean everything that relates to your fertility, from the physical mechanics (your organs, your hormones, your biological clock, your periods) to all of the related emotional issues, large and small, such as your feelings about having children, how your period affects your moods, and your feelings about specific matters such as menopause, hysterectomy, infertility, and so on.

Examining this question is a good way to gain a fuller picture of your health concerns, because for a woman, the reproductive system is central, even while it is often fairly unconscious. You can elicit relevant feelings and perspectives that might otherwise not get factored into your health decisions or your life decisions. By exploring your relationship to your reproductive system, you can bring complex feelings to the fore.

A good relationship is built on a healthy give-and-take and a sense of shared purpose. In relationships where there is good communication, the partners are less likely to be taken by surprise. They talk, they listen, and, yes, they argue—all to the good. They work in tandem toward mutual goals. So it should be with a woman and her reproductive system. The relationship exists on both the body level and the soul level. When you accept the partnership paradigm, you're less likely to see your system as an adversary ("Why won't this PMS give me a break?"), as a mystery ("I have no idea what's going on down there"), or conversely as something over which you have total control ("I think I'll have a baby when I'm forty"). Your reproductive system shouldn't be any of those things. It's part of you, and though it is hidden from view, it is capable of speaking in a voice that is loud and clear.

Dialoguing is a playful tool, providing us with an opportunity to hear that voice. It's a structured form of introspection. Your conscious mind poses a question, and you wait for an answer to come. Come from where? you may ask. From the usually quiet place within you, whether you think of it as your unconscious or your soul. It's just a you-to-you conversation, but with an intimate, perhaps unknown aspect of yourself.

If you choose to try Dialoguing with a female friend, taking turns, which is a great way to become familiar with the exercise, remember that the goal is simply listening, not discussing what comes up, not judging it.

Here's how Dialoguing works:

1. *Set the stage.* Find a quiet, private, and comfortable place to sit. Dialoguing doesn't require much preparation or ceremony. You don't have to close your eyes, although some women find they concentrate better if they do. The main idea is to be in a place where you can remain undisturbed, a place where you'd feel free to speak aloud if you chose to.

2. *Picture your conversational partner.* I don't mean that I want you to conjure up images of your female organs, nor of rising and falling levels of the hormones that regulate them. Rather, the idea here is just to set the scene. In order to have a two-way conversation, it's generally helpful to have some idea of who (or what) is on the other end of the line. When you feel ready, take a few moments to let your mind ruminate on being a woman: your body, your menstrual cycle (if you still have periods), your stage of female life. You just want to establish a general essence of your reproductive system as a presence with which you can interact. (That essence might take an anthropomorphic form or not; it doesn't matter.) You need only spend a few seconds on this, to create the space for the conversation.

3. *Begin the conversation.* When you feel ready, there are four key questions I want you to consider:

   • What does your reproductive system want to say to you?
   • Is there anything it needs from you?
   • What would you like to say to or ask your reproductive system?
   • Is there anything you need from it?

For each, accept the first answer(s) that come to mind. Ask follow-up questions that seem appropriate, such as "Why do you say that?" or "How long have you felt that way?" You can ask anything you'd like.

Approach the exercise with an open, even light attitude. For some women these questions feel awkward, perhaps vaguely absurd. And since your reproductive system is not a "person," it's perfectly natural to feel as if you are talking to yourself. In a way, of course, you are—your conscious mind is probing your unconscious mind. If you feel embarrassed or self-conscious about doing this (a common first reaction), you might be approaching the exercise too literally. Go back to imagining your system as an entity that works in tandem with you. You're partners, right? And as a partner, your reproductive system has its own perspectives. Suspend linear and critical thinking and ask again. See what kind of answers spring to mind. If you wait long enough, something will.

Remember, you represent only half of the conversation. Allow space for your system to "talk back" to you. For most women, the responses simply "come"; they pop into your head. Some women feel like they're making it all up. A few women actually "hear" a response. Any or all are great. Listen for the tone of the response, too. Like you, your system might be angry, sad, frustrated, or overjoyed.

Although you are quite conscious throughout this exercise, you might be surprised by the answers evoked. This is the "active imagination" at work. Candid conversations can reveal issues or feelings you didn't even know were there. Dialoguing can be a way to get acquainted, to repair damage, clarify misunderstandings, or rejoin long-standing disconnects. Sometimes the responses gleaned are obvious, but the mere act of focusing on them brings them more to the surface than they had been before the exercise began. That's all great. That's making it conscious.

Lorraine, 47:

— *"I didn't think I had anything to discuss. So the first thing I blurted out to my system was, 'Okay, if I'm going to go through menopause, isn't there a way to make it a little snappier? Rather than drawing it out for years so that I can't get my bearings? It's gotten so that I can't figure out if I'm getting my period, having my period, or recovering from it—can't you organize things a little better for me?' And my system responded by calmly saying, 'It is what it is. Be patient. You're not controlling the process. The journey will take as long* as it needs to mature into the next stage of your life as a woman.' Afterward, the intensity of the exchange surprised me. I hadn't realized that perimenopause was bothering me. I guess I have been upset by the prospect of 'the change' and trying not to think about it too much."

Afton, 21:
—"It said to me, 'Hey! Don't take me for granted. You're working me a little too hard here [sexually], kind of abusing me. Take better care of me!"

Wendy, 32:
—"My message was, 'It is still possible to be a mother. I'll try to work with you if you will work with me. I'm ready for what lies ahead!' "

Janet, 51:
—"I asked what my reproductive system had to tell me, and it told me, 'Stop fighting against me and receive the signals I have been sending you. I'm simply trying to get your attention. I'm trying to work with you, not against you.' "

Remember, Dialoguing is about bringing issues to the surface, not about finding solutions, although solutions often reveal themselves after the issue has seeped into your awareness.

I hope you will return to this tool again and again across the pathways of your life because it will allow you to become more conscious of how your concerns change over time.

Try It:

Use the Dialoguing tool alone or with a friend. The exercise can provide insights for any woman, at any age. Although I recommend that patients do it periodically, first-time users reap special benefits, because it helps set the stage for understanding where you are now and what kind of work you want to do to become more Consciously Female.

Nancy's Story: From Adversaries to Partners ⌒

Nancy was one of my fertility patients. She was thirty-nine and had been trying to conceive for several years. As she proceeded to try more advanced treatments, she mentioned that she felt angry and impatient but couldn't help it. While these are certainly common reactions, I suggested that we use Dialoguing to help clarify her feelings around the fertility treatments. The gist of Nancy's question to her reproductive system was, "Why aren't you doing what you are supposed to?"

The response she got surprised her. "My ovaries kept telling me, 'We're on the same side here. We're going through a lot, too. We're doing everything we can,'" she said. The Dialoguing experience began to change Nancy's relationship with her system from an adversarial one to an empathetic one. Over the course of her treatment I saw her go from being emotionally distanced from each procedure to greater engagement. Where each hormone shot once glumly represented that something was not working right, she became much more aware of the dynamics taking place in her body.

I've seen countless women with similarly antagonistic or disconnected relationships with their reproductive systems. The discord expresses itself in different ways, but it's a very repetitive theme. The reproductive system's message is "Nurture me. Take care of me. I'm working with you; please work with me. Attend to me." I think it's a comment on how disconnected modern women are generally, from both their bodies and their souls. Strangely, it's as if we're two separate beings, our everyday selves and our reproductive selves.

In a later visit, we repeated the exercise. Nancy's dialogue had totally shifted. Now she began by saying to her "poor little ovaries," "Thank you, I know I'm asking you to do a lot." The simple act of engaging her active imagination allowed Nancy to bring her soul and her body both onto the same page—and that unified outlook could not help but give her a healthier outcome, whether or not she would actually conceive.

TOOL 12: DREAMAGERY

This is my favorite tool in the Consciously Female tool kit, because once a woman understands how to use it, there is no limit to what she can explore about herself. I gave it its name by combining *dream* and *imagery,* pronounced "DREAM-a-jry." This is a tool of insight. It takes you one level deeper than the Dialoguing exercise. If imagery is the language of the unconscious, then Dialoguing was one of those learn-the-language tapes, and Dreamagery is a living, breathing translator, helping you make sense of the garbled and foreign. As with any translation, you might not "get" the meaning in plain English right away, but you will be much closer than before you attempted to get help with the task. It's like dreaming while you're awake, but with the added bonus of engaging both your conscious mind and your unconscious mind.

Use Dreamagery to explore specific topics in depth. You might choose a topic that you began thinking about while taking the Consciously Female Inventory, or a subject that you have been writing about in your journal and would like to explore further. Many women use it to confront or to try to learn something new regarding a specific health problem (infertility, a suspicious Pap) or symptom (hot flashes, pelvic pain), or to help overcome a roadblock in their health plan (remember Tamara, my patient in Chapter 2 who used visualization to explore what was holding back her attempts to lose weight). I often use this technique with patients in my office to get a fix on their general beliefs about an issue, or when I am at an impasse in diagnosing a problem. Sometimes, for example, all tests turn up normal and I'm unable to explain a particular symptom, such as severe cramps or fibromyalgia. Dreamagery can turn up additional information the patient and I might want to pursue.

Here's how it works:

1. *Create some quiet space.* You need a time and place where you won't be interrupted for at least fifteen to twenty minutes. Consider the same place you set aside for your other

Consciously Female work, so that you can more easily dive into a relaxed and focused state. But the beauty of this tool is that it can be done anywhere you won't be interrupted, even at work.

Then make mental space by doing some relaxation techniques. The 4/7/8 Breathing or Mental Muscle Relaxation (Tools 3A and 3B in Chapter 4) work well. Take as long as you need. No clock, no worries.

Allison, 29:
— *"Tracy introduced this exercise to me in her office."*

Delaney, 46:
— *"Once a week I've started to devote a whole hour just to thinking about becoming more conscious. I relax and I journal, and then I do Dreamagery."*

Paula, 42:
— *"I was sitting on a sunny patio when I learned how to use this tool."*

Rita, 56:
— *"A woman's group I belonged to worked on this exercise. We all took turns."*

2. *Find your safe place.* As your own tempo changes, slowing, becoming calmer, invite an image of a safe place to come to mind. It may be a place you have been before or a place you've only imagined. A favorite vacation spot, your childhood home, a setting from a book or movie, your bedroom or your patio, some fantastical made-up scene—it doesn't matter.

Notice as many details as you can. What do you see? Notice the details of the scene. How does it smell? What time of day is it? What is the temperature? Are there any sounds? Distinctive colors? Are you alone?

Revel in your pleasure at being there, safe and relaxed. Notice how you feel in that place. Spend a few moments enjoying the space and exploring your feelings. Don't rush. You might choose to return to this same imagined place each time you do the Dreamagery exercise. Or you may evoke a different safe place each time; either way is fine. The purpose of this place is to help you enter a relaxed and receptive state.

Allison:

⌒ *"A mountain meadow. It is peaceful, moist, and cool."*

Delaney:

⌒ *"This time, my safe place was on the sofa in my study. It's a room filled with windows and special objects from my life. So many memories are here. There are pictures of people I care about, my books, paintings on the deep burgundy wall. The room overlooks my garden."*

Paula:

⌒ *"I pictured myself at one of my favorite places on earth, a beach on Lake Superior. I spent a lot of time there as a kid. It's a beautiful, empty stretch of sand that also has smooth colorful stones and big pieces of driftwood. I concentrated on imagining the smell of the pines and the sound of the big waves breaking onshore. A good place to be alone with your thoughts."*

Rita:

⌒ *"I imagined an underground cave, deep in the Yucatán, that I visited recently. It's a mystical place, nourished by a system of underground rivers. I can hear the water, quiet as a whisper. It's so cool and peaceful there."*

3. *Invite an image to appear.* Once you are comfortable in your chosen imaginary place, invite an image of the topic you wish to explore to appear (for example, your reproductive system, your female soul, your fertility, your unborn child, your weight). Be patient and don't force the process. An image will come, even if you feel that you are willing it, creating an image just so that you can perform this exercise. That's fine. Give yourself and your image time.

Accept the first image that comes to mind, even if it's not what you'd expect or it doesn't seem to make sense. The image isn't always a big "wow"—it may be something quite mundane. It may not even seem to relate to your life in a direct or obvious way. Although the image might seem silly or strange or disappointing, squelch the voice in your brain that says, "That's dumb" or "I'm not doing this right." Let go. Be nonjudgmental.

For some women, especially those who are visual and intuitive, an image leaps quickly to mind. It's often simple and specific to the issue at hand. A pregnant woman may get an image of her womb or her unborn child. A woman in menopause may see leaves falling from a tree. It is equally likely, though, that women in such situations will get images that at first blush are entirely unrelated.

Imagery does not come easily to everyone. Less visual, more analytical individuals often need patience as they wait for an image to appear; these types of women often tell me they feel like they are "making it up." That's okay. That picture is still coming from within you, one way or another. Just be sure to accept whatever comes to you. Some women report they get more of a sense of something than a recognizable image. That's also fine. A picture isn't necessary; if this happens to you, concentrate on gathering as many details about the sensation as you can—how it smells, how it makes you feel, or what it reminds you of.

Once your image has appeared, do with it just as you did with the place that came to mind. Notice everything about it, all of the details. Are there colors? Smells? Sounds?

(The women in the examples that follow had invited an image of their femaleness, or what I call their "female soul," which can be a wonderful starting point because it is broad and rich with possibilities for exploration.)

Allison:
⌐"I saw my reproductive system, complete but tiny, a perfect miniature. I could hold it in the palm of my hand like a Happy Meal toy. Suddenly the little replica turned into a butterfly, a gorgeous monarch."

Delaney:

⌐—"I felt dumb, with no image, like I wasn't getting deep enough. Then suddenly I had an image of a bird, ready to take flight."

Paula:

⌐—"The first thing that popped into my head when I tried to think of an image of my reproductive system was a pink flannel blanket. It wasn't one any of my four kids had used. It seemed weird because it was so out of sync with the rugged outdoor setting I'd chosen. But there it was, quite clearly, this soft baby blanket. It seemed like a weird image to appear considering that my baby days are ending—my youngest child is three."

Rita:

⌐—"She came to me out of a maze, across Mayan ruins. She was dressed all in white, wisps of veils covering her face and hair. I could make out high cheekbones and a long, strong body—like a classical statue. She was wrapped in layers of white, fanned by an invisible breeze. I felt her presence like a buzzing energy source as she came closer, but I heard nothing."

4. *Visit with the image.* Then begin a conversation. Ask the image why it's there. Does it have anything to tell you? Wait to see what kind of response comes into your head. Why is it there? Is there anything it needs from you? Let the conversation go where it wants to go. Ask follow-up questions if they occur to you. Do you have anything you wish to say to it in return?

That's it—those are the main questions to get you going. Many women find that the interchange continues beyond these basics. A persistent back-and-forth is good; it means that you are engaged with the image and more likely to bring forward interesting information. If you can loosen up and go with it, you will most likely find the experience a good deal of fun.

The results are usually provocative, sometimes profound. Your image may "tell" you something you hadn't realized before. Or it may simply state the obvious, which itself can be interesting and lead you to wonder why, or why *now*?

Recognize that the stage at which you find yourself in your cycle or your life's pathway may well play a role in the kinds of images that appear. This kind of work may prove especially revealing at certain times, such as during the second half of the menstrual cycle (the luteal phase), during pregnancy, and around menopause, because these are times of heightened emotion when the veil between the conscious and unconscious is often thinner, allowing imagery to come through more vividly. The same phenomenon is true for me after I've spent a full day and night on call; sleep deprivation dulls the intellect and makes the instinct more accessible. The images at these times (however unclear their meaning) simply reflect what's going on in your life.

Allison:
⌐ *"I asked the butterfly why it had come. It wouldn't speak to me, but it seemed interested and listening. It flew in ever narrower circles before settling silently on my shoulder, and then the wings began to grow and elongate, like sheets of mother-of-pearl. The wings grew down my back until they became a cloak, wrapping around me."*

Delaney:
⌐ *"The bird said I was ready to take flight!"*

Paula:
⌐ *"I asked the pink baby blanket image what it had to tell me. It said that I was sad that I had decided to have no more children, wasn't I? And I realized that I was! I have always made jokes—'four and no more,' 'the end of diapers'—but in fact, I think I am very conflicted about bringing my baby days, and my fertility, to an end. They've given me so much pleasure. Somehow I knew the blanket didn't represent a desire for another baby—it was worn, not new. The blanket was there just for my own comfort, seeming to let me know that it was okay to give some recognition to this hard transition."*

Rita:

⌒—"A kind of light and warmth reached me long before the woman's arms held me. 'It is all good,' she said. And she was gone. I was still in the maze, the sun was still bright, and I felt more at peace in my body than I have ever been."

5. *Pay attention to what you've learned.* The final step actually happens post-Dreamagery. Think about what you have seen and learned. Allow yourself to float in it awhile. Resist snapping out of it to analyze right away. Talk about what you imagined, write about it in your journal, or mull it over in your mind (or do all three). Sometimes an image that makes no sense initially grows in meaning after you have stayed with it for a while.

Sometimes I am asked, "But how do I know if I'm interpreting it right? Maybe it meant something different!" It's not your job here to interpret—that's your head and intellect crowding in. Your job is to reflect and experience. The insights will reveal themselves when they are ready. They may come to mind subtly or when you least expect them, sometimes like revelations. Don't get hung up on interpretations as if you were reading tarot cards or conducting dream analysis.

Allison:

⌒—"I had been having a lot of unexplained pelvic pain and bleeding, and my doctors had prescribed the birth control pill to help manage my symptoms. I felt very demoralized, even obsessed about having all these gynecological problems. Over the last few weeks, sitting at my desk or on my bed, I found myself going back to my safe place in the mountain, consciously inviting the image of the butterfly cloak to return. I wrap myself in that cloak and reward myself with a feeling of peace about my womanhood."

Delaney:

⌒—"I guess I felt a sense of strength about my abilities. I had been thinking of starting my own business for years and that soaring bird made me ask, 'What's holding me back?'"

Giving Dreamagery a Chance

While the Dreamagery tool is one of the very best for bringing unconscious thoughts to the forefront, it is also the one that can be hardest for women to embrace. Many of us are not accustomed to using imagery of any kind, not to mention engaging in conversations with such images. All I ask is that you give it a try. Remember that what your image looks like is actually not the most important thing at work. It is very common for your conscious brain to butt in, criticizing or feeling embarrassed about what your unconscious brain is "seeing." Acknowledge those thoughts, and let them go; don't engage with them. Get back to the image, however odd or unrelated or literal it might seem. The dialogue that you have with that image is where the unconscious mind begins to unfold. Go with it.

I have worked with dozens of women in one-on-one Dreamagery sessions, and hundreds more in guided group settings. Almost everyone has gotten something out of the experience, and by far the norm is for the participant to come away with keener insights around a given topic.

In short, it might sound especially foreign to you, but it works!

Paula:
⟶ *"This was the first time I had done Dreamagery. So I had no idea what to expect. After the exercise ended, I found that I kept thinking about the baby blanket image I'd had. I realized that my transition out of pregnancy and babies had been a very private one—all of my friends had finished this phase some time ago, and my husband couldn't really relate. Yet it was a huge deal to me. I'd spent the past ten years being pregnant and nursing four babies! Instead of just moving on to the next thing—homework, soccer games, perimenopause— I decided I would take time for myself to get comfortable with the idea of bidding*

my fertility farewell. I mean, I still could get pregnant (maybe), but I'm choosing not to. That's a big deal, and I suddenly wanted to respect it as such."

Rita:
⌒*"My image was like a divine presence who came to reassure me that I am well and I am fine. Her image is one I hope never leaves me."*

Try It:

Do the Dreamagery exercise to get the feel of it. The first time you try it, invite the image of your femaleness, or your female soul, as the women in the preceding examples did. It's a great subject for a beginner, since every woman has one, and every woman's unconscious will have something to say about it.

Lin's Story: Surprising, Soothing Messages ⌒

When Lin, a thirty-two-year-old newlywed, began Journaling about her first period, she remembered that as a teenager, she had started menstruating late. At age fourteen, her worried mother—who had taken diethylstilbestrol (DES), a hormone once used to prevent preterm labor and miscarriage that has since been linked to birth defects—brought Lin to the gynecologist to see if there was a problem.

Lin had been anxious about this first gyn exam. She became even more concerned when the doctor muttered something about her being "too small." "He couldn't find a speculum small enough to fit me," she remembers. "There was some discussion about putting me in a hospital overnight to do the exam under anesthesia. I was terrified, sure I was abnormal." Her mother declined to do this, however, and Lin's first period appeared soon after. Subsequent gyn exams found nothing abnormal. But her anxiety about her reproductive system continued. "I was always worried something wasn't right with me. The DES thing haunted me. And you can't imagine what a basket case I was about having sex for the first time, worrying I was 'too small.'"

I suggested that she use Dreamagery to explore the old anxious feelings that her Journaling had unexpectedly resurrected. She invited an image of her reproductive system to appear. "I saw a simple line drawing of my reproductive organs, a quick pencil sketch in black and white," she recalls. "My first thought was that maybe it was too literal an image and I wasn't thinking creatively enough, but I decided to do what Tracy suggested and go with this first image. So I asked it simple anatomical questions: 'Are you all right? Are things normal? Is there a problem with your fertility?'

"It replied that being a mother wasn't about the physical part of having a baby. You can be a mom emotionally as well.

"That was so stunning because in my head, I had been so focused on the physical process, the specter of something being wrong with me that would hang over me all my life. But as the image and its voice floated into my consciousness, I kept hearing three words over and over: 'It's not physical. It's not physical.' It was as if the voice of my female soul was coming to me, telling me that I was too stuck in worrying that something was wrong with me anatomically. That I was missing the bigger picture—that I already have all that I need emotionally to become a mother. That my anatomy is my anatomy and it would be okay. Tears came to my eyes as I heard a voice, an actual voice that said, 'I will take care of you.'" The experience was profoundly, and unexpectedly, moving for her.

Lin's story is a good example of how you can start out thinking about one subject and be pulled in a whole other direction. What had begun as musing about her first period and what her female self had to say about that experience turned into what was really on Lin's mind, albeit buried: that she would never be a mother because her own mother had taken DES. And what she discovered, deep inside her, was the message that she should let go of her worries and have confidence that she had everything it takes to be a mother.

Misty's Story: Dreamagery over Time

Misty is a good example of someone who used Dreamagery repeatedly throughout a transition in her life—in this case, pregnancy. As often happens, one topic kept recurring session after session, but the imagery that the topic evoked kept evolving.

A thirty-four-year-old mother of two, Misty had had some difficulties with each pregnancy. After her first child was born, everything had seemed fine, but the placenta was not delivered. After waiting thirty minutes, the doctor had to give her extra anesthesia and do a manual extraction—put her hand all the way up into the uterus and peel the placenta off the wall of the uterus, then pull it out with her hand. In Misty's second pregnancy, she developed placenta previa, a serious complication where the placenta is attached to the uterine wall too low in the uterus, so that it partly or completely covers the cervix, blocking the baby's exit from the womb and putting mother and baby at increased risk for bleeding before or during labor. Because Misty had bleeding fairly early in her pregnancy, and because the second bleed is often massive and doesn't allow a woman enough time to get to the hospital before her or her baby's life is in danger, she was kept in the hospital on strict bed rest for the last three months of her pregnancy.

Once the baby's lungs were mature, he was delivered by C-section. Both mom and baby were fine, but it had been a long and difficult road, especially since Misty had a young child at home.

The risk of repeating the condition tends to rise with each pregnancy, and indeed, Misty was diagnosed with it again in the fourth month of her third pregnancy. After having a C-section, however, there is an increased risk of another condition, called placenta accreta. Because of the C-section scar, the placenta embeds itself right into the wall of the uterus, rather than being separated by a layer that allows the placenta to peel off after delivery, as usually happens. There was no way to know if Misty also had this second condition until the time of delivery. With placenta accreta, the mother very often ends up with a hysterectomy following the C-section.

"After finding out I had placenta previa again, I wasn't surprised, but I was very angry and very anxious," Misty recalls. "This would be the third time that the placenta didn't stick to its job of nourishing and helping my baby grow." Misty was referred to me by her ob-gyn in the hope that mind-body treatments might help reduce her stress and ease her delivery. I suggested Dreamagery to explore her upset feelings and help her create a healthy relationship with the thing she feared most.

"I tried to relax and pictured my family's lakeside home, a place that is near and dear to me," she said later. "When I invited an image of this pregnancy to appear, dozens of images flooded in—a bird, a smiling face, different pictures of babies. Finally one baby image seemed to linger. It said in a clear, sweet, non-baby-like voice, 'Mom, you need to eat and not worry so much about me. If you are taking good care of yourself, you will take good care of me.'

"This was revelatory for me because at that point I was not concerned about taking care of myself. I was completely focused on the baby's health. I had lost a lot of weight. I'd forget to eat or to take my prenatal vitamins. This conversation gave me permission to worry about me."

Misty continued to use the tool throughout her pregnancy. She saw the same baby almost every time, and it said, "Mom, you have to accept the fact that it's not just you and me in this process. It's also our placenta that's keeping us both alive."

Later, I encouraged her to use Dreamagery to explore her relationship with the placenta. At first no image came; then she saw a picture of an actual placenta, all blue veins and red tissue. "It didn't mesh well with the calm scene I had created for myself," she commented. She felt stuck. I encouraged her to continue doing the exercise weekly. Later an image came to her of her and the baby at a mom-and-tot swim class. "We were bouncing around in the water and an inner tube floated up— one of those life preservers you plop a baby into," she said. This was the first time she had had an image of the placenta as an instrument of safety, an indication that her relationship to it was beginning to shift. "Another time my image was of a little bird in a nest," she says. "My placenta was trying to show it was a life preserver for my baby, but my feelings were still mixed. I couldn't stop viewing it as an adversary."

After several weeks, Misty felt that her heart had opened enough to ask the placenta image if there was anything it needed from her. "It said, 'Have faith in my role in this process. I won't let you down. We are a trio and I am working for you and the baby, not against you.'"

Misty says, "I came to feel comfortable with my images of the placenta. I had been fighting it all alone, but it was reassuring me that I could rely on it and find it a trustworthy partner." By the time her due date approached, the true moment of partnership had come. "At one imagery session, my baby and I were performing a duet onstage and the placenta presented itself as the bright stage lights that are always trained on the soloist in a dance performance. The lights were bright and annoying, like the lights in an operating room. I was ready and able to connect the physical and metaphysical aspects of the birth soon to come."

As her labor began, Misty summoned her Dreamagery images to help her stay calm and focused. "I kept the images of me, the baby, and the placenta, all dancing together, present in my mind until the epidural began to work," she recalls. The delivery was complicated and dangerous. She began to hemorrhage and had to be given a massive blood transfusion—but she delivered a beautiful, healthy daughter. "Even deep under anesthesia, I believe that I knew that the placenta was my trustworthy partner in bringing Nellie to life, and it would do its part to make sure I could walk out of the hospital alive, with a healthy baby tucked under my arm." Afterward, Misty says she knew that her placenta had done what was needed—it had managed to sustain her baby all the way to term, for which she and the baby would be eternally grateful. They made a great threesome!

Jeannie's Story: Harvesting What's in Your Soul

I introduced Jeannie to Dreamagery when she was thirty-nine. She had occasional and sometimes persistent pain on the right side in her lower abdomen, which she associated with her ovary. She noticed that the pain was always worse when she was worried about a new setback for her chronically ill sister. A pelvic exam, sonogram, and other tests revealed nothing amiss. Because of this, and because she was under extreme stress caring for her sister, I suggested that guided imagery around the ovary might help her better understand her pain.

What she learned across a series of sessions over the next year was that the pain usually surfaced when she was totally neglecting herself. It was almost as if the pain was a way to get her attention. The message was that she needed to make space for herself no matter what else was taking place. In her very first session, she saw an image of herself as tall and obese (she's actually a tiny woman). "Fat Jeannie" was lying on a bed, unable to move or be happy. "Fat Jeannie" told her that she needed to pay attention to her, take care of her, or she would keep getting bigger and bigger.

By the next session, after she had taken that message to heart, "Fat Jeannie" reappeared—but about fifty pounds lighter. The time after that, she was her own size, floating blissfully alone atop a blue ocean. "It was very peaceful, with no sense of danger. No sharks. No worries about how to get to shore. No need to worry about sunscreen. I could just float on the water and retreat from the world."

The message, during this and other sessions, followed a theme: that she needed to protect a world of her own that was not consumed by the needs of others. Sometimes the characters she saw in the exercise provided practical tools and plans for how she might approach a specific problem. Once a session fell right before she made a long flight she was dreading but had to make because of another family crisis. "Suddenly a girl appeared, and she said, 'I *love* to fly! I love it when the plane moves! It's the best part!' That image reframed my fear of flying—that it could also be fun, 'the best part,'" Jeannie said later. "Now when I get on a plane I have this other image—this vivid girl is inside me enjoying herself. And I tolerate her, the way you let a child enjoy something even if you don't like it yourself, because you enjoy her happiness."

For Jeannie, the images almost always came fast and vivid. She became good at asking them questions until she felt like she had a sense of clarity around taking her next steps. Over time, her pain grew less and less frequent, but Jeannie continued the Dreamagery because she found it a useful tool for encouraging her to take care of herself and reminding her when she backslid. The imagery became a partner in her journey of self-discovery.

As you can see, the imagination is powerful. Remember that these tools aren't being used to conjure up a fantasy of how you'd like your health to be. This kind of imagery is rooted in the present. Dialoguing and Dreamagery harvest what is already in your soul, though perhaps not yet on your mind. It always has been part of you, just not a conscious part. Tapping in to it allows you to be more fully aware, more wholly present.

Now you have a full complement of tools with which to construct a workable approach to your health every day, every year.

Part Three

The Consciously Female Life:

How to Make It Real at Every Age and Stage

Chapter 8

Living the Conscious Life

What every woman needs, every day

"Changes that are loved into being are more likely to be permanent."

— CHRISTIANE NORTHRUP

I'm not big on blanket prescriptions: Take this. Do that. Eat these. One-size-fits-all health formulations are risky because there are too many variables. How could a single program be right for every woman? Such a diet or exercise program tends to be an unconscious plan, directed from the outside as opposed to built from the inside out.

I can, however, give you both a decision-making vehicle and some core information about the needs of your five Centers of Wellness that will help you develop a plan that's right for *you*.

In Part One, I laid the groundwork for the potential benefits of being Consciously Female and explained how bringing an active awareness to matters of health and healing can dramatically improve both your individual well-being and the health care system that treats you. In Part Two, I gave you some tools for coming into greater consciousness. They're certainly not the only tools a woman could ever use to gain insight into her body and her soul. They're merely suggestions, a framework for tuning in. Exploring your consciousness is a bit like exercising a muscle. For most of us, the link between body and soul is flabby from disuse. (Remember the woman who was too busy to go to the bathroom until she developed a kidney infection? Or that famous Roy Lichtenstein–style Pop Art painting of the businesswoman—fortyish, I'll bet—crying out, "Oh my God! I forgot to have a child!") The more you use the tools, the more tuned in you'll become. Remember, some tools will work better for you over time than others; collectively, though, they stress the deep linkage between your body and your soul that's already present and waiting to be listened to.

If we stopped there, however, you would only have learned how to become more aware. You would not have changed the choices you make in your life from day to day.

Part Three, beginning with this chapter, will show you how to craft a personal plan that works every day of your life. What's the secret to its effectiveness? It's built upon your own self-knowledge. It's built on your consciousness of what it means to live in the dynamic, changeable self that is you. That self-knowledge flourishes because you have made the space for it to do so. You have made an effort to understand how you've arrived at this place in your life. You have observed your body. You have observed your soul, bringing your inner wisdom to the forefront. Moreover, you have made yourself aware of how these two sources of information complement each other. When you're living consciously, they present a very full and textured picture, combining with the rest of your knowledge about yourself to make a vivid, realistic, dynamic 3-D portrait.

If a Consciously Female program is predicated on so much individuality, you might be wondering just what it looks like in practice. The short answer is that it looks like you. It consists of consciously made choices reflective of your individual needs and priorities. Your choices will be healthier for having been made in this way.

Every action you take involves a choice. Some are small but add up over time. What will you eat for breakfast? Will you jog today? Call a friend? Schedule that mammogram? How will you spend your free time this evening? By making the best choices for you, day after day, you can lose weight, avoid many illnesses and complications, shorten your recovery time, improve your muscle tone or bone mass, ease and enrich your transition through pregnancy or menopause—in short, feel your best in every area of your life.

And then there are the bigger choices that get made in each pathway of our reproductive life, from puberty through aging: Should I have sex? What kind of birth control should I use? Do I want to have a baby? When? At what point do I seek fertility help? Should I go on HRT? Just as with the small choices you make, you can certainly make these choices without awareness, but then your life remains disconnected from who you really are. It's driven by outside forces rather than your inner wisdom. When you make the choices that best correspond to your own inner dictates, the result is a sense of peace.

I witnessed a perfect example of the difference between conscious decision making and unconscious decision making when the NIH study on the long-term use of hormone replacement therapy came out in 2002. I (like every other gynecologist I know) was inundated with frantic calls from women wondering how this news affected them personally. Interestingly, those who had elected HRT as part of a conscious decision-making process—who had based their choice on internal data as well as the relevant medical facts—were concerned but notably calm. Those who had gone on HRT because "my doctor said I should" or "I read this was a good thing to do"—who had made the choice based only on external data about what somebody else said—panicked. About half of the women in each group wound up quitting HRT. But the difference in their reactions was stunning. When you're living in a Consciously Female mode, you know the data will change; that's a given. You understand that making choices is a dynamic process, so when new data come up your world doesn't turn upside down. You roll with it, reassess. Part of the panic felt by the "unconsciously female" group was triggered because they had put all their trust in an external thing, rather than in the process—of which the external data are just one part. As that study proved, nobody can give you an absolute answer about whether HRT is right for you. The answer is, "It depends." You have to make your own choice. What I call the Feedback Loop can help you do that.

THE FEEDBACK LOOP

The Feedback Loop is a decision-making cycle that enables you to arrive at choices that are mindful of your real needs. It's a very easy process to learn. The cycle consists of reflection, information, and action, and then begins again with re-reflection. If you run your choices through this cycle, you can't help living with awareness and intention, reaping the benefit of healthier choices.

Although the Feedback Loop may sound like a cumbersome mechanical process, the cycle of reflection, information, action, and then re-reflection quickly becomes second nature when you live it day by day. In fact, I can no longer *not* think in this way, I've grown so accustomed to it. It's a wonderful way to approach any kind of decision in your life, not just the health-oriented ones.

The cycle looks like this:

- *First, reflection.* That's another word for collecting your personal or internal data. It makes use of all the knowledge and insight gleaned from the Consciously Female tool kit in Part Two (Journaling, your health inventory, body checks, Dialoguing and imagery, and so on). Such data include your starting opinions, your emotions, your perceptions, your fears, physical evidence, and the status of your needs within your five Centers of Wellness.
- *Second, information.* That's learning as much as you need to know from external data. This might include medical options, statistical evidence, and the prevailing medical wisdom. Please note that this step doesn't mean that you must collect every scrap of data there is. How much to incorporate into your decision making is a very individual matter. For some women, hours of trolling the Internet and poring over medical journals are appropriate. For others, consulting a trusted physician would be sufficient. Decide how much you need to know and find out how to access it.
- *Third, action.* Take a step based on both the internal and ex-

ternal data you have gathered. It's vital that you collect this information *before* you take action, as it will inform what kind of step you choose to take.

- *Then, re-reflection.* Making a choice is not the end. You next reflect on the step you have just taken, beginning the cycle again. How do you feel about your choice? What are your body and soul telling you about this course of action? Does it feel right and good, or uncomfortable and disconcerting? This is new and important information. And you can continue the cycle. Gather new information if needed. Have any of the facts changed? What (if anything) will you do differently based on this new information? The cyclic nature of this process is essential. Without it, you risk slipping back into unconsciousness.

Making conscious choices is a continuous cycle, just like breathing—and just as fundamental. You breathe in (reflection, going inward for personal data), hold it a moment (the pause for the external information gathering), and then breathe out (take an action step out in the world). In-breath, out-breath.

The Feedback Loop is not something you do, it's a way you live.

Since we were talking above about conscious vs. unconscious decision making with regard to hormone replacement therapy, let's look at how to use the Feedback Loop to resolve this very complicated issue. Here's how I counsel a patient who is wondering what she should do.

First, reflection. I would urge her to make space in her life to explore her feelings and beliefs around HRT. Does she have preconceived notions or worries? What is her inner voice telling her? How does she feel about menopause? What are her fears or concerns? How do these relate to HRT? To access this information, a woman might journal about it and reflect on her health history—did her mother have an easy or difficult menopause? Does she know someone with breast cancer who believes it was associated with using HRT? She could try doing the Dialoguing and Dreamagery tools around this topic, and reflect on what kind of physical symptoms she is now experiencing. How disruptive are they? Is there anything particularly intolerable, and if so, why? Is there anything relevant in her health history?

Second, information. She needs to determine how much she wants to know. I would help her map out the options: different kinds of HRT, including bioidentical hormone therapy, with an overview of the benefits and risk factors of each, and also alternative approaches—mind-body therapies, lifestyle changes, and so on—to the particular issues she is concerned about. But many of my patients choose to use the information I give them as just a starting place for more in-depth fact gathering.

Third, action. All of this information leads her to a decision about what she would like to do, what options best fit her individual situation and needs. Then she can take a step and see what happens, knowing that this is not necessarily a final decision.

Then, re-reflection. Say she tried HRT for three months. How was that experience? What did she notice? If she did not feel much different on it, no better or worse, and the main reason she chose it was for short-term symptom relief, re-reflection might lead her to decide to stop the therapy and see what happens. If, instead, she had felt amazingly better—fewer and less intense hot flashes, improved sleep quality, clearer mind—then it might be easy to decide to stay on and reevaluate further down the road. Knowing that you are working within a continuous cycle helps to make the whole process much more manageable, much clearer.

Sometimes, especially when it's a matter of taking a step that can't be undone, I ask patients to not actually take the step, but to only imagine that they have and then reflect on that. For example, Darcy came in for a second opinion about having a large uterine fibroid removed. Actually, mine was to be the third opinion; one physician had urged her to have a hysterectomy, since she was not planning any more children, while a second felt that only the fibroid needed to be removed (a my-omectomy). Darcy's husband joined her at the consultation. Scheduled for surgery in four days, she was clearly very conflicted about what to do. I told them that the first choice was whether to have surgery at all. I asked Darcy to close her eyes and imagine that she had decided to have the operation, and to simply sit and live with that decision for a few moments. Interestingly, you could see her body tighten and her fists clench. She reported that she felt anxious, but also felt the surgery was "what I should do." I asked her to check in with her body: What did she notice, how did she feel? "Take a breath now and let that scenario go," I suggested. Next I asked her to imagine that she had decided not to have surgery. Even Darcy's husband remarked that he could see her visibly relax. Since the medical data did not indicate that either surgery was essential, her decision really boiled down to her own choice. What was right for *her*? When I pointed this out, the couple quickly agreed: She would cancel the surgery and take the next three months to make some lifestyle changes, then reevaluate.

In the chapters on the four individual pathways, you will see how the Feedback Loop can help make choices at each stage of life.

FIVE-CENTER BALANCE

You can see how the Feedback Loop helps you make conscious choices. But day-to-day healthy choices have to be made in the context of a core of good information about how to nourish your five Centers of Wellness. Together, these five centers add up to balanced well-being: Movement, Nutrition, Mind, Spirit, and Sensation. In Chapter 3, I explained why the concept of the whole person and all of her interconnected needs is one of the foundations of integrative medicine. In Chapter 6, I gave you a tool for checking in with these centers every day as part of your overall tool kit for tuning in. The five Centers of Wellness represent kind of a shorthand for how to think about total health. In this chapter I will give you some nuggets of information that you can use as a taking-off point for your own pursuit of information about how to keep yourself in balance each day.

To be sure, as you go through life you will face other decisions with regard to your wellness beyond these daily domains. But they are a huge part of the total picture because they are immediate and central. They are the key to optimizing your overall health and healing capacity.

Living consciously, it's best to take a step (or steps) every day within each of your five Centers of Wellness. You need to nurture all five Centers of Wellness every day to maintain healthy balance. That's because each supports the others. For example, stress can influence your food choices. Exercise can reduce stress. Simply becoming more mindful of the five centers will make it easier to use them as a structure for moving steadily and surely toward change.

Some of my patients moan, "Five things!" when I suggest this to them. Five things can sound like a lot. But it's not. Remember, *small* steps forge the most sustainable beginning. Use that power to propel you along. For example, here's what taking a step in each of the five centers might look like to a woman who already feels overwhelmed and is just getting started:

Movement: Take the stairs instead of the elevator once today.
Nutrition: Choose broccoli over french fries at lunch.
Mind: Do some relaxation breathing before a stressful meeting at work.
Spirit: Read a poem that gives you a feeling of spiritual connection.
Sensation: Wrap yourself in a favorite shawl.

None of these steps is particularly taxing. Their benefit is that they are moving you toward a new awareness and a new habit—not the specific habit of eating broccoli instead of french fries or walking the stairs instead of taking the elevator, but simply the habit of being more mindful about your well-being and making conscious choices.

Once you have made mindfulness an automatic part of your life, you may find that you are ready for bigger steps. Some women may be ready to take on major steps in one or more of the centers. A woman who has reflected and is ready to overhaul her Nutrition Center, for example, might choose actions that are more ambitious than simply eating a green vegetable at lunch. Maybe she's ready to realign her already reasonably good eating habits and shift to a more advanced program that will also help her lose weight. But she, too, has to start by taking a single step in that direction. She, too, will see her successes propel her on to still bigger ones.

I cannot tell you precisely what kinds of choices will be best for you. Only you know what you're feeling and experiencing and what works for you; only you know where you are right now. But I can offer some general guidelines to move you toward what's optimal. Use these ideas to inform your own day-to-day choices. You can apply these ideas or adapt them. Please realize that these guidelines represent my favorite nuggets of information—not the last word on each category. Within each center, your physician or other resources can point you to dozens of other suggestions. You'll no doubt hit upon your own favorites, too.

The guidelines presented here apply to all women, regardless of their pathway. In the following chapters I'll give more specific variations that apply to women who are on each of the four primary pathways of a woman's life: Cycling, Fertility, Transition, and Transformation.

THE MOVEMENT CENTER

Every day, find a way to integrate pleasurable movement or exercise into your life. That's often easier said than done. Movement takes time, for one thing. And many women have mixed feelings about it, either because of bad experiences in the past, guilt over their present routines, or a lack of clarity about what their bodies really want and need. But I can't say enough good things about the benefits.

Remember that movement can be virtually any kind of physical activity. Exercise is one dimension of movement and usually refers to more intense or sustained movement done for a specific reason. Explore both your internal body-and-soul messages (reflection) and what's known about exercise and women (information) to inform your choices (action).

- *Do something, anything.* There is no drug, vitamin, mineral, or herb that has as many health benefits as exercise. Women who move stay limber, burn calories, build muscle and bone mass, and work their heart and lungs. They live longer and better than their sedentary peers. To be more specific: They reduce their risk of osteoporosis, heart disease (including hypertension, coronary artery disease, and high cholesterol), diabetes, breast cancer, osteoarthritis, obesity, premenstrual syndrome, and depression, to name just a few! For example, the Nurses' Health Study, widely regarded as a reliable source of insights into women's health since it followed seventy thousand women over a period of years, showed that the most active participants had a 50 percent reduction in the risk of diabetes. And the protective effect of exercise was strongest in the people with the highest risk.

Another large long-term study (ten thousand women followed over twelve and a half years) found that sedentary women who became active—walking the equivalent of just one mile a day—decreased their overall risk of dying by 48 percent, their risk of heart disease by 36 percent, and their risk of cancer by 51 percent.

Medically, it's better to be overweight and physically fit than to be slender and sedentary. That's a tremendous reminder that, in terms of your health, the process is far more important than the package!

Being in motion is also a wonderful way of reconnecting your body and your soul. It triggers physiological responses that leave you feeling energized and uplifted, and it can be a buffer against stress and depression. A Stanford University Medical School study, for example, found that mild exercise can drastically improve mood; after only one day of walking on a treadmill, subjects began to experience improvements at the same level it took several weeks to reach on a standard antidepressant medication.

- *View exercise as a triangle.* Don't pursue one kind of exercise to the exclusion of others. Aerobic or cardiovascular training, flexibility training (stretching), and strength training (weight lifting) represent the three sides of the fitness triangle. You need to cover all three each week because each provides different physical benefits. Aim for sixty minutes of sustained heart-rate-raising exercise at least three to five times a week. That's the target advocated by the Academy of Sciences, though I know it can sound incredibly daunting. Other experts recommend thirty minutes. Either duration offers tremendous benefits in building bone, burning calories, and encouraging all-around feelings of energy, vitality, and strength. Stretch at least three times a week, preferably before other forms of exercise. Use resistance training (free weights, elastics, machines, etc.) on nonconsecutive days. Only 18.7 percent of American women do strength training (vs. 27 percent of men), according to the Centers for Disease Control. If you are not ready yet for the recommended amounts of exercise, do them half as often or half as long, or whatever works for you.

- *Use routine as reinforcement.* Research indicates that the most beneficial and easiest exercise habits to maintain are those you have made a part of your daily routine. For example, do them at the same time every day, so that you don't even think about whether or not to do them.

If you desire still more information about Movement, you can consult your doctor or the "Readings and Resources" section to point you to some suggestions.

Stella, 73:
⌐ *"Every morning before I get out of bed, I do my 'rolling pin' stretches. I stretch my arms all the way up and stretch my toes all the way down. Then I roll my body from one side to the other. It helps me feel in my body for the day. I love it!"*

Casey, 34:
⌐ *"I used to think I didn't have time for exercise. I was always signing up for classes at my local Y after work and then having to drop out. Then I took a dance class. I hadn't danced since I was in college, but I'd loved it then. Guess what? Now I look forward to going to class, and somehow I figure out ways to get there no matter what."*

Cora, 55:
⌐ *"I used to think I had to stick to my prescribed exercise routine no matter what. But when I check in with my body first, I've learned to heed what it's*

saying. I used to exercise right through a cold, but now if I feel one coming on, I step back. I might do stretching exercises instead of going for a swim. I think my colds don't last as long as they used to when I would try to fight through them."

THE NUTRITION CENTER

Find ways to bring meal-by-meal consciousness to what you eat, why you eat, when you eat, and how you eat. Conscious Nutrition begins with reflecting on your relationship with food. The goal is not to follow a "perfect" diet but to help you make mindful choices that support your physical and emotional needs, as well as your health goals.

A woman's relationship with food tends to be extremely complicated. We use food to nourish both our body and our soul. Food is fuel, food is social, food is visceral, food is sensual. Not only are our dietary needs highly dependent on (and influenced by) our reproductive status, but what we put in our mouths is also entwined with issues about body image, control, emotions, family history, sensual pleasure, and all sorts of unconscious issues usually held at bay. Food should provide the necessary nutrients while also being a pleasant experience free of guilt, anxiety, mindlessness, or fear. Yet it's often consumed with little conscious awareness (and little apparent pleasure).

Making choices around nutrition consciously, however, helps to crystallize what's taking place in your brain and on your fork. By bringing awareness rather than angst to the table, you can take Nutrition step(s) that better suit where you are today. It's an especially challenging center, not least because we face food hour after hour—at least three times a day at meals and usually far more often. Living without it is not an option. Still, the same approaches apply.

Following are a number of suggestions for making good choices in the Nutrition Center. You'll notice that the suggestions are more specific for this center than others. That's because far more research exists on nutrition, and because nutrition comprises so many different elements. (Because your nutrition needs change across your cycle and your reproductive life, guidelines for each life pathway are found in its corresponding chapter.) These guidelines, as well as the nutrition guidelines presented in subsequent chapters, are based on materials prepared by my friend and colleague Greg Hottinger, MPH, a nutritionist and consultant to the Duke Center for Integrative Medicine.

- *Tune in to your hunger and fullness cues.* Observe the way your body physically lets you know whether or not it needs nourishment. Rate your hunger on a scale of 1 to 7, 1 being "very hungry" and 7 being "very full." Your goal should be to eat when you feel 2 to 2.5 (moderately hungry) and to stop eating at 5 to 5.5 (moderately full). But most of us don't know what those states feel like. True hunger cues include a growling stomach, a feeling of emptiness, or headache.
- *Eat with body awareness.* Learn your eating triggers. For example, non-hunger-related cues that signal us to start eating include fatigue, the presence of an eating buddy we habitually dine with, and the clock ("It's dinner time...whether you're hungry or not!"). Potential triggers of overeating may include going too long between meals or eating something unsatisfying (so you continue foraging for something else).
- *Learn your patterns around eating.* Keep a Nutrition diary as a way to observe your present habits. Don't worry about making big changes at this point or making yourself sound good on paper; just keep an honest and complete record. Nutritionists believe that most women keeping food diaries underestimate their total calories consumed by as much as 50 percent. Not because they are trying to be deceptive, but because they miscalculate how many crackers they grabbed, forget that second spoonful of sugar in their coffee, or misjudge portion sizes—all signs of being mindless. Note everything you eat, when, how much, where, what you were doing, and how you were feeling at the time and afterward. Try to do this for a week if you can, or at least a day or two.
- *Experiment with mindful eating.* Chew one bite for five minutes. Yes, it's a long time! Notice everything about the food's taste, texture, and the way it makes your mouth feel. It's not realistic to eat every bite this way, but the exercise shows you the

difference between a big gulp and a conscious bite. I like to do it every so often as a mental jog—to remind myself to be more aware of the whole process of eating.

- *Use Dreamagery to explore childhood beliefs about eating.* Common holdovers from youth include believing that you must always clean your plate or that desserts are the best part of a meal. What were the messages you received about food as a child, both the conscious ones ("Clean your plate") and the unconscious ones ("Quick, grab your share before your siblings eat it all")? Were there times when eating was a joy? A battleground? Why? You might choose to do some imagery around one of these issues.

- *Cut down on portion sizes.* The supersizing of American cuisine isn't limited to fast-food joints. Regular restaurant servings, too, have grown ever larger. When women eat out often, they can lose an accurate perception of what a portion, as measured by nutritionists, really is. Reality check: One serving of pasta is about the size of your fist. Pause to focus on the *amount* on your plate before diving in. I know one woman who automatically divides her restaurant meal in half and puts it in a doggie bag *before* she eats the other half. Beware of home servings, too. Did you know that the standard Nestlé Toll House cookie recipe on the product's package in 1949 yielded one hundred cookies, but only sixty cookies today? It's not the amount of the ingredients that have changed; it's our perception of how big a cookie should be.

- *Know that the size of your stomach in its natural state is only as big as your fist.* Reflect on that as you fill your plate! You can also check in with your stomach; ask it how much it really wants.

- *See how you stack up.* Compare your diet with the Healthy Eating Pyramid, the revised version of the standard 1992 government-produced Food Guide Pyramid. It was based in large part on the Harvard Nurses' Health Study, which is nice to know since that means it was crafted from a large amount of data on women. This will give you a general sense of whether your diet needs an update. Then you can factor in the specific information below.

- *Think seven—at least seven servings of fruits and vegetables a day.* These foods are relatively low in calories but rich in nutrients and fiber. One thing that almost every diet plan, from Atkins to Ornish, agrees on is that vegetables are great. I make a game out of it: I keep a mental tally to see how early in the day I can get to seven, and if I get there, how many servings over that minimum I can go. A serving isn't enormous, so you don't need to worry about counting calories. But it does require conscious planning even to get to seven. Examples of a serving are half a banana, 1 medium fruit, 2 tablespoons raisins, or 1 cup raw or 1/2 cup cooked veggies. Depending where you are now on this score, your Nutrition step might as simple as adding one or two more servings a day to your diet.

- *Choose powerhouse fruits and vegetables whenever possible.* Ideally, your *daily* diet should include at least one dark green cruciferous vegetable such as broccoli (protective against an array of diseases), a leafy green such as spinach or chard (important sources of calcium and vitamin K, which protect bones), and one orange fruit or vegetable (rich in carotenoids, which seem to protect DNA). For your *weekly* diet you should aim for up to eight servings of lycopene-rich foods (tomatoes, red grapefruit, tomato sauce), as more than thirty-five studies have shown a significant inverse relationship between tomato intake or lycopene level and the risk of cancer. Be sure to include antioxidant-rich fruits (prunes, raisins, berries) and, if you tolerate them well, onions and garlic, which also possess antioxidant properties and are a good source of selenium, a component of the master antioxidant glutathione peroxidase.

- *Learn your fats and act on that knowledge.* It can be confusing—but it can make a big difference! Reduce *saturated* fats (cheese, butter, whole milk, ice cream, beef) to less than 15 grams daily. Replace *polyunsaturated* oils (corn, vegetable, safflower, soybean) with *monosaturated* oils (olive, canola, organic peanut). Try to avoid all *trans fatty acids* (found in Crisco, hard-stick margarine, tortilla chips, french fries, many commercial baked goods, and processed packaged goods). Information about trans fats, which was hard to find on food labels before 2003, is increasingly available and becomes mandatory in 2006. And add to your diet *plant fats* (nuts, seeds including flaxseed, avocado, olives, nut and seed butters such as peanut butter or tahini) and *omega-3 fats* (found in salmon, albacore tuna, mackerel, sardines, and herring). If the average woman reduced her daily saturated fat intake from 26 grams to 15 grams by substituting healthier fats, she would reduce her risk of heart disease by 42 percent. That's compelling evidence for a woman of any age.

• *Introduce yourself to flaxseed if you haven't already.* It's both a great source of omega-3 fats and a powerhouse of lignans, a phytoestrogen that contains promising anticancer properties. I recommend 1–2 tablespoons of ground flaxseed daily. You can buy whole flaxseed online or at health-food stores and keep it for a week in the refrigerator, grinding it as needed with a coffee grinder or blender. Sprinkle it on cereal, salads, or vegetables. Golden flaxseed has a nice nutty flavor and is an excellent source of fiber, nearly 12 grams per ¼ cup. That's quite an impressive amount of fiber packed into such a small container, especially when you consider that 25 grams is the generally recommended daily amount. You can use flaxseed oil on toast, on a baked potato, or as part of a salad dressing, but avoid cooking with it because heat makes it deteriorate rapidly. Caveat: Women who are taking tamoxifen or who have been advised against phytoestrogens should not take flaxseed.

• *Do a protein shift.* Move away from red meat and cured or smoked foods. (One beef hot dog contains half the recommended intake of saturated fat for a whole day!) In their place choose lean animal protein (chicken or turkey breast, fish, egg whites, low-fat yogurt, cottage cheese, low-fat milk), ideally organic or free-range varieties, which will lower your intake of hormones, antibiotics, and other chemicals. (But even the nonorganic varieties are a better choice than red meats.) Each week, eat at least three servings of an omega-3-rich fish. Also try to replace at least three servings per week of animal protein with soy protein, including soy-based veggie burgers, edamame (soybeans), soy milk, tofu, and tempeh. If that seems too ambitious, start by trying just one soy serving a week, or one meatless meal, and work your way up.

- *Swap out a white grain for a whole grain.* Fiber is one thing most women don't eat enough of. Fiber-rich foods include beans (ideal: four times a week), whole-grain breads (look for "100 percent whole wheat" on the label; you can't go by the brown color), and higher-fiber cereals (bran-based, oatmeal, whole-wheat-based). Most women already consume the same calories in low-fiber or no-fiber carbs, such as white bread, white pasta, white rice, bagels, pastries, baked goods, candy, ice cream, and soft drinks. Why fiber? Not only does it give all kinds of worthy benefits such as intestinal regularity, reduced cholesterol, vitamins, and antioxidants, but fiber intake may play a role in preventing breast cancer. Just a 5-gram increase in cereal fiber a day (that's half a cup of Grape-Nuts) is associated with a 37 percent reduction in the risk of heart disease in women. Since in many cases you need only swap one kind of product for another (brown rice instead of white, Grape-Nuts instead of Frosted Flakes), this often proves an easy step for women to take.

- *Take a sunbath.* Why is that a Nutrition fact? Direct sunlight triggers the synthesis of vitamin D, a nutrient necessary for calcium absorption. Women who live in northern climates and those who don't get outside much are especially vulnerable to vitamin D shortfalls. In fact, researchers at Nebraska's Creighton University found that people can lose up to 97 percent of their vitamin D stores between summer and winter. Ideally aim for ten to fifteen minutes of sun on your face and arms without sunscreen two to three times a week, in early morning or late in the day to minimize your exposure to harmful UV rays.

- *Stop after the first drink.* More than two alcoholic drinks a day (a drink being defined as 5 ounces of wine, 12 ounces of beer, or 1.5 ounces of hard liquor) increases the risk for malnutrition, stroke, hypertension, obesity, and many cancers. That said, red wine is a source of antioxidants (polyphenols), especially Pinot Noir. Drink consciously, if you drink at all.

- *Drink more water.* This is an easy step that most women neglect. A good goal is at least 48 ounces (6 cups) a day. Water reduces the incidence of kidney stones and gallstones and improves overall immune function. Ideas: Carry a water bottle throughout the day, buy bottled water instead of soda, or serve it with your meals. If you purchase bottled water, look for brands that are distilled, purified by reverse osmosis, or purified by carbon filtration.

- *Say yes more often to green tea and no more often to caffeinated coffee.* The benefits of reducing caffeine intake accumulate as you get older, so a woman of any age is wise to avoid or cut back a caffeine habit. Caffeine stimulates the central nervous system—and in high doses can mean insomnia, nervousness, gastric irritation, increased heart rate, and high blood pressure. A daily intake of 300 milligrams or more of caffeine (about 18 ounces of strong coffee or 6 glasses of soft drinks or tea) significantly increases bone loss from the spine, according to a study of 489 elderly women. Lesser amounts—1 cup a day—are considered safe. In contrast, green tea (whether caffeinated or decaffeinated) contains powerful polyphenols (a kind of antioxidant) that can slow potential cell damage and neutralize enzymes that advance cancer growth. One study found that Japanese green tea drinkers with breast cancer tended to have milder forms of the disease than those who drank black tea, and stayed cancer-free longer. The kind of polyphenol in green tea, flavonoids, also helps keep blood vessels healthy, providing protection against arterial disease. Try replacing a daily cup of joe with a cup of green tea.

- *Pop the right vitamins.* Start with a daily basic multivitamin—how's that for an easy Nutrition step? The nutrients in multivitamins are no substitute for food sources, but among their benefits, they can reduce bone loss. Ditto for calcium (500–1,200 mg) and vitamin D (400 mg). The National Academy of Sciences recommends 1,000 mg daily of calcium for women ages nineteen to fifty, 1,200 mg daily for women over fifty.

- *Plan your indulgences.* The foregoing advice steers you in the general direction of good nutrition. But since eating is food for the soul, too, you aren't going to be ultimately happy (or healthy) if you are following a diet that makes you feel cranky and deprived. Consciously build pleasure into your diet. For one woman that may mean whole-wheat bread and olive oil with a glass of red wine before dinner; for another, it's a weekly hot biscuit slathered with butter. As for me, my soul enjoys an occasional glass of red wine. I try to drink it mindfully, during intimate time with my husband. During PMS, I crave chocolate-chip cookie dough. Knowing that, I plan ahead so that I can make a batch with whole-wheat flour when the urge strikes. When you develop the habit of making conscious Nutrition choices, you'll find that your tendency to eat "bad" foods goes down and the pleasure you derive from the things you do eat goes up.

Meg, 47:
‎—"I realized that I was so busy taking care of my family and my mother that I skipped over myself. I would fuss over healthy lunches for the kids to take to school and make sure Mom had hot meals, but then I'd eat whatever I could grab on the run. My first Nutrition priority is to eat more mindfully—at least to start by sitting down when I eat!"

Kara, 25:
‎—"I hate fruits and vegetables. But I didn't realize that popping a vitamin didn't keep me covered—that you get other benefits from eating the real thing. So I am trying really, really hard to start by just having one fruit or vegetable

at each meal. I'm learning to really notice their beautiful colors and fragrances. When I eat them, I focus on the taste. And I'm realizing that there are some I really do like."

Jenny, 36:
⌐"I never linked what I drank to how I felt. It's not like coffee and wine are drugs or anything. But in a way for me maybe they were having that kind of effect. I would always have a glass or two of wine to help me wind down and fall asleep, then I'd have a cup of coffee to help me wake up in the morning, and keep pouring all day. Once I recognized this pattern, I didn't like it. To wean myself off caffeine and alcohol I'm switching over to decaf green tea after lunch and seeing if I can not have the wine automatically every day. I'm not ready to swear off coffee and go all morning without it, though!"

Lizzie, 27:
⌐"The image I got when I invited an image of my childhood binge eating during Dreamagery was of a gopher. That was pretty weird, but Tracy said to keep with it. So I asked the gopher why it was there—what did it have to tell me? It said it couldn't stop to talk, it had to keep burrowing. So I asked, 'Why?' And the gopher said, 'I have to keep digging because the dirt is there, and who knows when there might be such fine dirt again?' Even though this 'conversation' wasn't anything about food, I felt a pang of recognition. I guess I ate as a kid because it was there, like the gopher. My mother would always try to restrict how much we got at mealtimes—so we wouldn't get fat. Ha. Instead, whenever I was at a friend's house and a snack was served or I spent my allowance on something like a bag of chips, I'd snarf. Because it was there. Just like that gopher. Just in case I didn't get the chance again. Then I asked the gopher what I could do for it. It said, 'You could pet me.' I think the gopher wanted to take a break from tunneling. It wanted to be loved. That's when it hit me that my soul wanted a little love, too. It didn't want to keep binge-eating anymore than I did. And for the first time I felt a glimmer of what I want now, not what I wanted as a kid."

THE MIND CENTER

Find a time and a way, each day, to quiet your mind. I sometimes think of this as giving your mind the equivalent of sleep. Sleep restores the body and the mind, but the mind needs replenishment during the day, too. Although there are hundreds of ways to "do nothing," from five-minute meditations to two-week retreats, making this a priority can be one of a woman's most difficult challenges. Our lives are busy, our brains are busy; who has time to stop everything and unplug? In fact, I find that the Mind step is the first one patients cheat on, passing it by.

Realize that your mind has very different needs at different points in your menstrual cycle and in your reproductive life. Specific advice pertaining to those cycles and phases can be found in the following chapters. But the following suggestions are good at all ages and stages:

- *Center yourself.* Each time you move from one activity to another, take a few moments to center yourself. At the Duke Center for Integrative Medicine, we often preface meetings with a few minutes of silence to let participants shift gears and really be present. It's a practice that never fails to startle, and sometimes inspire, visitors accustomed to more rushed agendas. (The rushed part sometimes comes in once the meeting gets under way!) My husband and I like to join hands for a few seconds of silent reflection before a meal. Other examples might be taking a few mindful breaths before entering a colleague's office at work or doing breathing exercises before beginning an exercise routine. Allow yourself to focus on your breathing—not to alter it, simply to note your inhalations and exhalations. Then widen your focus to the sensations of your body. Finally, if you like, widen your scope once again to focus on everything around you.
- *Live in the present.* With so much crowding your mind, it is easy for your attention to wander. Thoughts about this evening's dinner intrude on this afternoon's meeting. Thoughts about the meeting earlier in the day invade

Run a Stress Check on Yourself

Become aware of what stress looks and feels like for you. Stress is most dangerous when we're unaware of it. The following checklist offers a quick way to evaluate whether you're dangerously out of balance:

- Check your heartbeat: Is it racing past thirty beats in twenty seconds?
- Check your breathing: Are you taking more than six breaths in twenty seconds?
- Check your feelings under the surface: Are you angry? Irritated? Impatient? Tired?
- Check your thought process: Are you dwelling on the same thoughts over and over?
- Check your voice: Does it sound tighter, higher, or squeakier than normal? Are your words rushed?
- Check your posture: Are your shoulders hunched near your ears? Does your upper back feel tight and constricted? Is your chin down?
- Check your hands and feet: Are they cold or clenched?
- Check your stomach: Does it feel knotted or relaxed?

If you answered yes to any of these questions, you know that stress is expressing itself. Although that's probably not a surprise, it's fascinating to realize how many different ways that message is being communicated.

tonight's slumber. When you notice your focus wandering away from the moment before you, call it back. It's okay to make plans—we all have to do that. And remembrances are sweet. Just monitor where your head is throughout the day so that it dwells for the most part in the present, not the future or the past.

- *Reflect on your stress points.* Your stress points are how your body manifests stress generally. In addition to the specific characteristics above that you might experience, there can be more generalized signs. For example, some women always get diarrhea when under duress. Others feel low back pain or become vulnerable to colds. We all have our own way that stress is manifested in our body. Learn what that is for you. When it does surface, you can recognize the real culprit and not just the symptom.

- *Be disciplined about relaxation.* This may sound contradictory, but it's not. Relaxation opportunities need to be scheduled into your day, just as opportunities for exercise and eating. Here's why: The body responds not to reality, but to perception. If you're sitting at the edge of the magnificent Grand Canyon yakking on a cell to a business associate about a project gone haywire, guess what happens? Your body doesn't react to the fresh canyon air and soothing kaleidoscopic colors. It reacts to the stressed reality in your brain: your adrenaline and cortisol (stress hormones) rise, your pulse quickens, your blood pressure increases, all the physiological consequences of what is collectively known as the *stress response.* It's automatic. Conversely, you can be in the middle of a stressful situation but make your body react in a relaxed manner simply by quieting your mind, which is known as the *relaxation response.* It's nothing short of magical.

There are many ways to activate the relaxation response, from yoga to meditation to walking, or any of the excellent ideas for creating inner space found in Chapter 4—whatever works for you. Many people pick just one that they like to use every day. Cardiologist Herbert Benson, who defined the relaxation response, has found that practicing meditation twice a day for twenty minutes, for example, brought significant reductions in blood pressure for many subjects. Meditative prayer, of course, is a component of almost all faiths, including Judaism, Christianity, Islam, Buddhism, Shintoism, Taoism, and Confucianism. Dr. Benson has found that repetitive prayer can elicit the same dramatic physiological changes as noted in transcendental meditation.

The relaxation response is not automatic, however. It won't happen unless you make it happen by making special time for it.

• *Avoid the stress response as your chronic mode.* What's wrong with stress? You've probably heard the answer before, but let me pile on some more facts. The stress response is useful to a human who's leaping away from a saber-toothed tiger or, to use some more modern examples, giving a speech or walking through a dark alley. It surges to prime your body for possible action and then recedes when the danger is past. The problem comes when stress is chronic. Your protective mechanism, the stress response, is overloaded. Your immune function is impaired. You fall back on poor habits (eating fatty "comfort foods," smoking, overworking, drinking too much, not exercising). High levels of cortisol are thought to shrink nerve cells in the hippocampus of your brain, which can result in memory problems. Even your shape can change, as elevated cortisol collaborates with insulin to store fat at the abdomen, rather than the hips or buttocks. As a *New York Times* report on a University of California–San Francisco researcher's work put it, even in slender women, stress, cortisol, and belly fat seem to go together. Prolonged stress has been also shown to weaken the immune system, strain the heart, slow recovery time, and damage memory cells in your brain.

• *Pay attention to sleep.* The average woman needs eight hours of sleep a night, although the exact amount is variable, depending on the individual. You might feel rested and alert on anywhere between six and ten hours of sleep a night. A Harvard study of 71,617 women found that those who got eight hours of sleep nightly were least likely to have heart problems. Those who slept five or fewer hours were 45 percent more likely to have heart problems, and those who slept nine hours or more were 38 percent more likely to have heart problems. Yet according to the National Sleep Foundation, women sleep an average of seven hours on weeknights. And one-quarter of us don't sleep enough to be fully alert the next day! Sleep restores the mind as well as the body, providing energy and alertness and nourishing the immune system. Sleep loss is cumulative. First you may notice changes in your mood or your ability to concentrate. Over a longer period, your reaction time and decision-making capabilities are affected. Sleep deprivation, especially chronic deprivation, causes as many fatal car crashes as drunk driving, by some estimates. Hormonal levels can influence the quality of sleep (specific information follows in the pathway chapters). So can your diet, illness, alcohol, and other factors.

- *Do something new.* People who try new things are healthier and happier than those who stick to familiar ruts, psychologist Ellen Langer has shown. A friend's octogenarian grandmother was famous for bringing home new products: "It's something new, I thought I'd try it," she'd explain. Was she already naturally adventuresome or did her explorations keep her spry? Probably both.

- *Redefine time.* When you're stuck in a traffic jam or a long grocery line, don't let it become a stress surge. Choose to spend the time doing 4/7/8 breathing or another kind of relaxation tool. Journal while watching your child's sports practice. I slip a book of poetry into my carry-on bag so that I can dip into it during airport waits. I'm not suggesting that you multitask to cram in Mind steps; rather, reframe the downtime moments of your life from stressful, boring, or idle ones to nourishing ones.

- *Invoke the automatic maybe.* We have a choice to say no to requests, even though we often forget it's optional! Women find it hard to say no. Guilt preys upon us, as do a sense of obligation and force of habit. Yet too often, we wind up taking on more than we can comfortably handle, and are stressed or resentful as a result. An action might be to never automatically say yes to anything. Make the commitment to yourself first.

Train yourself to respond, "That sounds great, but let me think about it and get back to you." Or "I'll check my calendar and let you know." The automatic maybe gives you the space to make your choices conscious. It's much easier to say no when you're not in the heat of the moment, after you've been able to give considered thought to the request.

- *Check the "Readings and Resources" section.* There you'll find good sources of specific Mind information. And use tools 3 and 4 from Part Two.

Amity, 35:

⌒ *"On my way home from work I stop at a park near home and just sit in my car for ten minutes doing breathing exercises, followed by meditation. I call it 'Amity time.' It helps me create a kind of safety zone between my busy work life and my busy home life."*

Suzy, 32:

⌒ *"When I am feeling angry or depressed, I write my heart out in my journal. That makes me feel better—but here is the best part. I bought a portable paper shredder that I keep on my kitchen counter, where I write. After I get it all out, I just shred the paper all up. It's out of my system, and I don't need to keep the pages. It's the process of doing it that I find calming and relaxing. I used to burn the pages, but the burns were making marks on my counter. This is neater."*

THE SPIRIT CENTER

Find a way every day to nourish your spirit. Spirit is what fosters a sense of connectedness between you and the larger world. It's a feeling that life is about more than you; you're part of a family, part of a community, part of a country, part of the incredible system of humanity, part of the vast universe. Spirit concerns having a sense of meaning and purpose in your life, whether you gain that from religion, faith, humanity, nature, or some other source. Both your body and your soul benefit when this center is nourished.

- *Reflect on what spirituality means for you.* We are all spiritual beings, whether or not you consider yourself "spiritual" in the conventional religious sense of the word. For you, Spirit might be your faith and your involvement in your religious community. For many women this is a powerful, bedrock source. In addition to this, or instead of this, other women find Spirit in their communion with nature, or in a one-to-one relationship with God or the universe. Spirit also refers to your human connections, your relationships to other living beings. Your family, your neighbors, and the personal and professional communities in which you operate can all play a role in stitching you to the world beyond yourself. (Pets count, too.) You can find spirituality in solitude also. There's nothing like sitting all alone on my back deck, focusing on a sunset, to give me an intense connection to the world beyond me. To be always alone is detrimental; to be occasionally alone can be incredibly nourishing. The important thing is to figure out what your particular Spirit needs are at this point in your life, at this stage of your personal development, and then to make choices to accommodate those needs.
- *Find your Sabbath.* In the get-you-thinking words of psychologist Joan Borysenko, who has written extensively about women, spirituality, and health, "Every person could kick their life into a whole new orbit by taking off one day a week as a real Sabbath. By this I mean to drink deeply at the well of faith, family, friends, joy, and rest, not a day to catch up on errands." What and when is your sacred time to connect with the bigger picture of life? All day on Saturday? Sunday mornings? The hour right after work? First thing in the morning? Committing to the importance of the pause of a Spirit step is the first action you should take. I recommend making at least one day a week a day for yourself.
- *Understand that connections count.* The evidence is compelling that people who feel connected boost their well-being. A study comparing populations in several cities found that the

individuals who were the least socially connected were twice as likely to die compared to people who were more socially connected, with the data controlled for health and lifestyle risk habits such as smoking, drinking, obesity, and a sedentary lifestyle. Studying women with metastatic breast cancer (the kind that has progressed to the rest of the body and is generally incurable), researcher David Spiegel found that those who were in weekly support groups and who were taught self-hypnosis lived twice as long as those who were not in support groups. While this finding has not been duplicated in subsequent studies, the quality of life for women in support groups has consistently been higher.

- *Express or rediscover your faith.* Don't overlook the obvious. Prayer works. As I mentioned earlier, the act of prayer has been found to trigger the relaxation response. Prayer and other mind-body interventions at the time of cardiac catheterization decreased adverse outcomes, including heart failure, repeat angioplasty, and death, by 25 to 30 percent.

  Interesting research has also been done on intercessory prayer—praying on others' behalf. Studies focusing on patients in situations as diverse as in intensive care units and undergoing in vitro fertilization have compared the outcomes of those who received prayer support (intercessory prayer) and those who did not. (The patients were not aware they were being prayed for, so their own belief systems were not engaged.) The ICU patients who received intercessory prayer experienced significantly fewer complications than those who were not prayed for, and the IVF patients had a 50 percent pregnancy rate, compared to a control group rate of 26 percent. No one knows how prayer intervention works, of course—is it God's hand or the power of the intention from the good wishes conveyed by concerned humans? Nevertheless, the medical impact of this kind of spiritual intervention is an intriguing area for future research. So if you already believe in prayer, use it.

  Another benefit to being active in a religious community is

that it affords many opportunities not only to interact with others, but also to help others. Whether you're building a Habitat for Humanity house, working at the church soup kitchen, or teaching Sunday school, selflessness is good for the soul, as they say. As much as I feel it's important to be attuned to yourself, there is also healing power in focusing on others.

- *Reconnect with the natural world.* Being in nature provides the dual benefit of triggering the relaxation response and stimulating a sense of connectedness to something greater than yourself. Especially if you live an urban or suburban life, it can require intention in order to commune with nature. Stargaze, noticing the scale of the sky; try to find the Big Dipper or the North Star. Grow something. Take a walk. Watch the birds or animals that share your habitat.

- *Explore your creativity.* There's a direct connection between artistic endeavor and the soul. Something is stirred. Even if you haven't picked up a paintbrush since grade school, consider buying a palette of watercolors and a tablet of paper. Take a pottery course. Set up a darkroom in the basement. If learning is your thing rather than doing, take a class in art appreciation at your local museum or community college. You don't have to think of yourself as "artistic" to find some facet of the arts that engages (and perhaps expresses) your spirit. Leafing through an art book, attending a concert, or going to a play all count as artistic endeavors that can provide profound connections. A Spirit action might be as simple as doing one of these things—provided it's done with wholehearted focus.

- *Schedule time alone.* It might sound counterintuitive that you can enhance connectedness through solitude. But many women are so accustomed to being with others that, while they do reap the benefits of those relationships, they sacrifice opportunities to find their inner peace.

- *Hone your communication skills.* Good communication can improve the quality of your relationships, increase your sensitivity to others, and ultimately improve health and longevity. Two common traps women fall into are a hostile-aggressive mode and one of passive compliance. The most productive communication style is healthy assertion: first you connect (i.e., you demonstrate an understanding of what the other person is saying) and then you request (i.e., you state your own request in a personal, specific, and nonjudgmental way). Example: "I know you're mad that I forgot to pick up the dry cleaning. But I ran out of time because I bought groceries and took the broken vacuum in for repairs. Let's figure out the best way to get it now." Consciously switching your communications to the people around you is a great example of a small step that sends out wide ripples of results.

Adriana, 28:

〜*"I got into studying Renaissance painters at a class. Now I can't quit. I can't explain it, but I fall into a kind of trance, delving into all that beauty. The time I spend in a museum is a time of grace."*

Frances, 36:

〜*"It dawned on me that I only felt spiritual on Sunday sitting in the church pews for an hour. And even then, I was still tense from the rush of getting three kids and myself ready, and I'd have one eye on them during the service and be thinking about what I was going to feed everyone for dinner. Our lives are so rushed. We have started taking a family walk together after dinner every night. It's just around the block, but it's a set thing. We all look forward to it. It feeds all of us."*

Debby, 44:

〜*"I started volunteering at the local Girl Scout Council. I don't have any kids, but I had loved being a Scout myself, and figured maybe I could help. It worked out better than I dreamed. They needed adult helpers, and I have developed all kinds of connections with the other women leaders at the council and with the girls that I work with. It's awakened something so satisfying and vital in me."*

THE SENSATION CENTER

Each day, take a step that supports your sensate needs. That is, find a way to support your senses and/or your sexuality in a conscious way. I call this center the last frontier of wellness. Most physicians do not include sensuality or sexuality in a woman's wellness plan. But I would argue that to be fulfilled with regards to Sensation is more than a "nice plus" to the other components of balanced health. Women are sensual and sexual creatures; it's part of our essential makeup. Our sensuality and sexuality are very real sources of vitality. Both are biological drives. A woman who exercises, eats right, relaxes, and has a strong sense of purpose would not be optimally healthy, in my book, if she were also unable to enjoy the free expression of her sexuality or sensuality. Both of those lapses indicate that something is wrong. She has needs that are going unmet, Sensation needs.

To be truly healthy, every woman requires an awareness of the richness of her senses and of her sexual nature, the ways they shift across her cycle and her life pathways, the ways that they nourish her body and her soul.

Sensuality and sexuality overlap. Sensuality is the appreciation and indulgence of the senses. As Mary Oliver, one of my favorite poets, expresses this concept, "Let the soft animal of your body love what it loves." Being in touch with your sensual side is to take nourishment from things that feel good to touch, to smell, to taste, to hear, to behold. Sensuality can exist wholly outside of sex—and sex can exist outside of sensuality—or they can feed each other. Interestingly, the vast majority of women I work with clinically have sex lives that have nothing to do with their sexuality or their sensuality. Sex is something they do, even enjoy, yet there is a disconnect between what their bodies are doing and how they feel inside emotionally. Most often, they are unaware this disconnect even exists. Beginning to explore the combined needs of your body and your soul within Sensation is central to wellness. It means not that you no longer care about your partner's needs or desires, but that you are fully conscious of your own. With this awareness, patients often find that something in their sexual encounters shifts, becoming more fulfilling to both partners.

I usually find this center to be the one in which women are most depleted. They tend to skip over the Mind and Spirit steps when rushed, but the Sensation step often doesn't even make it onto the agenda! The great thing is, it may not even require added time to complete this step. Often you simply tune in to activities you already are doing, but transform them by doing them mindfully.

Think about times when you've felt really healthy and alive. You probably also felt your most sensual, comfortable, and pleased with the skin you were in. That's because a conscious woman *is* a sensual woman.

- *Give yourself permission to live fully in your body in a sensate and sexual way that is a reflection of yourself.* Do some Dreamagery; invite an image of your sexuality in and ask what it has to tell you. Or explore this topic in your journal: If your female soul designed an ideal encounter, what would it look like?
- *Understand that sex takes place within many dimensions.* It's not just a physical act. All kinds of other things influence sex: your mind, your sense of connectedness, your mood, your day. Sexuality and sensuality are interwoven. Be aware of what's going on in the various dimensions surrounding lovemaking.
- *Take a walk as if this were your first day on earth.* What do you notice? Take in the sights, the sounds, the smells, the textures. This is a harder exercise than it sounds, but one well worth trying!
- *Recognize intimacy as a human need.* Whether you are sexually active or not is almost beside the point. Setting aside the obvious dimension of sex for reproduction, the desire for intimacy is a basic and acknowledged human need. That need isn't always explicitly or exclusively about intercourse. On a most basic level, it's about the power of touch, about physical and emotional contact with other human beings.
- *Understand your body's physiology.* Men and women have different sexual response times, for example. Physiologically, erection in a male and lubrication in a female are identical:

Arousal stimulates blood flow, which creates both a man's erection and a woman's vaginal lubrication. But a woman often takes longer to feel ready for intercourse. She may also face mental roadblocks her male partner may not consider. (*Might get pregnant. Might get an STD. Might not be thought of as a nice girl. Might look too forward.*) Understanding the mechanics of desire and human sexual response sounds elemental, but if you're wondering why you don't achieve orgasm, for example, it's utterly relevant. Educate yourself through books or videos (you can buy them online if privacy is an issue).

- *Don't be afraid to talk to your doctor.* Patients sometimes are hesitant to discuss sexual problems, whether it's a loss of libido, an inability to achieve orgasm, or vaginal dryness. There's a curious cloud of embarrassment that hangs over sexual matters—even in the privacy of a gynecologist's office. Some doctors are uncomfortable themselves. This shouldn't be! That's what we're here for.

- *Strengthen your PC muscles.* The pubococcygeal muscles connect the pubic bone with the coccyx (tailbone). They help to tighten the vagina and bladder, important for your overall sexual functioning. You can practice doing them at work or in the car—a Sensation action that no one will ever see! To do them, locate the muscle you use when urinating. Contract it for about ten seconds, then release. Do ten or twenty reps, and build up. *Caution:* Don't actually do this exercise while you're urinating, as you can cause urinary tract infections.

- *Be sexually adventuresome.* You have to come up with your own definition of what that means for you. But generally, creativity engages the mind and heightens your awareness. Experiment with different sexual positions or settings. Explore tantric sex, which is a way of experiencing a sexual relationship that's based on an ancient Indian yoga, focusing on an inner connection as well as an outer one.

- *Find ways to express your greater awareness of yourself as a woman in your intimate life.* More comfortable sexual expression is one of the greatest bonuses of being Consciously Female. It gives

Actions That Engage Your Senses

melling. Identify aromas that you love and bring more of them into your life. Open windows. Stop in the florist to smell fresh flowers. Sniff the cinnamon before you measure it. Wear perfume you adore even if you aren't going to encounter another soul all day long. They seem like insignificant steps, but each inhalation is a kind of salve. Aromatherapy is built around the premise that scents can soothe.

Touching. Ever watch a baby explore? She feels everything, with her tongue as well as her hands! Make an effort to be more tactile. I like to keep chenille throws around my favorite sitting places at home. Knead bread. Pet your cat. Caress someone you love or give a massage. Notice the textures of your own body, your hair, skin, limbs. Wear fabrics that feel good against your skin, such as silk, cotton, fleece, or angora. (One of my patients wears nothing but cashmere all winter long. She has a limited budget, but the fiber is so much more soft and pleasing to her than wool that she justifies its added expense as a mental health benefit—and she's right!) Find ways to be more aware of your sense of touch.

Hearing. The sound track to everyday life tends to not be particularly easy on the ears: traffic noises, raised voices, machinery, or—more typically—multiple sounds all at once. Think how different you feel when you put on some favorite music, or when you walk into a restaurant and the pianist is playing the perfect tune. Recall how relaxing it is to hear the sound of waves pounding on the shore or birds chirping on a mountain trail. Incorporate into your day moments of listening to chosen sounds *intentionally.*

Tasting. We all eat foods that taste good to us. But sometimes you can have experiences that transcend ordinary pleasure and are truly rich, stimulating sensations. Part of the experience is the food itself—yeasty fresh bread, Grandma's chicken soup, a complex gourmet dish—and part of it is your own mindfulness. Notice the textures on your tongue, the colors and smells of the food. Savor the flavors of each and every bite.

Seeing. Visually appealing objects and images can engage the senses. Visit a museum. Hang beautiful quilts or photographs in your home. Look out at a cityscape or landscape from your window. Simply notice. *See* what's around you. Make your noticing an active experience.

you permission to explore and express your female body and your female soul through intimacy. Both you and your partner will benefit.

• *Practice "conscious kissing."* That's a term physician and sex educator Lana Holstein uses to differentiate those unconscious pecks we give at bus stations and to boo-boos from the emotionally meaningful messages we share with our partner through our lips. Conscious kissing isn't about sex; it's about meaning. It's a sensual act.

Tina, 33:
⟶ *"My thing is moisturizer. I now make a ritual out of putting it on, in the morning and at night. I used to just slap it on, but now I make a point of noticing the smell and cool feel of it on my skin. I buy nicer stuff so I really enjoy it. I make a point of looking at my body and feeling my skin. It's such a sensual thing, but just for me."*

Kate, 44:
⟶ *"I stop at a flower shop on my way to work every morning. Usually I buy something small for a vase on my desk. Or I just look and smell. The colors are incredible. I used to rush by this place, but I have made it my Sensation thing to do now."*

The Number One Sensation Problem

The biggest complaint I hear from women of all ages in the center of Sensation is a lack of sex drive. "I just don't even feel like it," patients will say. There are many reasons behind the symptom of low libido, ranging from birth control pills causing a shift in the natural hormonal rhythms or natural postpartum shifts caused by childbirth to menopause. Often women are in their reproductive years, balancing work and marriage and young children. When your life is superbusy, why would you feel like having sex? But usually a huge piece of the puzzle that can cut across all pathways is a lack of intimacy. More specifically women often don't make time for intimacy. I tell such women that they need to create that time; the libido will follow.

Here's a little assignment that can help you recover intimate time. Agree with your partner to have sexual nonintercourse time once a week. Touch, hug, engage in sex play, but no intercourse. It's interesting what this does to your sex life. The focus becomes all of the other pieces that make up an intimate relationship.

As you become more conscious of yourself as a sensual and sexual person, you gain the courage not just to respond to what your partner wants, but to lead as often as you follow, to set the stage. That's a real shift for some women. But it can't happen until you have awareness of who you are and what you want, so you can bring that into the encounter. When you do that, it can transform not only the sexual experience but your entire relationship.

Hope, 48:
~"David and I went to a workshop on tantra-based sex as a lark. It turned out to be great on many levels. The breathing exercises and massages are very sensual; the different positions and new things to learn added a new level of intimacy to our relationship. Sex became about more than sex."

Sheila's Story: Beginning a Plan 〰️

Sheila's progression on creating her own Consciously Female plan mirrors that of many, many women I've counseled. Generally healthy but suffering from high blood pressure that seemed to be arising from some basic poor health habits, she needed to approach her life more consciously in order to make better choices. Initially, though, she was suspicious and full of rationales for not being able to do it. "I have a job, a social life, an extended family, and a long commute," explained Sheila, who is thirty. "Where's the extra time in my day? Maybe I could do something once or twice a week, but daily? You've got to be kidding." Not only was she intimidated by the fact that there were five Centers of Wellness she'd have to keep track of, but she wanted me to tell her what exactly it was she should do.

We started by looking for ways that she could make the space to begin. I suggested that Sheila first simply explore getting in tune with herself. I asked her to check in with her body with the Body Scan (tool 8) for a couple of minutes each morning, and to keep a journal of where she was in her cycle and how she felt each day.

Six weeks later, Sheila reported that she did feel slightly more aware of herself, although no less stressed out. We talked more about the Five-Center Review and how she could take her newfound awareness to a more specific level. I also suggested that Sheila use the information from her review to commit to making one small action within each Center of Wellness. Sheila agreed to (1) bring her sneakers to work so she could take a ten-minute walk at lunchtime (a Movement step); (2) change her breakfast from coffee and a bagel at her desk to high-fiber cereal with yogurt at home (a Nutrition step); (3) spend five minutes meditating before bed each night (a Mind step and a Spirit step); and (4) take time to notice and appreciate her body when she shaved her legs and applied oil after her shower (a sensation step). Small steps, to be sure, but at least they were something.

Her week began well, but by midweek Sheila got her period and didn't feel like walking at lunch; she had a pizza delivered to her desk so that she could read a magazine while she ate. A few days later, feeling better, she resumed the walk. Within a few days it stretched to a half-hour power walk. At this point, I calculated that Sheila was devoting about forty minutes a day to her plan (although she didn't notice it), scattered in small blocks throughout the day.

She stuck with it. After a few weeks, Sheila began experimenting with different action steps within the five centers. "The more I got used to checking in with the five centers, the more I wanted to think of ways to satisfy them," she told me with surprise. Three months later, she reported that the five steps had become a daily checklist for her. Some things she did routinely, such as meditation and the midday walk, while the Spirit, Nutrition, and Sensation steps varied from day to day. "It's become a game, deciding every day how I am going to take care of me," she says.

By her next annual exam, Sheila was upbeat and eager to share stories of her progress. She was on her third journal volume, had revamped her diet and exercise schedule, and struck me as a much more involved patient than in the past, full of questions and detailed feedback. I asked her how much time she thought she spent on her Consciously Female plan these days. "I have no idea," she replied after a moment. "It's not a plan for me anymore. It's just how I live my life."

A Consciously Female plan is that simple: conscious choices, begun realistically, made in a well-rounded and step-by-step way across your five Centers of Wellness, carried out deliberately with the help of the Feedback Loop, given the support to flourish, and moving forward consistently, the stumbles themselves becoming triumphs. I have seen it change so many women's lives. As with Sheila, it becomes a way of life.

Now you can turn to the specific life pathway that you are on right now and learn about making choices unique to your special circumstances.

Chapter 9

The Cycling Pathway

Able to conceive but choosing not to

"If you begin by loving the moment of life you are in right now, you'll find it easy to love the other moments, and even the ones you might have thought difficult or not worth paying attention to, will have their own gift."

—JOHN TARRANT

Most of us remember getting our first period. We may remember where we were, who knew about it, and how we—and they—reacted to the news. Such memories can be vivid because this first menstrual cycle is a pivotal event for females, changing our bodies and our lives forever after.

A girl's first period (menarche) is her official entry pass onto the Cycling Pathway. Although she may not actually ovulate for another couple of cycles or even years, she's on her way. For the next three to four decades until menopause, she'll leave this pathway only if she wants to try to conceive a child or "finds herself" pregnant (at which point she'll enter the Fertility Pathway). During her adult life, she may leave the Cycling Pathway, try to have a baby and/or do so, and then return back to Cycling afterward—once, twice, maybe more during her reproductive life. Eventually, typically sometime in her late forties, the Cycling Pathway merges, exit only, into the Transition Pathway. (Alternately, if she has her reproductive organs removed, a circumstance known as surgical menopause, she advances to the Transformation Pathway.)

The menstrual cycle is the central engine of the Cycling Pathway. It drives more than the pressing concern of which day your period will begin. It maps out the very rhythms of your body and soul. Every system of the body is affected by the dramatic hormonal fluctuations that occur within the framework of the menstrual cycle. Let me give you a few examples:

Your nervous system. Women often report being clumsier and more accident-prone premenstrually. That's because hormonal changes during these days slow neuromuscular coordination and dexterity, also delaying your body's response time. Migraines often worsen premenstrually, because estrogen is low. In fact, 14 percent of women with migraines have them only at that time.

Your muscles and joints. The hormone relaxin is highest in the middle of the luteal phase (days twenty to twenty-three in a twenty-eight-day cycle). This improves the integrity and quality of collagen but weakens the tendons and ligaments that support your joints. (The same thing happens during pregnancy, when relaxin stays high.) More women have injuries at ovulation, when estrogen surges and relaxin increases.

Your digestive system. It's not your imagination that your reactions to food change from day to day. Appetite decreases around ovulation, and gastrointestinal function slows during the second half of the cycle.

Your sexual responsiveness. Our sexuality differs throughout the cycle, too. Estrogen is lowest just before and during menses. That means desire and sexual response time can plummet premenstrually. They peak around ovulation, which reproductively makes perfect sense.

Your immune function. Even our odds of getting sick have a cyclical component. CD4 cells, which help fight infection, are elevated in the first half of the cycle and decrease in the second half. We're therefore more vulnerable to viral infection premenstrually. Tumors tend to grow more aggressively then, too. Meanwhile the body is routinely at greater risk of uterine or vaginal infection every month at menses, because of menstrual flow. So our bodies employ several neat protective mechanisms. Vaginal epithelial cell secretions (in the lining of the vagina) kill bacteria premenstrually only. And antibodies in cervical mucus are highest during menses.

Your moods. Increased estrogen is associated with feelings of well-being, elevated progesterone with negative mood. Progesterone, of course, begins to rise after ovulation and peaks right before menses. That's part of the reason that moodiness, depression, anxiety, and weepiness happen premenstrually.

Given that your moods, your energy level, your sexual desire, your resistance to disease, even your breathing change over the course of your menstrual cycle, it makes perfect sense that how we care for our bodies and souls should be every bit as dynamic.

When it comes to the intricate workings of the human body, the menstrual cycle is a masterpiece. Not that you'd know it by the way the cycle—or more specifically, menstruation, the part we tend to fixate on—is regarded by women individually and by the culture at large. "The curse." "*That* time of the month." Or my all-time favorite, "OTR" (for "on the rag"). From that first period (age twelve is the American average, although anytime between eight and sixteen is considered normal), girls often plunge into a new world of whispers, embarrassment, shame, and myth. Even today's more enlightened mothers and body-conscious young women often have a sketchy grasp of the physiological details surrounding "the facts of life." Periods tend to be presented as problems to be cleaned up as efficiently as possible once a month, or avoided altogether. Although so much is happening right there within them, many women have little conscious reaction to the whole production, other than what they've decided they dislike about it.

It's a big loss.

Women aren't the only ones turning a blind eye to the intricacies of the monthly cycle. It's endlessly fascinating to me that in medicine, by and large, little attention has been paid to health and disease in relation to the menstrual cycle. And yet there is an increasing array of evidence that cyclical changes do have an effect on the rest of the body. For example, certain chronic problems such as asthma, migraines, digestive disorders, acne, and rheumatoid arthritis can worsen premenstrually. And an exciting new branch of research known as chronotherapy is investigating the implications of a woman's cycle on the timing of medical tests and treatments. Large-scale studies have raised the possibility that breast-cancer surgery in the luteal phase of the menstrual cycle (days fifteen through twenty-two) reduces recurrence rates and increases survival rates. It's also been found that mammograms are most accurate in premenopausal women (having the least likelihood of false positives) when they are performed before ovulation. And it's already common knowledge that mid-cycle is best for a Pap smear, because the cervical mucus is thinnest around ovulation and therefore provides an optimal cell sampling.

We need much more information about how such changes in things like immunity, stamina, appetite, disease risks, and mental states change not only across the menstrual cycle but across the different phases of a woman's life, such as pregnancy or menopause. Part of the problem is that, traditionally, women's health overall has not been deeply investigated as different from men's. It's always been felt that it was simpler and less risky to do health research on men because they can't get pregnant and have no dynamic cycles to complicate findings. While that's true, it's also the very reason women need to be looked at separately.

If you're on the Cycling Pathway, you owe it to yourself to understand exactly what's taking place within you. I see three clear benefits:

- You'll gain a deep appreciation for the marvels of the female body—*your* body.
- You'll see how virtually every aspect of your body and your soul are affected in ways both subtle and dramatic.
- You'll be able to make choices that best support these systems and the needs that they create.

Making your best choices means being attuned to your daily changes. And that means really understanding—on a day-by-day basis—what's going on in your body each month. Because we are dynamic beings, what's best for you is likely to shift as you do.

Alexi, 32:
⁓Three days before her period: "I know that I blew it today. I went to talk to my supervisor for my review and everything she said made me want to cry.

She said it was only constructive criticism, but you know that feeling when if you blink too fast, a tear will run out the corner of your eye and embarrass you totally? That was me today. I felt totally unprofessional."

Pam, 26:
⌐ *"My hormones are chasing me. I could probably go through the last ten years of my journal and chart my gloom-and-doom phases on a monthly calendar. Then I get my period and the dam breaks—till I ovulate again. Two weeks like a normal person, two weeks descending into paranoia. I'm certain it's a physical thing. But I must try to control it better."*

WHAT'S HAPPENING NOW: THE PRIMAL CYCLE

Let's sketch a picture of the menstrual cycle and what's really taking place here. Far from being an abstract event that happens *to* you, it's a fundamental component of *who you are*. Every single day—whether you are aware of them physically and psychologically or not—changes are under way, fueled by dramatic fluctuations in your hormonal makeup. And since every day of life on the Cycling Pathway is a day in a menstrual cycle, you're continuously affected by these events.

Not all women have the same cycles. Some run as short as twenty-one days, others as long as thirty-five. (You count the length of a cycle from the first day of one period to the first day of the next.) The length of your cycle will vary across your reproductive life. Typically they are shorter and more consistent when you are younger, and become longer and more variable as we age. The phases within them are variable, too. The standard cycle is considered twenty-eight days, although only a minority of women fit that exact pattern. The cycle is divided into four main phases:

- Menstrual phase: days one through five
- Follicular phase: days six through twelve
- Ovulatory phase: days thirteen through fifteen
- Luteal phase: days sixteen through twenty-eight

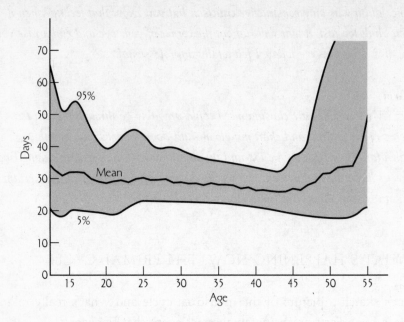

Variability of menstrual cycles from onset to menopause

The first day of the cycle is the first day bleeding begins as your uterine lining is shed through the vagina because there is no pregnancy requiring its lush protective presence. This *menstrual phase,* a.k.a. your period, generally lasts three to five days (though up to eight days is not unusual). Estrogen levels are now one-tenth of what they will be at their peak. As bleeding ends, a hormone known as FSH (follicle-stimulating hormone), secreted from the anterior pituitary of the brain, stimulates several ovarian follicles to develop, only one of which will fully mature. The growing follicles release estrogen in increasing amounts, causing the lining of the uterus to begin to thicken again. This is the *follicular phase,* which is fairly variable, lasting anywhere from five days (in a twenty-one-day cycle) to twenty days (in a thirty-five-day cycle).

As the chosen egg approaches maturity inside the follicle, it secretes progesterone in addition to the estrogen. Then FSH is joined by LH (luteinizing hormone, also secreted from the anterior pituitary) to signal the ovarian follicle to release a single egg. (Or, rarely, two or more eggs, which if fertilized would result in multiple gestations.) This is ovulation, occurring midway through the cycle, or on day fourteen of a twenty-

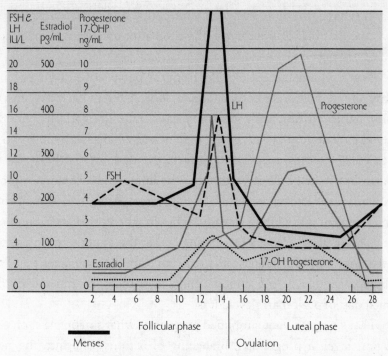

FSH & LH IU/L	Estradiol pg/mL	Progesterone 17-OHP ng/mL			
20	500	10			
18		9			
16	400	8		LH	Progesterone
14		7			
12	300	6			
10		5	FSH		
8	200	4			
6		3			
4	100	2			
2		1	Estradiol	17-OH Progesterone	
0	0	0			

2 4 6 8 10 12 14 16 18 20 22 24 26 28

Follicular phase — Ovulation — Luteal phase

Menses

Hormone levels across the menstrual cycle

eight-day cycle. Thus begins the *ovulatory phase,* when the greatest chance of conceiving occurs. Most fertilization takes place while the egg is on its several-day journey down the fallopian tube en route to the uterus.

After ovulation, the uterus goes into full gear to prepare for a possible implantation of a fertilized egg in the uterine wall. This is the *luteal phase.* Once the ovarian follicle releases the egg, its structure and function are transformed and it is now called the corpus luteum, whose job is to secrete hormones, primarily progesterone, to help prepare the body for pregnancy. Estrogen, LH, and FSH decline and progesterone rises sharply. Progesterone is forty-times higher now than it was at its lowest point.

If the egg is fertilized, estrogen and progesterone will continue to be produced, and soon the embryo itself will begin producing a hormone called HCG (human chorionic gonadotropin), which is the substance a home pregnancy test detects. If the egg is not fertilized within about fourteen days of ovulation, progesterone drops along with the falling estrogen. The corpus luteum shrinks and is reabsorbed, the uterine lining breaks down and is shed—and another period begins.

In general, the time between your period and ovulation is referred to as the first half of your cycle; the time after ovulation is the second half of your cycle.

That's what a cycle looks like from the perspective of the egg. The ovary and its follicle, or corpus luteum, look different each day, and the hormonal levels also shift, on some days quite dramatically. Another way to look at your cycle, to help understand what's happening within, is to consider the process as it affects the endometrial lining of the uterus. In the first half of your cycle, the lining is thickening, or proliferating. This is known as the *proliferative phase*. After ovulation, if there is no pregnancy, the lining is ready to be sloughed off. This is known as the *secretory phase*. What's fascinating is that the endometrium changes every single day. So distinct and predictable are these changes that from a biopsy sample of the endometrium, a pathologist can tell exactly which day of a woman's cycle it is!

That's a somewhat simplified portrait of what's happening on a biological level: a progressive branching of actions, one into the next, working together to ready your body for a new life. And then, should pregnancy not ensue, the process starts all over again. On any given day, not only do the levels of the various hormones differ, but other aspects of their functioning vary radically as well, including how fast and how frequently they are secreted, and how much of each is released into your bloodstream. For example, LH (the hormone that triggers ovulation) is secreted in pulses every sixty to seventy minutes before ovulation; that rate slows to every two hundred minutes just before your period. And the amount of LH secreted in each pulse changes 300 percent across the course of the cycle.

The menstrual cycle isn't merely an isolated, automatic function of your reproductive system, though. A great deal may be happening "down there," but it's not happening in isolation. What's going on in the rest of your body and in your life plays a huge role in determining how you're influenced by the ever-changing hormonal cocktail circulating within you each day. And the place where that interface between your cycle and the rest of your life is mediated is an organ that resides deep in the center of your brain: your hypothalamus. The hypothalamus is fascinating because it is your body's connection between the outside

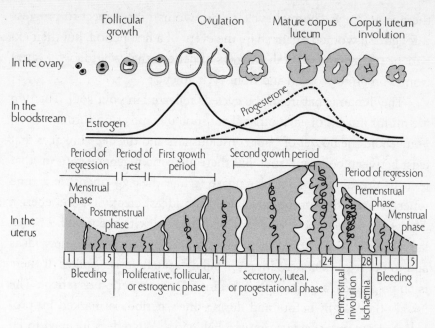

Follicular growth · Ovulation · Mature corpus luteum · Corpus luteum involution

In the ovary

In the bloodstream

Estrogen · Progesterone

Period of regression · Period of rest · First growth period · Second growth period · Period of regression

Menstrual phase · Postmenstrual phase

In the uterus

Premenstrual phase · Menstrual phase

1   5   14   24   28 1   5

Bleeding · Proliferative, follicular, or estrogenic phase · Secretory, luteal, or progestational phase · Premenstrual involution · Ischaemia · Bleeding

Cyclical changes in the ovary, bloodstream and uterus

world and the body's own inner world. The entire process of hormonal secretion is regulated from the hypothalamus, and stress, anxiety, poor nutrition, depression, illness, grief, and other circumstances can all influence it, thus altering normal hormonal function. And of course the reverse is true, too. Rest, relaxation, joy, pleasure, good eating habits— these also have effects. It's the hypothalamus that releases gonadotropin-releasing hormone (GNRH), which determines the levels of FSH and LH. (Gonadotropin-releasing hormone is a long but appropriate name, since FSH and LH are gonadotropins.) Stress, poor nutrition, and poor overall health can all affect the pace and volume of GNRH pulsations. The hypothalamus determines the levels of FSH and LH through the control that GNRH exercises over the pituitary gland, which is located just below it and secretes FSH and LH, as well as other hormones. The hypothalamus also regulates the adrenal gland, which secretes stress hormones such as cortisol. And this is just a partial catalog of the hormones over which the hypothalamus has control.

Because of the many variables affecting hormones, and because the rise and fall of hormones affects so many other systems in the body, there is no single "normal cycle" every woman can expect to progress through. All women might share the event of a first period, but their experience of it—and of all the dozens of periods that will follow—varies from woman to woman and from cycle to cycle.

The dynamic nature of the cycle is reflected in your soul. The two are mirror images of each other. That should come as no surprise when you behold the power of your consciousness and the deep linkages that exist between body and soul. But there are certain general patterns that tend to prevail. The follicular phase (while the egg ripens) is a time when women tend to be most ripe with ideas, creativity, and energy. They tend to be upbeat, outward, and engaged with the world. At ovulation, many women find themselves especially receptive to new ideas and to other people. Sensation (including sexual desire) spikes. If there is no pregnancy, a woman then begins to enter a period of retreat. The luteal phase, right before and during one's period, is marked by progressively more reflective, inward behaviors. We're less inclined to be "out there," more inclined to tears, fatigue, and contemplation.

Christiane Northrup likens a woman's cycle to the cycle of the moon, which in addition to honoring an apparent biological link makes for a vividly memorable analogy. The two cycles are of the same duration, one month, and share the same pattern of waxing and waning. Day one of the cycle is the new moon; the moon grows bigger, rounder, and fuller (the follicular phase) until it peaks at day fourteen with the full moon (ovulation). And then it begins to wane (the luteal phase). "Women, too, go through a period of darkness each month, when the life force may seem to disappear for a while [the premenstrual and menstrual phases]," Dr. Northrup says. That darkness, however, is only a metaphorical one. Although a woman is in psychological retreat at this phase, it's very much a time of regathering, reevaluating, and re-reflection.

The experiences within the body (as hormones rise and fall) and within the soul (as emotions surface and retreat) are not a cause-and-effect relationship. It's not that progesterone *makes* you moody or that estrogen *makes* you more upbeat. Rather, the hormonal fluctuations of your body create different environments, and in some of those emotional environments you have greater access to the workings of the soul.

It's true that there is some kind of mechanistic relationship between hormones and their effects on our bodies and our souls. For example, the surge in estrogen at ovulation may be the cause of physiological changes that trigger desire. But in general, the connection is corollary, not causal. You are not your hormones.

Once you recognize the dynamic relationship *between* your hormones and your emotions, however, you can choose to see the days leading up to your period (in the luteal phase) as a span of time during which feelings may surface that are most likely to be authentic expressions of your deepest reality. They are the same emotional realities that are always there within you—how you feel about your life, your dreams, your wishes, your goals—but you can see them more clearly because the veil between our unconscious and our conscious is thinner at such times. Conversely, there are times (the follicular phase, from your period to ovulation) when the veil is thicker, and the defense mechanisms keeping us from these inner truths are layered more thickly over the soul.

When describing this repressive mechanism, my friend Steve Forrest uses the analogy of a border guard. We all have this little guard who stands on the border between our conscious and our unconscious. It's useful to have him there. He keeps the scary, overwhelming thoughts from getting out of the unconscious and into our conscious mind, so we can go about our day. If we never kept out any of this repressed material, we'd go crazy and never get anything done; in a way, that's what some mental illness is. So for the first two weeks of the cycle, our crossing guard is sharp, his senses alert for intrusions, keeping the unconscious at bay. In the second two weeks, though, he gets increasingly tired. He begins to take longer catnaps. He's still able to catch the big things, but the other stuff he normally stops at the border now slips through. Of course, the metaphor isn't entirely apt because the unconscious thoughts on the other side of the border are not the enemy; they are us. Though they can be scary at first, getting to see them and spend time with them periodically is an opportunity to visit with a deeper dimension of yourself, to learn something new.

Let me repeat, though, you are not ruled by your hormones. Remember that old claim that a woman could never be president because she couldn't be trusted not to fall apart once a month with PMS? That's cockamamie, of course! Yes, we have certain patterns that are common to us as women. But it always gets back to the choosing. You can choose to use the luteal phase to explore what's in your heart, to journal, to wallow in tears and see where introspection takes you. Other times, you choose to override it because you have papers due or meetings that require a less bared soul. You choose. But, of course, you don't have the choice if you aren't conscious in the first place. Because of this ability to reflect and intuit deeply if we choose, I would argue that this would be a significant *advantage* to a woman president!

If a woman is oblivious to the tremendous changes the menstrual cycle brings, it's partly because they are internal: out of sight, out of mind. Only the menses are visible and therefore acknowledged. But a bigger reason, I think, is that many women have never considered this dynamic dance within them. We're unconscious of its import because the whole culture around the menstrual cycle is designed to enable us *not* to focus on it. We'd rather make short work of the whole business with superefficient tampons or period-erasing continuous pill taking. It's a social convention—and a social construct—that a woman's period is an annoying, useless holdover from the premodern days when we could not "control" a woman's body and therefore had to endure its fluctuations. The value of the changes brought by the cycle is ignored. The dismissal of the idea that the menstrual cycle may have value beyond its role in reproduction was captured well in a 2003 *Newsweek* report on the testing of Seasonale, the birth control pill that reduces the number of periods per year to four. After examining the cons of menstruation and the pros of oral contraceptives, the report asked the seminal question: "Why, then, have monthly periods?" To which a physician responded, "There's really no benefit." That, in a nutshell, is the problem with how the menstrual cycle has traditionally been viewed. The idea that there might indeed be pluses to the existence of this very natural cycle is never even considered. Such thinking is a perfect illustration of the loss of the connection between body and soul. The body is viewed in isolation—which sounds fine, except for the pesky little reality that there is no such thing; the body is *never* in isolation from the soul!

By paying closer attention to the subtle shifts brought by the menstrual cycle,

What If You're on the Pill?

The natural waxing and waning experienced during the menstrual cycle can be affected by hormonal methods of birth control, which include not just oral contraceptives (a.k.a. the Pill), but also the patch and the vaginal ring. This is because the Pill—and the others—by design override your own hormonal cycles. The exact effect is very individualized. A few women will continue to notice the same cyclical changes. Others will feel their effects in a blunted way; that "veil" between the unconscious and the conscious becomes thicker, less translucent, but not entirely opaque. And for many women, all sense of mood shifts is erased completely; nothing gets past the veil. Ironically, this is why the Pill is sometimes prescribed—to flatten out the symptoms of PMS. Before prescribing it for this reason, though, I would counsel a woman to first increase her consciousness around her cycle, to gain an awareness of what might be influencing the severity of her symptoms. And I'd point out that she can use those extremes to her advantage, as opportunities that can be mined rather than as problems to be medicated away. These things can be done in combination with other approaches for easing premenstrual symptoms, found at the end of this chapter.

Obviously these drawbacks to the hormonal contraception don't outweigh the benefits that make it so popular—effectiveness and convenience. The Pill has also been shown to decrease the risk of ovarian cancer. I'm certainly not dismissing it; indeed, I often prescribe it. But I'd like for any woman choosing it to do so consciously, aware of both the gains and the potential losses.

If you find it difficult to recognize and access soul-level insights because you are taking hormonal contraception, make an effort to create your own cycles of introspection. Mimic the progression of the natural cycle, and use the luteal phase to consciously invite more reflection time into your life. It's not exactly the same, since you have to work a little harder to mine your unconscious, but it's definitely possible, and a very nurturing thing to do.

you can better track what your body and soul need—and then tailor the choices you make each day to best meet those needs. That's no small gift. Remember that the dark moon is also known as a new moon.

Lindsay's Story: No Tick, Tick, Tick? No Problem

Lindsay, twenty-seven, was engaged to be married and thrilled about it. This new patient was worried, though, about one thing: She did not think her biological clock was ticking as loudly as it should be. Lindsay felt that because she was nearing her thirties and not yet interested in procreation, something might be amiss hormonally. "I don't gush over friends' babies. I don't look at my boyfriend and think about what a great father he will make," she explained. "Do you think there is something wrong with me, or am I just selfish and immature like my mother says?"

Her health history indicated nothing unusual. Her periods did not seem to be a major issue in her life; Lindsay rarely experienced any PMS symptoms and treated her occasional cramps with ibuprofen (Motrin). We then spent some time exploring her feelings around sex and about reproduction with the questions in the Consciously Female Inventory (tool 6).

It became apparent that Lindsay was simply not yet ready to move from the Cycling Pathway to the Fertility Pathway. I explained that she might get there in the next few years, or she might never get there. Both alternatives are completely normal. Just because you can have a baby now doesn't mean you have to or that it is right for you. There is a difference between knowing that you are capable of reproduction and being ready to encompass the responsibilities of motherhood—so long as you're conscious of which side of the seesaw you're really on.

I explained how living in a more Consciously Female way would help Lindsay to stay in touch with her thoughts about this issue. By creating a space in which she could define her own femaleness, she'd be able to make choices that weren't determined by anyone else's opinions or by conventional myths about what it means to be a "normal" woman.

LANDMARK: PMS

Landon, 19:
— *"I feel like a crazy person. Face breaking out. Throwing things. Arguments with everybody. A couple of days of wanting to pull the covers over my head and be left alone. I'm sorry, but this doesn't seem normal."*

Carolyn, 36:
— *"Look, I'm a lawyer. I have this successful, busy life. I don't need to be turned into some kind of fly-off-the-handle, cry-in-the-bathroom demon every month. I can't afford it!"*

Sue, 43:
— *"When I get my period, I give myself permission to draw inside myself. For a day or so, I don't force myself to be the most vivacious, efficient person on the planet. I take a break from what everyone wants of me, and I do what I want instead."*

Amy, 31:
— *"I can't stop eating just before my period. I want salty, I want chocolate. I can't stop. I'm not a binge eater normally, but for a day or two there, I'm out of control! My breasts hurt, my jeans are tight, my skin is a mess, and I just want it to be over. Isn't there something I can take so I don't feel like crawling into my cave for two or three days each month?"*

Identifying PMS and PMDD

It's the distinct pattern of when symptoms appear, more than the nature of the symptoms themselves, that is the key to diagnosing PMS. The symptoms begin to develop after ovulation, increase across the luteal phase, usually peak right before menses, and disappear at or soon after the start of bleeding. (In very severe cases, a woman's distress can be prolonged so that she feels like she's in near-chronic PMS, but she can usually remember that when symptoms began, they fit this cyclical pattern.) Note that a woman who has painful periods (dysmenorrhea) does not necessarily have PMS. It is possible to have PMS without experiencing cramping and other physical forms of pain. PMS can be manifested in either the body or the soul or both, as the following list shows.

Symptoms vary from woman to woman, and can change over time in an individual (often worsening, if unaddressed). The "classic" symptoms include some combination of the following:

- Abdominal bloating
- Acne breakouts
- Alcohol intolerance
- Anger
- Anxiety
- Asthma flare-ups
- Backache
- Breast tenderness, swelling, or pain
- Bruising
- Confusion
- Cramping
- Crying
- Depression
- Fainting spells
- Fatigue
- Forgetfulness
- Food cravings or binges
- Headache or migraine
- Hemorrhoid flare-ups
- Impatience
- Insomnia
- Irritability
- Joint pain or stiffness
- Loneliness
- Mood swings
- Nausea
- Night sweats or hot flashes
- Panic

- Sadness (pervasive)
- Sex drive changes
- Sinus problems
- Social withdrawal
- Suicidal thoughts
- Swelling or water retention (edema)
- Tension
- Tremors
- Vaginal dryness

If women think at all about the menstrual cycle (aside from the period part), it's most often in terms of premenstrual syndrome (PMS). Seventy-five percent of women report some PMS symptoms, and for 3 to 4 percent of women, the symptoms keep them out of work or severely limit their lifestyle. PMS is referred to as a syndrome because it encompasses a wide range of physical and emotional symptoms that tend to predictably occur in the luteal phase of the cycle, usually disappearing abruptly when the period begins.

Each woman experiences PMS differently. And the severity of symptoms can change from cycle to cycle. These symptoms cover a huge list, with more than 150 different experiences identified in the literature (see box). A more severe form of PMS is PMDD, or premenstrual dysphoric disorder. It's basically the extreme end of a continuum, although with intense emotional symptoms accompanying the physical discomforts. These can include significant anxiety, depression, withdrawal, extreme fatigue, a feeling of being overwhelmed, and difficulty concentrating.

PMS and PMDD are real. By tuning in to every single day of your cycle—not just the days that PMS symptoms tend to show up—you can better anticipate the changes and respond to them accordingly.

As with all the common issues that women face along the Cycling Pathway, you can use the Consciously Female tools and techniques to make choices about these issues that reflect who you are and what you need right now. Remember that making conscious choices, large or small, involves using the Feedback Loop formula, as described in Chapter 8: reflection, information, action, and then re-reflection.

First, reflection. The first thing I do with patients who complain of PMS symptoms is to talk about the whole concept of shifting the paradigm for how they perceive the condition. I try to help them reframe. What if instead of seeing the hormonal, emotional, physical, and behavioral changes they experience as a negative to be dismissed ("Oh, it's that time of the month for me. It will soon be over"), they saw these shifts as messages? Emotions are close to the surface right now—so what are they saying to you? What are the fears and wishes and other thoughts in their heart and soul now? This is a time when a woman should be doing more and deeper exploration within all five Centers of Wellness, not less. It's an opportunity for insight. For most women, it's a huge "ah-ha!" moment. It's a complete shift in the way they have always looked at PMS. (It certainly was for me.)

Once you understand this framework, you're ready to explore it personally a little more. Any of the tools in Part Two—Journaling, Dialoguing, Dreamagery—can help you get there. What happens, exactly, during your PMS? Keep a chart of your symptoms, noting which day in your cycle it is, for a couple of months. Also keep a record of your feelings, moods, and physical sensations, such as appetite, sexual desire, energy level, and sleep, and see what you notice about how they are affected.

Think about your cycle across time, too. Has it been worse at some times than others? Over the course of your life, what else has been going on when PMS flared up? The condition is almost never completely consistent from month to month; sometimes it's mild, sometimes severe. (These differences over time also can be more marked for some women than others.) Think of a time when it was really bad. What else was going on in your life around that time? Most women, when asked, begin to say, "Well, now that you mention it..."

Reflect on the past six months. Are there certain issues that you tend to focus on more when you are premenstrual (or PMS-sy, as I like to say)? Maybe, for example, right around your period you begin to question your marriage. An unconscious response is to say, "Oh, I'm just being premenstrual! I shouldn't worry so much about that. Of course I married the right guy!" Well, not so fast. Let's pay attention to what's coming to the fore. Explore what it is about your marriage that is troubling you; face that information rather than deflecting it. If you don't, it's apt to come out anyway in an unconscious expression, such as in the form of increased fights with your husband, or as ever-worsening premenstrual symptoms.

I have had severe PMS myself. Over time and across my process of becoming more conscious of how it has manifested in my life, I began to remember that as a teenager and young adult, I would become completely overwhelmed with worries about my parents before my period. My parents, whom I loved deeply, had issues of their own that sometimes spilled into our family life. My father battled problems with alcohol. My mother had periods of severe depression. While my upbringing in many ways was your average happy childhood, I know that what my parents were going through often became a huge burden on me. Kids see everything. I knew that alcoholism and depression colored my parents' behavior in ways that were, if not overtly damaging to me, nonetheless distressing. Most of the month I kept those issues well under control. But once a month, for days at a time, they would overtake me. Later, the stress of college and medical school made my symptoms worse. The PMS symptoms are messages; you need to pay attention.

While I don't look forward to the cramps and mood changes I still sometimes experience from month to month, I have now learned to anticipate the changes that my cycle brings. I actually find myself looking forward to seeing where my insights are going to take me. Even more surprising, perhaps, my husband looks forward to this time, too. He's learned that he will see a different, more vulnerable side of me. Connecting during these times deepens our relationship—even though there are moments when I can't believe he could want to be around me! The severity of my distress eased tremendously once I began to approach my PMS in a Consciously Female way, because I was able to take steps to minimize my discomfort and accommodate my needs in a much more fine-tuned way.

That's not to say that PMS can be entirely eliminated. The estrogen and progesterone receptors throughout our bodies are going to respond to rising and falling levels of these hormones, and many of us are going to feel the effects very keenly. The resulting symptoms can and should be treated to optimize your body's ability to weather them. However, hormones are not solely to blame. Stress and other environmental effects seem to worsen PMS, studies have shown, working through the hormones (by way of the hypothalamus). You can think of hormones as the language of stress as expressed in both body and soul. If you learn to pay attention to them, you can help things calm down.

Second, information. Be sure to learn about ways you can physically ease symptoms of PMS. (See the Centers of Wellness Modifications for Cycling, later in this chapter, for some suggestions.) Talk to your doctor. Get as much information as you feel you need. But remember, you can't just rely on this step alone. PMS is very much a syndrome of both the body and the soul.

Third, action. Once you are aware of your patterns (physically and emotionally) and your history, you're empowered to make choices about how you wish to interface with the landmark of PMS. Sometimes you will want to really delve into it and see where it takes you. Create space for yourself to do that. Maybe a premenstrual day falls over a weekend, and you're able to surrender to the day, allowing yourself to feel what you feel, to be alone, to cry all day if you feel like. Alternately, maybe you have a lot going on that particular weekend and can't go delving into your inner soul. That's fine, too—so long as you have made a conscious choice to override those messages this time around. In that event, you might look for ways you can better support yourself during this time, ways you can show yourself a little tenderness to accommodate your soul-level needs right now. Maybe that translates to making an effort to eat better, to get more rest. Maybe it's allowing extra time when you travel so that you don't become so unraveled by the inevitable delays. When you consciously override the messages of your soul and nurture it as best you can, it's soothing. When you unconsciously ignore those messages, you wind up snapping at colleagues or your spouse, feeling tighter and more upset.

Then, re-reflection. Don't forget that you should always filter your choices back through the loop again. How do you feel when you make an effort to surrender to the messages of the soul in the premenstrual phase? Conversely, how do you feel when you override those messages? Are the steps you take to give it a little space and tenderness working? Are there other things you could try to do? You can really get to the point of looking at your calendar in terms of your cycle and preparing yourself accordingly.

Painful Periods: Dysmenorrhea

Many women report painful uterine cramping at the time of menstruation. Called dysmenorrhea, this condition can occur either as a component of PMS (that is, you have painful cramps along with other PMS symptoms) or by itself, with no other symptoms. It's usually treated easily with a pain reliever like Motrin. (Other therapies that show promise include supplemental magnesium and an increased intake of omega-3 fatty acids. There has also been one small but methodologically sound study indicating that acupuncture can greatly ease dysmenorrhea.)

Because it's so effectively treated with pain relievers, I rarely see women who present dysmenorrhea as a problem that interferes with their life—unless of course they also experience other PMS symptoms along with the cramping. If this is the case for you, work through the advice given for PMS.

Rhiannon's Story: "I'm Not Myself Half the Time!"

I see patients like Rhiannon quite frequently: intelligent, beautiful, vibrant, confident—for two or three weeks out of the month. Starting soon after ovulation, though, and with gathering intensity up to her period, a different Rhiannon appears. She experiences despondent moods, withdraws from others, is short-tempered, and cries uncontrollably. Her breasts hurt and her cramps become quite severe in the first few days of her period. Between the physical pain and the emotional roller coaster, she says, "I just don't feel like myself half the time. By the time the cramps and everything else is gone, half the month has gone by. I can't live like this!"

The first thing I assured her is that of course we can take steps to level out some of her most severe symptoms. Debilitating PMS symptoms are very real. Before I outlined the medical interventions that can help ease those symptoms, however, I urged Rhiannon to reframe the way she *perceived* her cycle. She was skeptical ("Really, I just want you to give me something to make it go away and give me my life back!") but open-minded.

After I described the Reflection exercise (outlined above), her reaction was one I have seen over and over again: A lightbulb goes on. "Wow, I never thought of it that way before," she admitted. That conversation alone makes everything that follows different.

Rhiannon agreed to begin writing in a journal around the topics that came up for her during that black half of her cycle. Doing so is a way of acknowledging her emotional needs rather than just writing them off as something that was attacking her. At the same time, she went through the process of evaluating her Center of Wellness needs, and we agreed to make some adjustments. She went from taking no vitamins or supplements to taking a regular daily multivitamin, plus additional calcium, magnesium, B_6, vitamin E, and chasteberry. An avid runner, Rhiannon had been training hard for the first two weeks of her cycle, fighting it but continuing to run during the third week, and then giving up in week four. Instead, she decided to try continuing with some form of exercise throughout her cycle: two weeks of intense running, a week of a lighter run plus increased weight training, and then weights and stretching during her tough week.

When I saw her three months later, Rhiannon reported a slight shift in her symptoms and a significant shift in her ability to deal with them. When she was feeling stressed, she still had black days, but during cycles when she was able to pay close attention and nurture herself, she noted improvement. "I feel like I still have a ways to go," she told me. "But the big thing I learned was that it is okay for every day to be different. There is no one 'right' day. That is just a whole different way of thinking for me. Now I go with the flow, to use a bad pun."

LANDMARK: CONTRACEPTION CHOICES

Shelby, 25:
⌐ *"Even though I have been taking the Pill for six years, I can't seem to get used to how it makes me feel. I feel blue, bloated, and queasy almost all the time. I think my libido is lower, too. But it's so easy, I wouldn't even consider not taking the Pill."*

Katie, 23:
⌐ *"I've figured it out. If I take my birth control pills continuously, I never have to get my period again until I want to get pregnant. Whoopee and thank you, medical science!"*

Suzanne, 45:
⌐ *"I am so tired of messing with diaphragms but am afraid to take a more drastic step. I am through having kids, but maybe I should just wait it out until menopause."*

Bess, 32:
⌐ *"My girlfriend told me about the fertility awareness method. I like the idea of not messing with pills or condoms, and I like that it's low-tech. She was raving about it. But I still don't know if it's a good idea for me. How do I decide?"*

Being Consciously Female means accepting that your body is specially designed for bringing forth new life. But it doesn't mean you have to use your body that way. Women who are on the Cycling Pathway are menstruating but not interested in getting pregnant. And that means they need to use some form of contraception, to avoid any unplanned or unwanted pregnancy.

All contraceptive options are useful and effective, although to varying degrees. There are basically four categories of contraceptives: devices (diaphragm, condom—male and female, IUD, cervical sponge), hormonal methods (the Pill, the patch, rings, rods, injections), surgeries (tubal ligation, vasectomy), and external monitoring methods (fertility awareness method, rhythm method, abstinence or periodic abstinence). What's right for you depends. And what's right at any given time can change across your Cycling years.

It's so interesting to me how often contraceptive choices are made unconsciously. You'd think that because a woman actually had to make a decision, it was therefore conscious. Not so. It's amazingly common for patients to make choices without truly processing them. They select a birth control method with less consideration than they use to select a new sofa or a pair of shoes. Whether you are choosing a contraceptive method for the first time, coming back to it after time away, or wishing to change your current method, the process is the same:

First, reflection. The starting place is to consider what's important for you.

- Ask yourself why you need it. It's that old "for-the-sake-of-what" question. Do you want birth control only, because you're in a monogamous relationship with no concern over sexually transmitted diseases? Do you need protection from STDs as well as from pregnancy? What brings you to investigate contraception in the first place?
- How do you feel about the various options themselves? Where do those feelings come from? Your friends' recommendations? Your mom's? Your partner's? Something you once read? Previous experiences? It's not enough to trust your first reaction. I have seen young women who wanted to go on the Pill continuously (blocking menstruation) because that's what all their friends did. Once we talked through the why, it would emerge that they saw their periods only as big negatives. In such cases I would encourage work on exploring those feelings. Sometimes the woman would stick with her initial choice as truly the best option for her; other patients would decide that when they reframed how they viewed their cycle, they didn't want to quit having those soul-heavy moments. Another big area is the IUD. Because of problems

with the design and manufacture of the old Dalkon Shield model, which was withdrawn from the market in 1975, many women who are in their forties and older have a strongly negative impression of this method. Yet today's IUDs are perfectly safe, effective, and problem-free, and can be a good choice for just that age group. If you stop at your first reaction, you won't get a full or true picture of how you feel given all of the information.

- How do you feel about hormones? Some women say, "I just don't want my hormones messed with." They have very strong feelings about that issue. Or they have tried the Pill before and had a negative experience. In some women, for example, oral contraceptives cause depression, loss of libido, or headaches. Other women see the Pill or patch as being full of advantages, such as ease of use, and aren't bothered by the mechanism involved. Among the noncontraceptive considerations around hormonal birth control are the effect of hormones on complexion, PMS, dysmenorrhea, and the risk of ovarian cancer or breast cancer. (Birth control pills lower one's risk of ovarian cancer but raise the risk of breast cancer. For a woman with a big fear of cancer or a strong family history, this should definitely enter into the decision.)

- What about delivery system? Within the arena of hormones are still more choice points, around the method of delivery. Some women know they won't remember to take a daily pill or don't want to be bothered. Some won't remember to change a patch or are troubled by the cosmetic effect or the public nature of it (feeling that even if strategically placed, there's that chance it could be seen in the locker room or in the bedroom, and others would know). Other women can't bear shots.

- How at ease are you about interacting with your body? Some women are very comfortable touching their bodies in an intimate way. Using a diaphragm, for example, involves this kind of touch. Using the fertility awareness method requires you to feel your cervical mucus. If you don't like this kind of intimate contact, you're likely not to be sufficiently consistent or careful in practicing your contraceptive technique.

- How do you feel about your relationship? A woman who is very secure in her relationship and who can plan ahead or call time-out to insert a diaphragm is in one place. A woman with a new partner might be less comfortable with such a lack of spontaneity.
- How permanent do you wish your choice to be? Are you certain you are finished with your childbearing, or is there a possibility you will want to have a child? If you think you might want pregnancy in the future, how far off? Soon? In ten years?
- How devastating would pregnancy be in your life? If your answer is very, you'll want to choose the most reliable method, not natural methods with lower effectiveness rates.

Use the tools in Part Two to arrive at your answers. Spend some time on this step.

Second, information. Work with your doctor to learn about the choices available. Getting the facts from a reliable source can also help you separate myths from facts. About half of all unintended pregnancies are the result of contraceptive failure. That's why fully understanding your choice is crucial.

- Learn about their relative effectiveness. If you absolutely, positively cannot afford to get pregnant, for example, the Pill and IUD (both with fewer than one per hundred users becoming pregnant) are better choices than one of the fertility awareness methods (three to thirteen per hundred users become pregnant). Effectiveness rates can vary not only according to proper usage but in relation to other factors as well. For example, the cervical cap and sponge are more effective in women who have not previously had children.
- Understand what's involved on your part—an office visit to

insert an IUD or have a shot? Taking a pill every morning? Major abdominal surgery? Think about how this choice fits into your life. If you forget to take a daily multivitamin, a daily oral contraceptive may not be for you, for example. If you or your partner dislikes the feel of condoms, you may be less likely to use one every time.

- Are there any limitations based on your health situation? For example, do you have high blood pressure or migraines? Do you smoke? If so, hormonal options are probably not the best choice for you.
- Compare the relative costs. For example, you might want to consider whether your health insurance covers contraception. If you pay out of pocket, do you have a preference for a monthly payment (e.g., oral contraceptives) vs. a one-time-only cost (e.g., tubal ligation)? Something like a diaphragm requires an office visit for a fitting, and the cost of the device itself, but then the only added cost is the occasional purchase of spermicide. Cost should not be your primary consideration in choosing birth control, but it's important to have this information. Finally, remember that all of this information can't stand alone. You need to filter your reflections through this data to come up with what works best for *you*.

Third, action. Once you align your choice with where you're at in your life, it will be the right choice for you.

Then, re-reflection. Except for surgery, almost no contraceptive choice is permanent. Once you've made your choice, live with it for a few months and then run the choice back through the loop. How does it make you feel? Physically? Emotionally? What do you notice? Do you need to make a change? Or has anything changed in your life that would seem to require a change in your choice? For example, a new mother who is breast-feeding but had been on the Pill before her pregnancy will want to resume with a new formulation compatible with nursing, or a different form of contraception altogether.

Skipping Periods

There's a current vogue for taking birth control pills continuously (either skipping the sugar pill week in a multiphasic formulation or using an extended-cycle formulation designed to skip over periods, such as Seasonale). I'm not necessarily against this practice. At certain stressful or complicated points in your life, taking a vacation from periods can be a welcome idea. I know many medical residents who do so regularly in order to avoid premenstrual symptoms and/or cramping on top of the sleeplessness and physical exhaustion their schedules require. Cutting back on ovulation is thought to possibly reduce the risk of fibroids and endometriosis, as well as ovarian and uterine cancers. It may seem "unnatural," but keep in mind that modern women have three times as many periods (450 over a lifetime, therefore more ovulations) as our ancient ancestors. Owning to modern medicine and contraception, we bear far fewer children, spend less time pregnant or nursing, and live longer—which you could also call "unnatural"!

What I don't support is using this form of contraception unconsciously. I think that a woman who uses hormones to negate this aspect of her femaleness for extended blocks of time—so that she won't have to deal with mood swings and menstruation—may be missing something extremely important. By eliminating her cycles completely, she may risk denying herself the opportunity to tune in to her intrinsic, authentic self. I foresee a time when a young woman could go from a chemically regulated, cycle-free life straight to pregnancy or fertility drugs. A modern breakthrough making life neat and orderly—or a perilous disregard for the natural order of things? And that question is quite apart from the question of potential physical risks, because there is not yet a lot of data about the long-term effects of suppressing menstruation altogether, as with the continuous Pill.

Jenny's Story: Changing Contraception Needs ⟵⟶

Jenny, now forty-two, began taking a triphasic pill when she first became sexually active at twenty-five. Her first and only partner was Adam, whom she later married. "I considered all of the options, and this one just seemed the easiest and most reliable," she remembers. "I was not at all comfortable with the idea of groping around inside my body or having anything inserted. Popping a pill was something I could relate to." The only time Jenny quit the Pill was during each of her three pregnancies. She breast-fed each child for three to six months, and during those times she switched to a progestin-only formulation that would not interfere with breast milk.

Jenny's periods had always been regular and uneventful. The Pill gave her a pretty predictable twenty-eight-day cycle, although in her late thirties she began noticing that the amount of time she bled was getting longer. She also was anemic, a condition that had begun during her pregnancies and probably was not being helped by the long periods. Her ob-gyn (not me) tinkered with the kind of pill she was taking, adjusting the amounts of hormones being delivered, and eventually she fell back into regular cycles.

By the time she met me, Jenny had begun questioning whether the Pill was best for her. "I never had any complaints, but the more I worked through the Consciously Female process, I realized that I didn't like taking oral hormones," she noted. "It's funny, my husband used to say, 'I would never put something like that into my body!' But it didn't bother me because it worked so well." Now, given her age-related risks, such as blood clots, heart attack, and stroke, all of which increase on the pill in your forties, and her out-of-nowhere bouts of acne, plus concerns about low libido and eventual perimenopause, Jenny expressed an interest in changing her contraception for the first time in seventeen years.

I asked her to reflect about her gut-level reactions to the various options. I also presented information about which options were suitable to her circumstances (monogamous relationship with no STD concern, desire for something simple, not hormonal, finished having children). A vasectomy is often a good choice for women in Jenny's situation. But her husband refused, saying, "Why don't you have surgery instead?" I do see women in this situation automatically electing surgery themselves, by default: *He won't, so I guess I will.* Here's where the reflection and information steps come in handy. I see a lot of women going into a tubal ligation who are really mad at their husbands because "he doesn't want his family jewels cut," as one woman put it. I encourage them to process those feelings more before we schedule surgery, because those feelings can affect both their surgical experience (complications, recovery time, etc.) and their relationship afterward. It's also useful to review the data: Vasectomy is a simple outpatient procedure involving local anesthesia. A tubal ligation requires general anesthesia; it's invasive abdominal surgery with the usual associated risks. Also, while it is sometimes possible to reverse it, a woman should not choose such a procedure if there is even the remote possibility of changing her mind later.

Jenny didn't want her tubes tied any more than her husband wanted to have his snipped. So they went back to the drawing board to consider other options. He was willing to use condoms; she found them, like the diaphragm, bothersome. I asked why she had skipped over the IUD in her considerations. "The very word sounded scary," Jenny admits. "I just had it planted in my mind because of the old problems with them that they were a bad option." (All kinds of IUDs stopped being sold in the United States for years after manufacturing problems with one particular model, the Dalkon Shield, although problem-free brands never stopped being made or being popular in Europe. Today's versions are associated with extremely low health risks.) I explained the facts about IUDs today and how she was, ironically, an ideal candidate. Women who have previously had children tend to tolerate the device with few problems, unlike those whose uteruses have never had anything in them before.

So she agreed to try it, with the provision that she'd monitor how she felt and what she noticed, body and soul, and reevaluate in three months. The IUD proved to be comfortable and easy, and after an initial few weeks of being worried about its effectiveness and safety, Jenny reported she soon forgot it was even there. So she decided to keep using it.

It's Not Just About
Contraception Anymore

Consciousness around contraception requires cultivating an awareness about more than just birth control. Unfortunately, here in the twenty-first century you also have to be aware of sexually transmitted diseases.

In the good old days, we used to think STDs were something that only "loose women" got, not nice, smart women like us. The fact is, if you're sexually active, even with just one partner, you have to worry about them. Everybody, except the very few who have been in trusting monogamous relationships in which neither party has had other sexual partners in the past. But two groups I see are especially vulnerable to ignoring this dimension: (1) teenagers and young women who are just beginning to be sexually active, who tend to be flush with the heady thrill of sexual overdrive, and feel invincible about most matters of life or death, and (2) women who are reentering the dating scene after divorce or the end of a long-term relationship and who last were in the dating mode ten or more years ago, when the specter of AIDS and other STDs was not so harrowing as it is today.

It's not enough for these women to say, "I'm on the Pill, I'm safe." The Pill offers no protection against disease. Many women choose to use condoms with the Pill, or perhaps even more popularly, to switch to a barrier method, such as vaginal condoms or a diaphragm, which appear to reduce the risk of STDs because they protect the cervix, although not nearly as well as male condoms.

I wish I didn't have to hammer this message home, but after you've given a woman the word that she is HIV-positive, you don't ever forget it. Why give yourself a possible death sentence—or even a nuisance disease that disrupts your lifestyle—over a choice that is within your control?

LANDMARK: UNPLANNED PREGNANCY

Stacie, 23:

~—"I was sure that I was just sick. Being pregnant never crossed my mind!"

Yasmin, 33:

~—"Now what? I can't believe this is happening to me!"

A woman who is living consciously on the Cycling Pathway needs to start with the general awareness of the possibility for pregnancy, even though by definition it's a circumstance she is trying to avoid. I see so many smart, wonderful people who totally repress the very possibility. They're so petrified that they could be pregnant, they ignore every signal their soul is sending out ("It seems like I see pregnant people everywhere I look; funny I never noticed so many before"). They ignore the body signals, too ("I'm sick to my stomach; must be the flu." "That speck of blood sure was a light period—I'm sure it's fine").

It's absurd, but believe me, I see it all the time. Elaine came into the office saying, "I don't think it's really possible that I'm pregnant, but I missed a period and thought you should check it out." "Well, are you sexually active?" I asked. "Well, yeah..." The most extreme example of the unconscious female, which every ob-gyn has seen more times than she cares to believe, is the woman who presents in the emergency room with abdominal pain. She's in labor! Full term! And swearing that there is no way she could be pregnant! You have to be pretty darn unconscious to ignore every hormonal effect, every fetal kick, and every external change of pregnancy. Every time I see it, I think, *This can't be happening!* But humans have an amazing set of skills when it comes to repression.

So the place to start coping with this landmark is, frankly, anytime when there could be a *possibility.* You will be caught much less unaware should it happen, putting you ahead of the game when it comes to making a conscious choice about what to do next. Ask yourself, what if? What if you are pregnant? At least you have put the issue on the table and can get more information. Don't torture yourself trying to push it out of your consciousness. You can take a pregnancy test. Home tests are very reliable; you don't even need to go to a doctor. If it's negative, it might still be too early; you'll want to retest again in a few days. You can't be sure you're not pregnant until six weeks after your last period began. Confront it. And if it's positive, well that's a piece of information, too.

Okay, so now you know you are. Then what? The Feedback Loop.

First, reflection. Allow yourself a tremendous—I repeat, tremendous—amount of space to explore this matter. You do not have to do anything in the first week after confirming your pregnancy. Neither outcome (continuing the pregnancy, terminating the pregnancy) will be affected by a week's delay. In fact, doing an abortion too early decreases its success rate. This provides a natural window for reflection. The biggest mistake I see women make with an unplanned pregnancy is to make a hasty, knee-jerk reaction: "I would never have an abortion, and so I will have to have the baby!" Or "I would never have a baby, so I need to get an abortion!" Or "I could never give a baby up for adoption, and I can't keep it, so I'll terminate." Recognize that first impulse, acknowledge it, and then set it aside for a moment.

Even though the impulse is to "do something" right away, the reality is that what you really require is a great degree of consciousness. Gaining that insight is not an immediate thing; it's a deliberate process. Why so much caution around this particular issue? Because you can't change your mind. You can't decide after the abortion is over to have the baby. You can't decide, when you're six months along, not to go through with this pregnancy. (You can decide you want to give the baby up for adoption, but that's a whole other issue for reflection.) Your challenge is to live with the uncertainty of what you'll do even while part of you just wants to get it done with.

Give yourself permission to truly explore the issue: "This is not what I planned, but how do I feel about it?" Separate your initial reaction from the feelings that might come later. Use the tools in Part Two. Dreamagery is particularly effective now for dredging up deeply held beliefs. Journaling or talking to a nonjudgmental listener can also be effective. But be sure it's someone who will listen rather than render opinions. You're trying to uncover what *you* really want, not what someone else thinks is right.

Second, information. While your ob-gyn cannot make this decision for you, you should use this resource to further understand the ramifications of your choice. Learn what the abortion procedure is and how it works. For women in the first trimester, the options are a mechanical procedure (a suction D & C to make sure the uterus is empty) and a chemical choice (RU-486, a medication that causes you to expel the fetus—that is, miscarry). After the first trimester, abortion is a much more complicated procedure at higher risk to the woman. Learn what an abortion costs, whether mechanical or chemical. Discuss optimal timing for it. Learn about what pregnancy would entail from a health perspective.

Consult with a clergy member if that feels appropriate to you. Also consider the effect of a baby on your lifestyle—the practical ramifications in terms of your job, your home, your budget. The decision to bring forth new life should never be a mere cost comparison, since there are incalculable costs whatever you choose. But all information helps you make a better choice.

Explore the possibility of adoption. How does it work? Call an adoption agency to learn more; remember that gathering the information is entirely different from making a commitment. It's just gathering information. But the more external information that you collect, the better you can filter all of these realities through the important soul-level work to come up with the best choice for you. Also, having all these facts can have a galvanizing effect once you have decided; you can move ahead with confidence.

Third, action. Women who go deeply and really explore an unplanned pregnancy wind up with a profound sense of peace and clarity about their choice. It's still a complex, painful choice. It still involves grieving, whichever way they go. But the act of processing the choice leaves them feeling far better about the decision than if they had not done so. I see this all the time and it's remarkable. The women who make their choice unconsciously very often wind up experiencing unexpected repercussions at every step of the route they took. If they have the baby, they seem to be the women who have worse morning sickness, more difficult labors. If they have an abortion, they are back in my office six weeks later looking for antidepressants, their PMS worsens, they get insomnia, their relationship falls apart.

Then, re-reflection. Once the decision is made, it's *essential* to reflect on how it is for you. What comes up? How are you feeling now and what do you need now? *Do not* take the perspective that what's done is done and so further reflection is pointless. In many ways it's even more important now. Whatever your choice was, it was momentous, and it will always be a part of you. Whenever I hear a woman tell me that she had an abortion and never gave it another thought, I believe she has likely tamped down her feelings about it and they are still percolating within her. Re-reflection is necessary in order to come to terms with it and provide yourself with the information and support to help you feel comfortable with your choice and be able to move ahead in the healthiest possible way.

Emergency Contraception

Women today have the possibility of terminating a pregnancy almost before it's begun. The morning-after pill gets its name from its timing: high-dose birth control pills (estrogen and progestin, or progestin alone) given for a few days immediately after unprotected sex. The catch is that you must begin taking them within seventy-two hours of unprotected intercourse. So you can't wait until you miss a period to know whether you are definitely pregnant before you take the pills. The exact mechanism of how they work isn't known. But the pills apparently change the lining of the endometrium, creating an environment that is not conducive to the implantation of a fertilized egg, so a woman is unlikely to sustain a pregnancy. It's still possible, but not likely. Effectiveness hovers around 75 percent, though one review of ten studies found rates ranging from 55 to 94 percent, making this method less effective than oral contraceptives. You're treating the *concern* that you may be pregnant. You'll never know whether you were or not. (Most women who take them, in fact, were most likely never pregnant.)

The alternative is to wait a few weeks to see if you really have conceived. Then you can run a Feedback Loop on that reality and decide how you want to proceed—bear the child (and keep it, or let it be adopted) or terminate the pregnancy.

There's a difference between fearing the possibility of pregnancy and making a choice based on that fear (emergency contraception, or not) and knowing that you're pregnant and making a choice based on that knowledge. A lot of women choose the morning-after pill to avoid the possibility of the latter dilemma. Popping a few pills now may seem easier than having to wait to find out the reality a couple of weeks later—and then possibly having to make a choice about termination. Women who are against abortion, for whatever reasons, convince themselves that "this is different." Indeed, the American College of Obstetricians and Gynecologists and the National Institutes of Health consider emergency contraception to be a contraceptive, not an abortifacient, since it works prior to implantation. Whatever the point at which you define the beginning of pregnancy, my feeling is that taking morning-after pills to avert pregnancy "just in case" tends to be the unconscious, avoid-the-hard-questions route.

Of course, there are circumstances in which consciously choosing not to face the question of pregnancy may be a form of self-care. For example, for a woman who is raped there could be an additional level of emotional trauma in having to deal with being pregnant on top of having to deal with having been raped. Here's a case where it can be better not to know; emergency contraception is the kinder, gentler option under these circumstances. I would argue, though, that dealing with the possible consequences of an act of violence against you is very different from having to make a decision about the unintended pregnancy resulting from unprotected intercourse.

I do prescribe emergency contraception for some situations other than sexual assault based on the in-depth conversation my patients and I have about their situations. But generally I find that now that RU-486 is available, providing a quick and noninvasive early abortion, it makes more sense to see if you actually needed to do anything in the first place. Then you can make a conscious decision about what's best, with all the information in place. It's always better to be conscious proactively.

One thing I do frown on is using the morning-after pill as a routine form of contraception. I sometimes see women who ask for it serially; these aren't just rare big-time mistakes, but a pattern of not being conscious about contraception in the first place and then falling back on the morning-after pill as a result. There's a potential health risk to this kind of behavior: These are high-dosage pills. The effect of repeatedly dosing your body with high levels of hormones (much higher dosages than in regular oral contraceptives) has not been thoroughly studied. If the effect is significant enough to prevent a pregnancy, you have to wonder what else it's doing to your body! Use sparingly, if at all.

Rita's Story: "More Ready Than I Thought" ⟋

At twenty-seven and married for three years, Rita was "shell-shocked" to learn she was pregnant. She was genuinely torn about what to do. She had no strong feelings against abortion; it was mostly something she had never considered in a personal way before. Nor did she have an immediate sense of joy about having a baby. And she couldn't imagine having the baby and giving it up for adoption. She and her husband, Tony, had discussed children before they married, but their plan was to wait while they established their Internet business and bought a house—something they guessed might happen by her early- to mid-thirties.

I can't tell a patient what to do. Choosing to terminate or continue a pregnancy in these circumstances is a personal choice, not a medical one. So I encouraged Rita to take a week or so to really explore her feelings and her options. "Isn't it better to have an abortion as soon as possible?" she asked. It's true that you don't want to wait past ten to twelve weeks from your last period to do this procedure. But there's no need to rush out the next day; the first-trimester window should still allow adequate time for mindful reflection. Repercussions for the woman can be so huge, I explained, that it's especially important to give yourself the time to do reflective work. If you don't spend this time coming to terms with your decision, it is very likely that the abortion will come back to affect you in some unexpected way down the road. Even women who find the decision easy to make should spend this time to affirm their choice.

Not quite a week later, Rita called to make a prenatal appointment. She had spent a lot of time talking with Tony and reflecting on what a baby meant to her life now. "We realized that we are ready to shift around all our plans to accommodate this baby. It means working through a lot of logistics and psyching ourselves up, because we had always thought of it as something for 'later.'" At her exam, she confided that she had realized she'd been "forgetting" her diaphragm with increasing frequency, and that that information had been very revealing to her. "I think I was more ready than I thought I was," she said.

Anya's Story: Reversal of Impulse

When I first met Anya she was a scholarship student just beginning medical school. It was, she said, "the absolute worst possible imaginable time to get pregnant." At the same time, she held strong personal convictions against abortion. She simply did not see that as an option for her. Although a cousin had given up her baby for adoption and felt comfortable with this choice, Anya worried about struggling to carry a child to term while keeping up the grueling schedule of a med student.

My job is to be the facilitator in choices like these. There's no medical "best" choice, and my personal preferences and politics are irrelevant. Before she finalized her decision, I encouraged Anya to explore the situation from every angle, to weigh what was in her soul, her practical considerations, and so on. (I would emphasize this step whichever way a woman was initially tilting.) She reflected that she did not believe in abortion. She had another cousin who had had several, almost as a form of birth control, and Anya strongly disapproved of that. Anya was not in a serious relationship; if she had a baby, she would raise the child alone. She was also afraid that if she chose adoption, she would not be able to give the baby up after delivery. She had worked very hard for a scholarship in a program that was only in its first semester; could she continue that as a single mother? How might her life change? These are all extremely difficult and personal considerations.

I encouraged her to "try on" each decision—terminating the pregnancy and continuing the pregnancy—and live with it for a few days. How did it feel? Only she knew what felt right for her.

In the end, Anya chose termination. It was a very poignant experience. She grieved. She also felt a sense of relief. But, important, the process of confronting what had happened, and what it meant to her, did not end with the procedure. Anya then continued to work through her feelings (re-reflection) and not bury them. She wound up a top graduate of the program, and although I don't know what happened to her, I think of her often. I like to imagine her with her own successful medical practice and a cluster of children as well.

CENTERS OF WELLNESS MODIFICATIONS FOR CYCLING

Follow the general suggestions in Chapter 8, but with the following adjustments unique to the needs of the Cycling Pathway. Recognize that these are generalities that affect the majority of women on the Cycling

Pathway. You will want to observe and learn your own individual patterns. Then you can further fine-tune your choices to your specific needs on any given day.

ℬ Movement

Have you ever noticed how some days you can't wait to exercise, and other days you can hardly bring yourself to throw on your sweats? How on some days you easily go the extra mile (figuratively or literally), while on other days your body feels uncoordinated or sluggish? Both your physical abilities and your mind-set about exercise and movement alter cyclically. In general, your needs around movement shift from a greater emphasis on body-nourishing activities in the first half of your cycle to soul-nourishing activities in the latter half.

Especially if you are a regular exerciser, these shifts may become obvious to you once you stop and think about them. If you're not sure, keep an exercise diary for a couple of months, noting what kind of movement you undertook each day and how you felt about it beforehand and afterward. Also record the progression of your cycle. Then see how your individual phases match up with your exercise needs. (You can do this within your Consciously Female journal, on the pages of your daily planner, or wherever it's simplest for you.)

The goal should be for you to align your activities, their pace, and the setting of your Movement choices to correspond with where you are in your cycle. The more they mesh, the more likely you are to maintain momentum and have a sustainable Movement plan that supports your overall well-being rather than pitting you against yourself.

In the first half of your cycle: Right after the heavy days of your period, you're most likely to feel energetic, competitive, and physical. This is the waxing time, when your body is gearing up, full of preparation and promise. It's a good time to:

- *Push yourself.* If you are working on increasing the distance that you walk, run, or swim, or the length of time you work out, or the amount of weight that you lift, you may find yourself more successful at this point in your cycle.

- *Do the hard stuff.* Examples of movements that tend to feel best now include running, team sports, lap swimming, kickboxing, spinning—in general, aerobic activities that make you work hard.
- *Start a new class.* You'll be more receptive to new ideas and learning fresh movements at this phase, making it a more productive time to sign up for that new class at the gym or even to embark on a new exercise regimen.

In the second half of your cycle: As your cycle reaches the luteal phase, especially right before your period begins, the mood turns inward, retreating, waning. It's not sudden, like flipping on a switch, but rather a progression along a spectrum. You may feel less inclined to hard physical activity and more in need of movement that feeds your soul. At the cycle's midpoint, your body also produces more relaxin, the hormone that tells your muscles to stretch and relax. It's a good time to:

- *Pay extra attention to stretching.* You'll feel more mentally inclined to focus on staying limber and loose, actions that make you feel calm and content in your body and soul.
- *Take it down a notch.* You won't want to quit exercising altogether for two weeks. But you can pull back a little before revving up again later, in your next cycle. Good examples of exercise downshifts as your period approaches include individual sports, low-impact aerobics (instead of high), walking (instead of running), slow walking (instead of power walking), yoga or tai chi (instead of kickboxing), gentle cycling (instead of spinning). Experiment with movement options that nurture you physically rather than challenge your limits.
- *Stoke your soul.* Find ways to build satisfaction into your workout beyond an emphasis on achieving a goal in distance or output. For example, you might switch your daily run to a more scenic location even if the course is not as long, or walk-run instead of jogging all the way, in order to better tune in to

your surroundings. You might wear your favorite soft old clothes during a step class and also switch from high step action to milder marching moves sans the step. Skip a tough class if you don't feel like going, and substitute a leisurely swim or an afternoon of gardening.

In general:

- *Consider your exercise needs across a whole month.* Construct a workout routine that looks past the strictures of a given day or a week. I'm not suggesting that you should completely abstain from any activity on any given day. Rather, you might find your routine more satisfying and productive if you put a greater emphasis on aerobic efforts in the first half of your cycle and on stretching or weight-bearing activities in the second half.

- *If you are an athletic competitor, note where you are in your cycle when competitions are scheduled.* Then you can prepare yourself accordingly. For example, if you're premenstrual, you might want to give yourself extra preparation time and be especially vigilant about your nutrition and sleep needs; meditate and visualize more.

- *Run a Body Scan (tool 8) before you exercise.* Let it guide your choice of workout intensity and focus. Use it to help identify the places that need more attention, such as stretching.

- *Use Movement therapeutically.* Remember that even moderate exercise can release the feel-good endorphins that help to ward off mild depression. Exercise can also trigger the relaxation response, transporting you out of stress mode. As you assess your Five-Center Review each day, listen for signals from your Mind Center that might influence the Movement choices you make. Aim for a fluid, need-based Movement program, rather than one that's rigid and unchanging from day to day. (You'll not only feel better, you'll like it better.)

☙ Nutrition

Do you crave chocolate or chips right before your period? Binge on a particular food even though you didn't mean to? Find protein and leafy greens totally appealing one week and less so the next? Your nutritional needs and preferences—indeed, even the way that food makes you feel—change over the course of your cycle. Women with premenstrual syndrome, for example, have been found to have poorer diets overall than those who don't have PMS. (Although whether this is because of their diets or because their PMS leads to a poor diet is a chicken-or-egg–first question.) Your hormones affect your cravings, and your food affects your hormones and how you feel—yet another cyclical pattern of women's health.

In the first half of your cycle:
- *Put your vibrant feelings to good use.* This can be a great time to launch dietary improvements or make changes, because you're feeling open and revved up.
- *Watch the processed foods.* It was once thought that curbing salt throughout the cycle helped alleviate PMS. Although cutting down on salt may slightly reduce the tendency to retain water, it won't stop symptoms. But it's still smart generally to pay attention to hidden sources of salt, especially in processed foods and junk food.

In the second half of your cycle:
- *Take added calcium, magnesium, and vitamin B_6,* to curb severe PMS. If you have PMS, be sure to take 1200 milligrams per day of calcium with meals, split between two doses. A large study found that individuals taking this amount of added calcium had significantly less pain, mood swings, food cravings, depression, and back pain, with an overall 48 percent reduction in symptoms. It's also important to be on calcium for the prevention of osteoporosis. Increase supplemental magne-

sium from 200 milligrams at the beginning of the cycle to 400 milligrams daily, beginning on day fifteen of your cycle and continuing until the onset of menstrual flow. (The maximum can be raised to 400 to 800 milligrams as needed.) A good study in 2000 found that adding 200 milligrams of magnesium per day, along with 50 milligrams per day of vitamin B_6, significantly reduced anxiety-related PMS symptoms such as nervous tension, mood swings, irritability, and anxiety. The fact that chocolate is high in magnesium—who knew?—may be part of the biochemical explanation for why many women crave chocolate in the last half of the cycle. The mood-elevating effects of chocolate, however, are believed to operate through a serotonin mechanism, so don't be surprised if your cravings don't completely disappear when you supplement with magnesium. (Note: Take supplemental magnesium only under a doctor's supervision if you have liver or kidney disease.)

Vitamin B_6 binds to estrogen and progesterone receptors. Taking 50–100 milligrams per day with meals has been found to help reduce breast pain and swelling associated with PMS.

• *Add chasteberry.* The botanical chasteberry (*Vitex agnus-castus*) appears to regulate several key reproductive cycle hormones, lowering levels of luteinizing hormone and progesterone, as well as decreasing prolactin (via dopamine), a hormone that is a possible contributor to breast pain. In one study of more than sixteen hundred patients, after use in three cycles, 93 percent of women reported that their PMS symptoms decreased or went away, with no serious adverse reactions. (One symptom it does not seem to relieve is bloating.)

• *But choose other botanicals with care.* St. John's wort, one of the most popular botanicals around, is often used for depression, but it does not have similarly promising evidence of effectiveness for PMS; there is also a possibility that it can inhibit the effectiveness of oral contraceptives. Other botanicals that are often used but which I don't recommend for treatment of

PMS symptoms include black cohosh (not well studied for PMS), evening primrose oil (not shown effective), the Chinese herb dong quai (not well researched), and kava (or kava kava, associated with liver problems).

- *Indulge yourself, mindfully.* When a sweet tooth or craving for fatty foods hits and you know it is a few days before your period, succumb to it (in moderation) without beating yourself up. Plan for this eventuality, with gentle boundaries. Choose your treat intentionally and try to eat it mindfully. You'll feel more satisfied and be less apt to have your splurge turn into a major binge. You may need to do this for several days in a row before your period, or more than once a day. That's okay—if you're conscious about what's going on and why.

In general:
- *Soy it up.* There is good evidence that premenopausal women who have diets rich in phytoestrogens have a decreased risk of breast cancer and heart disease. Soy products (tofu, tempeh, soy milk, edamame) are great sources of phytoestrogens. Aim for 25 to 50 grams per day.
- *Rely on flaxseed.* I've recommended this rich source of alpha-linolenic acid, an omega-3 fat, for all women, but the additional fiber from just 2 tablespoons a day of ground flaxseed is particularly helpful in easing constipation and cramping in women who experience these symptoms during their cycle.
- *Reduce or eliminate processed foods containing refined sugars.* Research shows that women with PMS show a significant increase in carbohydrates consumed, especially in foods with simple sugars, such as cake or dessert. This can contribute to mood swings and overall lethargy. For some women, an easy way to do this is to avoid white flour and white sugar. If you focus on whole, natural foods, you're more likely to avoid mood swings.

❧ Mind

Please don't neglect taking Mind steps during this phase of your life. Women on the Cycling Pathway tend to have power-packed lives, studying, building careers, falling in love and forging relationships, perhaps managing families. I've seen again and again that when women are really busy, the Mind step is the first to get jettisoned from their lives. In fact, it's one of the best secret weapons I know to keep you grounded, calm, and actually *more* productive.

In the first half of your cycle:
- *Focus on making space for Mind steps.* You're apt to feel energetic and gung-ho, but that doesn't mean you don't need downtime. This is a good time to use meditation and breathing to feel centered and ward off stress. It's an especially good time to introduce new relaxation or breathing tools.

In the second half of your cycle:
- *Explore issues in deeper detail.* Women seem to glean the most from Journaling (tool 4), Dialoguing (tool 11), and Dreamagery (tool 12) after ovulation. Take advantage of the open window between your conscious self and your unconscious self at this time to explore what's on your soul right now. When you take time for this kind of consultation with yourself, the emotions that tend to be more raw at this point in your cycle are able to find expression and nurturance.

In general:
- *Practice relaxation techniques.* Here's a no-cost, no-risk strategy to relieve PMS. One study examining the effect of inducing the relaxation response for fifteen minutes twice a day for three months, compared to women who read for the same amount of time and women who simply charted their symptoms, found that 58 percent of the women in the relaxation response group had improvement in their symptoms, com-

pared to 27 percent for the reading group and 17 percent for the charting group.

ℬ Spirit

The need to nourish Spirit remains constant throughout every pathway of life. The main differences are the kinds of support that you seek out at a given stage of life. On the Cycling Pathway, you will probably notice that you are most receptive to socially interactive expressions of Spirit during the first half of the cycle and more inclined to solitary or one-on-one expressions during the second half.

In the first half of your cycle:
- *Go outward.* Find Spirit connections that mesh with your increased energy and enthusiasm to engage with others. This might include long walks or runs with friends, group activities through your place of worship, or volunteer work.
- *Extend yourself physically and mentally.* Spirit expressions that might appeal now include ambitious, connecting things like an overnight hike or camping trip, making a gallery tour or day of antiquing with friends, or undertaking a big project like running the church tag sale or helping to build a Habitat for Humanity house. (Remember: It's not that you can't do such things at any point in your cycle, only that you are more apt to feel up for them because they mesh better with what's going on right now in your body and soul.)
- *Stoke your friendships.* You may have more to give during this phase, making it a great time to plan long gossipy lunches or weekend getaways.

In the second half of your cycle:
- *Go inward.* Find Spirit outlets that mesh with your more reflective mood. This might include yoga or other meditative exercise, prayer, stargazing, reading philosophy or poetry, and so on.

- *But reach out, too.* You may find yourself more emotionally vulnerable in the week or so before your period. Be aware that you might need more support from friends and loved ones—don't be afraid to reach out for it. This is the time to call the friend to whom you can say anything, to have a cozy coffee conversation rather than a big party.
- *Explore any issues that come up around your life path.* This is an especially ripe opportunity to delve into your feelings around work choices (Where am I heading? Do I love what I'm doing?), relationship issues, and personal existential questions (Why am I here? What is my purpose?).

In general:

- *Consider your schedule.* Realize that you may be more up for an activity that involves group effort during the first half of your cycle, and less so later. If you have any flexibility about activities that involve your Spirit needs—such as which days each month you act as a Big Sister in a volunteer program, or when a major church retreat is planned—timing is a useful consideration in making your plans. What seems thrilling and exciting the Saturday after your period might feel like an overwhelming chore the Saturday before.

☙ Sensation

You already know that your sensuality and sexuality are meant to be accessed every day, not saved for special occasions like your fine china and fanciest lingerie. You may find, though, that you are more inclined to (or need to) indulge your sexuality in the first half of your cycle, and your sensuality more in the second half. Generally, a woman feels more energetic and adventuresome in the first half, making her more open to and interested in sex play; by the second half of the cycle, as she draws inward, she wants to be nurtured and cosseted. What's more, hormonal changes are directly linked to sexual responsiveness, including desire. At ovulation, when progesterone rises, many women report they are most likely to initiate sex. Other women feel sexier just before their period arrives. The kind of sexual activity you prefer can shift as well, from more direct and more passionate encounters in the first part of the cycle to, premenstrually, those involving more cuddling or more gentle, loving touches.

This is not to say that you shouldn't have sex in the second half of your cycle or indulge your sensuality in the first half, of course! It simply means that you'll probably be more in the mood for one or the other at different times in your cycle.

In the first half of your cycle:
- *Persist with Sensation steps even if you don't think you need them.* Take the time to continue nurturing your senses of smell, touch, taste, and so on. You might feel that you get less out of the experiences—that is, that you need them less—now than later in your cycle when your appreciation is richer. But they still serve a nurturing function, even if you notice the effects less.
- *Explore your sexuality.* When you do make time for sex in the follicular and ovulation stages, you'll be more up for pushing the envelope. Creative sex play, fantasy, new positions, bringing out your dominatrix side—all are activities that may appeal now more than at other times in your cycle. You might crave orgasm more than intimacy.

In the second half of your cycle:
- *Respect your sensuality even when you don't feel sexual.* Focus on sensual pleasures ranging from hot baths to massage to extra self-indulgences.
- *Don't overlook your intimacy needs.* I often hear complaints of low libido from women on the Cycling Pathway. Busy Cycling women often ignore their Sensation needs at every point in the cycle.
- *Cosset yourself.* Take advantage of Sensation actions that make you feel nurtured and supported. Whatever comforts you— mint tea, soft sweaters, jazz, your favorite perfume—this is the time to be sure to use it.
- *Indulge your sexuality.* This stage of the cycle finds women feel-

ing more mysterious, deep, and sensual, bringing out their romantic or introspective sides. Massage, mutual masturbation, or really soulful lovemaking that reaches the most intimate places of you and your partner may be particularly appealing now. You might crave intimacy more than orgasm.

- *Try not to shut out your partner.* Women have a tendency to withdraw when feeling blue and PMS-y. But you can reframe this vulnerable time as an opportunity to connect and, in so doing, deepen your relationship.

In general:

- *Tune in!* Women tend to be least aware of their needs in this center and how they change across the cycle because we're the most repressed about sexual and sensual matters. Really make the effort to listen.
- *Make your partner aware of the rhythms of your cycle.* It's easy for couples to fall into sexual patterns and routines. You develop certain habits concerning positions, games, who initiates, and so on—and these patterns tend to remain the same throughout the cycle, even though your interests and responsiveness change. If your partner is aware that your sexuality and sensuality have a cyclical ebb and flow and you both adjust your time together accordingly, you're both apt to benefit.
- *Learn to be conscious of how your contraception coexists with your sexuality.* The pharmaceutical contraceptive choices give you freedom from worrying about pregnancy and allow greater spontaneity for your lovemaking, but they may have some negative effects, too.

For example, some women who take oral contraceptives or Depo-Provera experience a decrease in their libido; the magnitude of the impact varies from woman to woman. Devices such as diaphragms and condoms don't affect body chemistry, but there is a trade-off in terms of spontaneity. Use tools such as Body Monitoring and Five-Center Review to observe the impact of your contraception method across your centers. Then use that information to help guide your choices.

Chapter 10

The Fertility Pathway

A baby, maybe

Trust yourself.
You know more
than you
think you do.

— BENJAMIN SPOCK

Do you want to have a baby? Are you trying to conceive? When a sexually mature woman desires pregnancy or finds herself pregnant, she moves onto the Fertility Pathway. She might be a bride, an adult woman in a committed relationship, an adult woman without a partner, straight or gay, eighteen or younger, forty or older. Some women choose never to enter this pathway, deciding that it is not necessary to have a child to make their lives complete. And of course some women enter this pathway quite by accident—unconsciously—but embrace it once they find themselves on it.

The Fertility Pathway is an exciting place because unlike the Cycling Pathway, where life tends to settle into the predictable framework of monthly cycles, suddenly everything is strange and new. When should you try to conceive? How long will it take? What will that feel like and how will you know? Are you ready? What should you be doing now to optimize your chances of a healthy baby? What will pregnancy be like? What do you need to do along the way? How will your life change during pregnancy and after? What will labor be like? And what if you don't get pregnant right away? What are your options? How do you feel about them? How long should you keep trying?

Ideally, if time permits, a woman should log up to six months on this pathway before actively trying to conceive, in order to get her body and soul in optimal shape for motherhood. Not every woman who chooses this pathway conceives. Many face choices about whether to become a fertility patient and how (and how long) to pursue such efforts. Many women conceive and then miscarry, a painful landmark that brings them back around to the beginning of the pathway, reevaluating whether to continue with a new attempt to bear a child or to move back to the Cycling Pathway.

At first glance, a woman who is not pregnant and one who is might seem very different. Certainly there are physical differences. But in terms of their consciousness around the matter of having a baby, they share many similar needs. For example, my nutritional counsel to a woman intending to become pregnant is about the same as to a woman in her first trimester of pregnancy. A woman struggling with infertility and a woman struggling with a newborn have similarly intense Spirit needs in terms of finding a supportive community for their very specific experience around childbearing. Fertility is a continuum that starts before conception; leads to conception, fertility treatment, or adoption; and in the case of conception proceeds through three distinct trimesters of pregnancy (or to a branch, miscarriage) and a postpartum phase. After recovering from childbirth, some women return to the Cycling Pathway, while those who immediately desire more children remain here.

WHAT'S HAPPENING NOW: BEFORE CONCEPTION
TO AFTER DELIVERY

You probably have a general sense of what happens in this pathway. Let me review some of the highlights, if only to fix in your mind what a dynamic and multidimensional route it is.

Conception is the moment when sperm meets egg. But let's back up. To create an optimal environment for conceiving and maintaining a pregnancy, it's a good idea to plan ahead. Although I like to see my pregnant patients ASAP (and ideally for a preconception checkup), the typical ob-gyn's first prenatal appointment isn't until one, two, or more months after conception. The reason I recommend seeing a doctor even before conception is to learn about changes you can make to support a healthy pregnancy for both you and your baby. You might want to make adjustments to your diet, such as taking supplementary folic acid, for example, or kick dangerous habits such as smoking. You could learn how pregnancy will interface with any preexisting medical conditions, such as anemia, diabetes, high blood pressure, an STD, or obesity. And you might take certain medical steps, too. A woman who has not had rubella (German measles), for example, should have an immunization three to six months before she tries to conceive. You can also use the time before you actually abandon birth control to plan for a more conscious conception (see box, page 273) and to begin to prepare yourself mentally for parenthood.

At ovulation, one of the two million to three million eggs you were born with is swept into a fallopian tube. If within the next twenty-four hours one of the 350 million or so sperm in a typical ejaculation manages to travel up through the vagina, the cervix, and the uterus (often out into the tube) to meet the egg, *voilà!* Conception. If it sounds a little complicated, well, it is. And it isn't, in the sense that this biological sequence unfolds almost automatically. You can't do much about it other than help make sure that the timing for the egg and sperm union is felicitous. And at the same time, that's what can make it a bit of a challenge.

You can learn to identify when you are going to ovulate by observing your cycle and your body. It typically falls at midcycle, or around day fourteen in a twenty-eight-day cycle. But since everyone's cycles are different—even a woman with a twenty-eight-day cycle is apt to experience occasional variations—pinpointing the day isn't always easy. You have other clues as well, though. Your estrogen levels begin rising sharply during the days leading up to ovulation, causing marked changes in your cervical mucus. Where it's usually scant and sticky, it becomes increasingly plentiful and thick. The texture becomes slick and slippery with long strands (called spinbarkeit), like an egg white. These changes are nature's way of helping the sperm get to the uterus, protecting it against the acidic environment of the vagina. (Sperm is alkaline, the opposite of acidic. Of those 350 million sperm in the race to the egg, only one in a thousand can make it through the vagina, and only four hundred or so will make it as far as the fallopian tube.) Right after ovulation, the cervical mucus goes back to its sticky, less abundant state. Since active sperm can live for up to five days, you have a window of time in which conception can take place that's broader than just the immediate hours around ovulation.

Estrogen also spurs desire, so you may feel more lusty around the time of ovulation. Some women who are incredibly in tune with their physiology can even feel the actual moment of ovulation as a slight pain in the lower abdomen (a.k.a. *mittelschmerz,* or "pain in the middle"). This is the follicle rupturing and releasing that month's chosen egg. Don't worry if you have never noticed this, though; most women don't. You can rely on other signs—not just the amount and quality of your cervical mucus, but the feel of your cervix, your basal body temperature, and/or a home ovulation detection kit.

Monitoring your cervix is challenging and not the best indicator of ovulation. Generally, though, it dips down slightly and feels no longer flexibly firm like a nose, but softer, mushier. The feel of the mucus is a much better indicator. So, too, is your basal body temperature—your temperature the very first thing in the morning, even before you get out of bed—though this indicator is more short-lived than cervical mucus, offering you a briefer window of opportunity to conceive. Here's how it works: Your usual temperature (before ovulation) is about 97.0 to 97.5 degrees F. Before ovulation, your temperature dips slightly and then, as progesterone levels shoot up over the course of a day or two, leading to the moment of ovulation, it rises to between 97.6 and 97.8 degrees F. By tracking your temperature across a cycle, you can begin to understand your own cycle and when you typically ovulate.

For roughly one in ten couples, conception does not occur easily. The problem may be as simple as mistiming intercourse. Normal aging plays a role in both women and, it is now believed, men. Or the problem might be an underlying disease or disorder in the woman (a thyroid problem, a history of endometriosis or fibroids, a past STD, etc.). Or the problem might be an underlying disease or disorder in the man (a less than optimal sperm count, previous urogenital surgery or injury, etc.). Stress and lifestyle conditions can also be major contributing factors.

Whether conception occurs naturally or with medical assistance (assisted reproductive technology), the pregnancy proceeds the same way. Unless she miscarries—which happens surprisingly often, in as many as two in five pregnancies—a woman will experience three trimesters, each roughly three months long, and then a three-month postpartum phase. Each segment features distinct characteristics.

The first trimester sees the fertilized egg (called a *zygote*) advance from a minuscule cluster of cells (called a *blastocyst*) to an apple-seed-sized ball (called an *embryo*) to a two-inch-long tadpole (now called a *fetus* until birth) whose heartbeat can be heard through a fetoscope or Doppler stethoscope. All of your baby's organs and body systems develop during this phase. Your hormone levels, especially progesterone and hCG (human chorionic gonadotropin), are in overdrive—hCG doubles every two days in the early weeks! And all that inner activity takes a toll on the host mother. Early symptoms (as early as the week after conception) include tender breasts, an aversion to certain smells, nausea, increased urination, and fatigue. Some women spot-bleed a week after conception, when the fertilized egg is implanted in the uterine wall. The surest signs are a missed period and a positive pregnancy test. Your emotions can range from awestruck joy to apprehension, fear, outward ambivalence—or all of these! Those early responses can intensify as the weeks continue. Some women get so sick and worn out that their overall health is at risk, making it especially important to carefully monitor your body/soul needs on a daily basis and respond accordingly.

By the second trimester (week thirteen, counting from the date your last period began), things suddenly calm down. As hormones from the placenta take over, hCG levels plummet. Many women describe this point as a sudden lifting of clouds, an almost overnight vanishing of their irksome symptoms. This tends to be the most peaceful, pleasant, sparkling time of a pregnancy. You feel great and look great. Glowing skin tone (thanks to increased blood volume) and a high energy level (thanks to no more hCG or fatigue and nausea) add up to the characteristic "bloom" of pregnancy. You first feel the baby move within you.

Although nausea-making hormones ebb by the second trimester, your overall hormonal profile remains incredibly dynamic all through pregnancy—and at magnitudes that help to explain why this state is like nothing else you'll ever experience. By your ninth month, for example, relaxin levels are ten times greater than they are in a nonpregnant woman. Your cardiac output doubles.

During the third trimester, slowdown sets in. Ever-increasing girth affects how your body moves and feels, and tends to truncate your activities. It may be difficult to tie your shoe, for example, let alone enjoy intercourse or stay on your feet all day at work. The recommended weight gain is twenty-five to thirty-five pounds, depending on your starting point, health, and risk levels, but it's not at all unusual to pack on as many as fifty or more. Women report feeling tired, and tired of being pregnant. Sleep is more challenging, as the weight of the uterus against the bladder keeps you making bathroom trips. And it's just more difficult to get comfortable, whether you're sitting, standing, or lying down. Even simple daily tasks like walking become challenging, as the bones of your pelvis actually begin to separate in preparation for childbirth. Combined with a shifted center of gravity, many women get a very wobbly or waddling sensation. As the due date nears, so do fears about labor and worries about impending motherhood.

The exact mechanism by which labor is triggered is not fully understood. It's thought that some kind of signal passes from fetus to mother. Whether this is because the fetus is at last fully formed or can no longer thrive in the womb is unclear. At any rate, a cascade of hormonal triggers sets labor in motion. The baby's head drops lower into the birth canal, the thick mucus seal that has protected the cervix comes out (the "bloody show"), the membranes that contain the amniotic fluid may break, and contractions begin. A contraction is the involuntary tightening and relaxing of the long muscles that wrap around the uterus. When the muscles contract, they shorten, allowing the cervix at the base of the uterus to dilate and eventually enabling the baby to exit the birth canal. No two labors proceed exactly alike. Although there are many things a woman can do to optimize herself for the challenge and pain of labor mentally and physically, she can't control every part of the process. Some things can only be determined by either her medical team, her baby, or the powers that be.

After delivery, the body gradually works its way back to its prepregnant state. This can take as much as six weeks, for the immediate physical recovery, or six months or longer, for the complete adjustment to new motherhood. Physically, your body is bouncing back from the extreme effects of pregnancy, during which your blood volume doubled, the capacity of your uterus expanded a thousandfold, and almost every major organ and blood vessel was either squished around or working overtime. (A woman who has had a C-section must also recover from major abdominal surgery.) The emotional and practical realities of your life are about to be even more dramatically altered. Your priorities, routines, identity, relationships, and budget are affected. Sleep deprivation (because of a newborn's round-the-clock needs) and breast-feeding can be added challenges. The postpartum transition to motherhood—often ignored by our culture as the collective focus shifts to the newborn—is as seismic a time as puberty, pregnancy, and menopause in terms of the dramatic nature of the shift taking place within both the body and the soul.

LANDMARK: THE BABY QUESTION

Kim, 25:
— *"I'm here to talk about quitting the Pill. All of my friends have babies. I've been married for five years. I'm not getting any younger. It's better to be a younger mother, isn't it?"*

June, 33:
⌐ "I was walking to the mailbox alone and I heard myself say out loud, 'I want a baby.' Just like that. I realized it suddenly felt like the right thing to do."

Krystle, 29:
⌐ "I'm the last person any of my friends ever expected would want a child. I guess I'm not the maternal type. But my clock is ticking, you know, and I want to plan this out just like I've planned out my degrees and my career. Now I have to find a good father."

If this landmark had a shape, it would be a doorway, because it's a world you choose to enter—or shut the door on. Are you ready for motherhood? For most women, the decision is not sudden or simple. There are myriad, complex factors to consider. Here's how I recommend approaching them, with, as always, the help of the Feedback Loop.

First, reflection. Ideally, this is an issue on which you should check in with yourself on as many levels as possible, beginning in your Cycling days. A truly Conscious Female learns to view her life itself as a cycle with seasons; by being aware of them, she develops a sketch of what they might look like for her. To be conscious is to hold a sense of your past and your future, as well as a sense of what's unfolding right now. That ability to look backward and forward helps inform how you make choices in the present.

If anyone ever says to me, "I'm ready to have a baby, I have no reservations whatsoever," a warning bell goes off. A complete lack of reservations says to me that she most likely has not done all the necessary work, because nobody ever has all parts of her life align perfectly toward motherhood. For most women, one part feels ready ("I'm thirty, my clock is ticking") but other parts do not ("I just started law school," "I'm single," etc.). There are almost never all green lights or all red lights. Many women recognize the conflict and then just leave it at that. Dwelling on it might complicate their lives, they decide; easier to let it rest. *But you've got to go there!* If the baby question can never be all green lights, the onus is on you to explore your readiness in multiple dimensions, to weigh the reds and the greens, and then consciously decide what adds up to go for you.

- Explore your soul-level readiness. What are your feelings around children and motherhood generally? Why do you think you want children, if you are sure you do? What are your fears? Dialoguing with your reproductive system can be very useful. Doing this kind of work during the premenstrual part of your cycle can be especially productive.
- Explore your relationship. Are you in one now? How strong is your relationship? How do you imagine your partner as a father? Have you discussed parenthood? What are your partner's wishes and fears? How would a child affect your relationship?
- Explore your career. It's a fact of modern life that the majority of mothers and would-be mothers work today. How will a child affect your career? What might change? What are the implications of those changes, in terms of income, personal satisfaction, ambition, stress, logistics, and other factors? This is one area where you can't know until you're there how you will really feel—that is, you can't make concrete plans at this abstract point about whether you will quit your job, be a working mother, or try working part time. If you are financially secure enough to have the luxury of choice in this matter, you will have to do the decision making later, but thinking about it now can help "till the soil," so to speak.
- Explore your health. Are you physically ready for the demands of pregnancy? Are there particular things you should do first to get ready? Do Body Monitoring and the Five-Center Review to help give you pictures of your status now. How does your body feel?
- Explore your stage of life. Do you feel "too old" to have a baby? "Too young"? Women who get to forty and have trouble conceiving but have always been conscious that conception might be difficult if they waited too long are in a vastly

different place from those who have never considered the implications of waiting, never acknowledged that fertility wanes as the years go by. It's still hard, still painful—but it's not a total life crisis. A woman who waits until forty to even think about babies and then has trouble conceiving tends to experience the disappointment much more harshly.

Second, information. Now gather as much information as you feel you need about the relevant medical concerns and check it against your inner reflections. Discuss with your doctor any possible implications for quitting your current method of birth control and how that should best be done. Learn about ovulation and how you can monitor its timing. Take your age into account. Fertility declines with age, while the risk of having a child with birth defects increases. Prospective mothers or fathers with a family history of genetic problems or prospective mothers who will be over age thirty-five at the time of delivery can benefit from talking to a genetic counselor about their specific risks. You'll also want to discuss any preexisting medical condition with your doctor and talk about how pregnancy may or may not affect it. Many chronic conditions often improve in pregnancy (such as seizure disorders, rheumatoid arthritis, irritable bowel syndrome). Other problems, such as cardiovascular conditions and hypertension, may worsen or even be life-threatening. Still others, for example diabetes, will require special care approaches.

Third, action. Few women wind up "stuck" after going through this process. They almost always come out of it on one side ("Yes, I'm ready") or the other ("No, not yet").

Then, re-reflection. Before you actually do anything, know that you can make a choice and live with it. Try it on and see how it fits. If you have decided to try to conceive, pretend for a day or a week that you are doing so (but don't toss the birth control yet). What does that feel like? Do you have a sense of excitement and readiness, or of fear and trepidation? Ditto for the other route.

Conscious Conception

So you've decided to try to get pregnant. Do you toss your pills and go to it? You could, but you'll be starting from a more advantageous place if you bring some awareness to the business.

Get to know your body, if you haven't already. Become familiar with your cycles so you have a sense of when you ovulate. Try taking your basal body temperature for a cycle or two, or use a store-bought ovulation kit. I like these processes because they are fun ways to explore your body. Some women, though, hate that kind of thing. To them it feels overly mechanical. If it serves you well and you enjoy it, great. If not, work instead toward developing a general sense of when you're fertile from the length of your cycle and the signs from your body.

Next, get conscious about how much sex you're having! The old school of thought, which many obstetricians still espouse, is that you should avoid intercourse for three days (or two or five, depending on the method) immediately before and after ovulation. The idea is that the strongest sperm will then have a sure shot at the egg. But for a doctor to counsel a patient to time intercourse around ovulation doesn't make sense without consideration of your lifestyle. No formula works for everyone.

A better approach relies less on formula and more on knowing yourself. If you become aware of when you ovulate and have sex more frequently around that time, it becomes a far more natural process (and therefore more apt to work). The couple who has intercourse only once a month (or once a week) can simply make a point of having it within the two-day window when the woman is most fertile. The couple who has sex every two or three days doesn't have to worry at all, because there's always sperm around.

Finally, just as you pay attention to what your body needs in order to conceive, take the needs of your soul into account, too. For example, I've heard patients half joke, "No wonder we're not pregnant. All we seem to do is fight." No wonder indeed. Find ways to feel right and receptive around ovulation time. For many couples, this happens quite easily. They articulate their hopes and work together to make this time a calm, loving, and, yes, *welcoming* time. You don't have to go out and do fertility dances and create fancy rituals (unless that happens to suit you). But do consider this component; it's a unique opportunity.

Meredith's Story: It's Time—Isn't It?

The biological clock is a fascinating concept. Say the words, and every woman of every age has a picture of it, ticking off the minutes of her available time on the Fertility Pathway. Women hear that *tick, tick* at different ages. For some it's strong and loud; for others it's low and very much in the background. However you imagine it, the concept is very real. Everybody needs to pay attention to it, whether you choose to try to have a baby or not.

For Meredith, the clock sounded at what seemed to her an unlikely time. She was thirty-seven, in the middle of establishing her own floral shop after years of working for others. She was not in a relationship. "I never gave much thought to having children because I was single," she explained, almost apologetically, at our first meeting. "But now that I'm inching closer to forty, I have begun thinking about babies all the time. I see them everywhere, at the mall, at the park, on the street. Where were they before?"

Meredith came to me because she wanted to explore conceiving a child through a sperm donor and becoming a single mother. She wanted to make sure "everything is in working order" and get some ideas about how she might proceed. We went ahead with the exam because she was due for an annual checkup. But before she proceeded with the sperm banks, I suggested that Meredith spend a little bit of time exploring her feelings about her biological clock and single motherhood. Because it was such a big step, she readily agreed.

After spending a couple of weeks reflecting on the subject, Meredith reported that she felt more sure than ever that she wanted to have a baby. She felt financially secure and confident that she had a lot to offer a child. She felt very clear about why she had not wanted a child in the past (not being in a permanent relationship) and why this had changed now (because she felt she didn't need to wait for a partner, her window for fertility was more limited, and she was comfortable going it alone because she had a lot of other support systems).

Unfortunately, Meredith's two attempts at artificial insemination failed to result in pregnancy. After each try, she went back through the Feedback Loop to reevaluate her decision. The second time, she felt that she faced another choice: to take the next step on the medical side (IVF), to pursue adoption, or both. Meredith went back into reflection mode, studying each of these options. She also began collecting information about what each option entailed, medically and financially.

I was surprised when she called one day to say she had decided to do nothing. "Even though I would be enriched by a child, and have a lot to offer a child," she said, "I just don't think I want it that badly to spend a lot of time and money in much more complicated pursuits. If I were married, I might feel different. Or if I were independently wealthy, I might be more inclined to take the risk. But I am okay with my life as it is right now."

Because this was a dramatic change from her inclinations only a few months earlier, we explored her feelings further. As she continued her reflections, Meredith felt that her desire for a baby had been based more on her fears about getting older and never having thought about children in a conscious way than it was about actually becoming a mother. She decided to stick with her decision to take no further steps toward pregnancy at this time, but to continue Journaling and doing Dreamagery, recognizing that these feelings and what was right for her may or may not shift.

LANDMARK: OUTSIDE FERTILITY HELP?

Ali, 39:

⊸*"I got my period today and I started weeping in the ladies' room. I've been trying to get pregnant for six months. Nothing seems to be working."*

Felicity, 26:

⊸*"Today is our second wedding anniversary—and the first anniversary of when we started trying to have a baby. That means we're infertile, right?"*

Pru, 39:

⊸*"After three years and I don't want to even think about how many dollars, I know everyone wonders why we don't give up. I have been poked and prodded and injected and studied. And then there's what Ben has gone through. But I just can't bring myself to stop. I keep thinking,* Maybe next time. *I keep hearing about new things they're doing. I tell myself I'm not even forty. It has become the number-one goal in my life, so how can I stop now?"*

If you don't conceive right away, the natural question that forms in a modern couple's mind is "Do we need help?" Technically, the medical indication for a fertility workup is a year of unprotected intercourse that has not resulted in a pregnancy. But deciding that it's time for you to get outside help is a very individualized matter. You may want to wait less than a year, or more, depending not just on your age, but on your feeling of emotional urgency. But if you do decide to seek fertility counseling, be aware that it's a significant threshold to cross, given what's involved.

From my first exposure to infertility protocol back in medical school, I believed that there is little we handle so badly from a whole-person viewpoint. Our treatments and diagnostic tests can be humiliating, painful, and depressing for both women and men. These expensive and time-consuming tests invade the most intimate part of a couple's life with very little apology. Once a couple starts down the fertility treatment branch, it changes everything in their intimate life (and often a great deal about the rest of their lives as well). Instead of making love, they are conducting a science experiment. They may postpone other major decisions in their lives, put career advancement on hold, become isolated from friends and family, go into debt, grieve. Yet until recently there has been little emphasis on emotional care during this traumatic time. I'm speaking from both sides of the fence here: as an ob-gyn who sees many women struggling with fertility problems, and as a patient who has herself experienced infertility workups and IVF.

A couple who is centered and feels good about each step of the process can find the patience and humor to persevere until they are pregnant or until it no longer feels right. A couple who begins making choices unconsciously isn't sure how they really feel. They may at some point find that if they had stopped and asked themselves, they would have realized they didn't really want to continue any further but were propelled along anyway by doctors' suggestions, their old dreams, and their own inertia in the face of the fertility machine. An unheeded change of heart can then turn around and express itself as major marital stress; many marriages dissolve over the dynamics catalyzed by infertility. The marital stress comes on top of the intimacy-sapping mechanical nature of the process, financial stress, and the stress of grief over the absence of a hoped-for child, which tends not to be honored by the culture at large.

Here are the considerations around choosing fertility assistance.

First, reflection. Before anything, get clarification for yourself on these issues:

- Consider your age. Are you still in your twenties or early thirties? Regardless of your youth, you might feel ready for a fertility workup, or you might feel concerned but still optimistic and willing to wait and see. Are you nearing or past forty? You may feel that time is of the essence and wait six months or less before seeking help. Or you may decide that you are so ambivalent that you are willing to just put the situation in God's or nature's hands.
- Consider your anxiety level. Check in with all of your

Centers of Wellness for evidence of stress in your life. How are your concerns about fertility shading your lifestyle and health habits? How has your relationship, including your sexual relationship, been affected? What is your partner's anxiety level, and how does that affect your own? Your anxiety can drive the sense of urgency you feel about getting help, though it should not be your only motivation.

- Consider your feelings about infertility. Is the subject one of hope and optimism for you, or an admission of "failure"? How does your reproductive history color your present feelings (e.g., do you have a family history with infertility, or have you had an abortion or a miscarriage?). Continue using the Dialoguing tool with your reproductive system—which can be more useful than ever in these circumstances. What does it want to tell you? What do you want to tell it? What does it need from you?

- Consider your feelings around fertility treatment. Many couples tend to think that their doctor or a fertility specialist can "fix" whatever's wrong; there's an assumption of immediate results once help is enlisted. Explore your expectations. What are your feelings generally around assisted reproduction? Are there certain procedures that make you more comfortable or uneasy than others? At this point, you're not deciding anything. You're simply putting on the table as much data as possible to make a conscious decision.

- Consider the what-ifs. What if you started fertility treatment? Live with that experience for a few days. How does it make you feel? Then imagine you have decided against treatment, and live with that. Compare your reactions.

Second, information. Don't say yes to treatment without a good understanding of what's involved. Depending on your circumstances, you may have a number of options. Learn what will happen first if you decide to go ahead. The typical first step is a fertility workup, intended to help identify where the problem lies. This can include, for the woman, a laparoscopy, a surgical procedure to evaluate the pelvic organs; a hysterosalpinogram (hSG), a test that injects dye into the reproductive tract to illuminate tubal or uterine abnormalities; and blood tests to confirm that you're ovulating and to identify possible hormonal problems. The man will undergo semen analysis (providing a sample in a cup to be tested for sperm concentration, motility, pH level, and so on).

Depending on what's found, there are many possible treatment branches, growing ever more complex. But it's important to note that no cause is found in up to 40 percent of fertility patients. The range of options is constantly expanding, including such procedures as artificial insemination and IVF (in vitro fertilization) to the use of donor eggs and donor sperm. What are the success rates for a couple in your situation? What are the risks? What are the price tags (no small consideration, since insurance often does not cover fertility treatment, and one cycle of IVF can run $10,000 to $15,000)? It can be hard to get straight information, given all of the variables involved. Fertility clinics are understandably reluctant to make promises and want to keep hope alive, so you may need to work to pin down the facts. Ask a lot of questions. Learn as much as you need to know to feel comfortable.

Explore both conventional and alternative treatments. Your approach doesn't have to be an either-or proposition; many CAM therapies work with conventional ones. A study of 160 patients who received acupuncture twenty-five minutes before and after embryo transfer, for example, found that they achieved a pregnancy rate of 43 percent, compared with a rate of 26 percent among women who did not receive acupuncture.

Make a point to also explore venues for dealing with the emotional stress. In a 1993 study, Boston psychologist Alice Domar found that many infertile women are as depressed and anxious as cancer patients, although they had been mentally healthy before fertility treatment began. What's more, there is good evidence that cognitive therapy during fertility treatment doubles the success rate; those who get psychological support are twice as likely to wind up with a baby. Clearly many fertility problems are based in physiological snags (low sperm counts, endometriosis). But this is one place where you need all the help you can get to break a classic vicious circle: Stress can affect fertility, (through the hypothalamus) and the whole fertility process itself is stressful. Investigate at the outset what kind of support and counseling are recommended. Learn how it works.

Third, action. Weigh internal and external data together to decide whether to advance to fertility treatment or to the next steps in fertility treatment. Because you need both an egg and a sperm to procreate and because you are going to need all the support you can give each other through this challenging process, it is essential for your partner to undergo a similar process of conscious choice-making.

Then, re-reflection. Know that your choice to get help or not is reversible. For example, it is totally legitimate—and indeed best—to reassess your choice after having your first appointment for infertility. See how you feel. For some couples, it feels the same; they are still ready to proceed. In fact, many couples will feel excited and hopeful once they are taking concrete steps. For others, the actual experience of starting the process makes them feel unsure.

Fertility treatment is *not* a conveyor belt of no return. Many people I counsel tend to believe that they can't get off once they've stepped on it. It's easy, once you immerse yourself in the new world of tests and procedures that are unfamiliar and possibly intimidating, to go unconscious fast, to surrender to the process. Don't! Keep checking in. Do the Feedback Loop. There's a lot of breathing room between getting pregnant and exhausting every possible option. Only by being really conscious every step of the way will you really know which point is the best for you.

I can't emphasize enough this need for ongoing reflection. The quest for conception takes on a life of its own—not necessarily the new life the prospective parents are hoping for, but an insidious life of hope run amok. It's precisely because the stakes are so high that emotions run high, too. What's more, these strong currents of emotion are occurring at a time when you may feel your life spinning out of control. You're having to acknowledge your inability to reproduce naturally (a central aspect of your identity as a woman), and having to endure an invasion by strangers into the most intimate dimension of your life. Believe me, when your husband's sperm is put into your vagina by another man (or woman), you can be sure that the act will be loaded with emotional triggers!

Hanna's Story: Choosing Support ⌒

My colleague Hanna, a happily married thirty-year-old, had a crushing first-term miscarriage a year ago, a traumatic and frightening experience for a first-time prospective mother. It was a difficult miscarriage involving significant blood loss, the kind where the discouraged mother is sick enough to be kept overnight in the hospital for observation. But Hanna recovered and returned to work with no lasting medical concerns as far as she knew.

Since the miscarriage, Hanna and her husband, Jim, had been diligently trying to make a baby. Something wasn't working. By conventional medical standards, this young healthy couple was now labeled as "infertile" and was slated for an infertility workup. To Hanna, this was a depressing prospect. She didn't feel infertile, even though she had been trying to get pregnant ever since the miscarriage. Because she had gotten pregnant once before, she knew that she could conceive; this fact reassured her greatly. Was it really time for her to cross the threshold into high-tech medical intervention? On one hand, she was concerned that if she waited too long to get help, she could lose her best chance to address a fertility problem that might be easily solved. On the other, Hanna worried that the constant monitoring, prodding, and analysis would degrade her sense of wholeness, both physically and in her relationship with her husband.

After a few days of uncertainty, Hanna politely said no to the recommended infertility workup and treatment protocol. She would just wait and see what happened. A young woman with great faith and positive energy, she decided that this course felt most comfortable for her at this point. Mindful of the risks and benefits, Hanna had her own vision of what her body needed.

Both as a physician and as a friend, I respected Hanna's decision and supported her in every way I knew. But I also knew that shrugging off medical suggestions has its own risks and can be a hard road for a young woman to travel. I admired her for making the decision based on what was right for her—a conscious decision.

The next months weren't easy for her. Hanna didn't instantly get pregnant, as she had secretly hoped. Each month when she got her period she felt devastated. Had she made the wrong decision? Jim tried to bolster her. "It's okay," he'd say supportively. "We'll try again next month."

As the months went by, "it" became a problem between the couple. Focusing on conceiving became a central issue in Hanna's life, but she avoided talking about it to Jim, not wanting to hear his well-intentioned pep talks. She dreaded disappointing him, because she felt so down herself. She began carrying the burden alone, not letting Jim know when her period came, not allowing him to see or support her misery.

Often I could tell just by her face when she came into the office exactly what was going on in her reproductive life. Though I wanted to be helpful, I felt slightly uncomfortable about crossing the professional line. But I have seen this scenario too many times. "Look," I told her, "you have to let yourself grieve each month, even if you think you aren't supposed to. Let yourself consciously articulate your fear that you are never going to get pregnant, that maybe you should have been doing the whole infertility treatment thing. You don't have to start treatment; you just have to allow yourself to admit your uncertainties. Once you can consciously state your worst fears, you can move on to the next step.

"Next," I continued, "you have to let Jim into the process. This is something that affects both of you. Don't carry it all upon yourself as if ovulating or getting your period is a secret shame or a private burden. Teach him how to know where you are in your cycle," I suggested.

One day, Hanna came in and whispered to me that she was so happy. No, she wasn't pregnant yet, but her husband had asked her the night before, "Isn't it about time for you to ovulate?" He had become her partner in the process, and her burden seemed much lighter. He had also become conscious of the cycle of her femininity, aware that where she was in her cycle had great impact on his life as well as hers.

The next six months were a little better. Things were smoother at home, and Hanna was more philosophical when her period arrived. She felt calmer, less discouraged. Importantly, she kept checking in as to whether it felt right to continue without medical intervention. It did. Finally, the morning came when she walked in beaming and told me that yes, she was "late." I was as excited as she was. I immediately started calculating due dates and writing prescriptions for prenatal vitamins. All is now progressing just as wondrously and boringly normally as Mother Nature intends.

Rachel's Story: Getting Off the Conveyor Belt

Because I practice integrative medicine, I see patients while they are simultaneously working with a fertility clinic. I also get many patients who come to me as a kind of last resort after having worked exclusively with fertility specialists. Rachel was such a patient.

Two years ago, at age thirty-nine, she and her husband, Joe, had embarked on their journey, beginning with the initial steps of an infertility workup by her regular ob-gyn. They went through the usual battery of tests and sperm samples. It was discovered that Rachel did not ovulate regularly; some cycles were anovulatory. So she went through several cycles on Clomid (clomiphene citrate), an oral drug that stimulates ovulation, without success.

"I knew when we started the treatments that I was ready to go that far," Rachel recounted. "But I had not thought much past that to anything more invasive." So when she was referred to a specialist who suggested IVF, Rachel and Joe went along with little forethought. IVF is a complex treatment that requires administering shots daily, getting multiple ultrasounds, and a minor surgical procedure to retrieve eggs. It's also expensive. There is a 10 percent to 20 percent success rate per cycle, depending on the cause of the infertility.

What happened to Rachel—what happens to many fertility patients—is the escalator effect. The doctor says, "Well, that didn't work, let's try again." Or "Let's try this other thing." Focusing only on the prize—a baby—the couple follows along willingly, although not necessarily consciously.

"I woke up on my forty-first birthday feeling really, really blue," she said. "That's when I decided, *This isn't working! I need to try something else!* I heard about the Center for Integrative Medicine and figured maybe you have a different procedure we can try."

In fact, I did. But it wasn't exactly what Rachel and Joe had in mind. What they needed was not yet another fertility treatment, but a chance to catch their breaths. For two years, the couple had tried procedure after procedure without coming up for air. I suggested that they pause and use the Feedback Loop: reflect on how they felt about where things stood, regroup with the facts about their success to date and new information I could share about alternative approaches, and then decide whether they wanted to go forward or not. Many couples, when they finally get conscious about their situation, decide that the fertility quest no longer feels right; they look into adoption, or decide to leave the baby question up to fate.

We paid a lot of attention to emotional healing, using tools such as Dialoguing, Journaling, and talking. Although Rachel had no regrets about what she'd undergone so far, she realized that she had not fully acknowledged what a high price she'd been paying. After making some space for that process, I gave her information about various alternative techniques, such as Chinese medicine (acupuncture, tai chi and other movement therapies, and herbals) and mind-body therapies that have been showing promise. I told her about a fertility support group, since women with this kind of support benefit in mind and spirit, and also stand to improve their fertility success rates.

Ultimately, Rachel did decide to try some alternative therapies, including acupuncture; she wasn't ready to give up her dream for a baby yet. But from here on, she would go through a re-reflection step at the end of each cycle, in order to be walking consciously through each try, rather than passively zooming along on the conveyor belt.

Adoption

Adoption is not a biological matter and therefore falls outside the role of an ob-gyn. But it's a choice that many women arrive at after they have spent time as a fertility patient. Deciding whether you are ready to adopt (whether you have had fertility issues or not) ideally follows the same conscious-choice process described for having a baby.

As with any choice, it's important to acknowledge any loss you may be feeling around dreams or wishes that you may be letting go of. Run your possible courses of action through the Feedback Loop, making yourself conscious of all the thoughts, feelings, biases, and many choices within this process. The degree to which you will fully embrace the adoption process, and your adoptive child, will in large part depend on how consciously you transition to this choice.

LANDMARK: PREGNANT!

Patricia, 38:
— *"At first it was like the most prolonged case of PMS I ever had in my life. I thought, 'If this is what being pregnant is all about, how am I going to stand it for eight more months? Why did I ever want this in the first place?' But by the end of the third month, a fog lifted. I have never felt so alive!"*

Gillian, 32:
— *"I felt my baby kick today for the first time. It's like I've joined a secret society that I never knew existed—all the other mothers in the world."*

Sam, 35:

⌐"My pregnancy wasn't that hard—or maybe it was. I don't even know. I was so busy that I didn't really pay much attention. I would look down at my belly and say, 'Wow! What's happening to you?' And then I would go back to work and forget all about it. Until I went into labor, I had compartmentalized the entire nine months so it felt more like an intellectual exercise than a physical or spiritual one. Labor was different, though—hard to ignore that! I felt off-kilter, and the pain was awful. After the baby came everything was out of whack, too. I wasn't prepared for the emotional surges, the new division of labor in the house, the endless nursing. I feel like I spent nine months on the sidelines of my pregnancy and then labor threw me into the game. My regret is that I didn't get into the whole thing from the start."

Leigh, 25 (who had a previous miscarriage):

⌐"Tracy first asked me to imagine a safe place where I felt totally comfortable. I pictured a sunny room. Once I felt comfortable, she asked me to invite an image of my baby. So quickly that it surprised me, I saw a picture of a blond, blue-eyed girl, about four years old, dressed in white.

" 'What do you want to say to the image?' Tracy asked.

"I almost blurted out, 'Don't leave me.' And I started crying. I knew I was acknowledging all of the unconscious fear that I had suppressed all during my pregnancy. The little girl did not instantly reassure me. She just smiled and looked at me. I can't say that I knew right then that everything would be all right with my delivery, but I knew that I had made contact with my baby, with my own inner self."

Laura, 25:

⌐"If I'm supposed to be so happy, why am I crying all the time?"

So you're going to have a baby. Because this landmark is viewed culturally (and often personally) as a joyous event, we tend to rush to congratulate—and the mom-to-be, in turn, puts a thrilled smile on her face. But being pregnant is a very big, very loaded transition. You may already have been wanting a child for some time. Or you may not have planned your pregnancy, and have skipped right over from the Cycling Pathway to land here, mid-Fertility. Perhaps you struggled with infertility or suffered a miscarriage before conceiving this time. To whatever degree you are happy or psyched about being pregnant, you would not be human if you did not feel a spectrum of emotions (yes, joy, but also trepidation, fear, panic, anxiety, ambivalence, detachment) that change from day to day.

First, reflection. You're entering a new cycle—three trimesters, birth, and postpartum recovery before circling back to not being pregnant. Just as you felt different throughout your menstrual cycle, you will feel different every day of this cycle. On every level—hormonal, physical, spiritual, emotional, social—across all your Centers of Wellness, significant changes are afoot. A menstrual cycle lasts an average of twenty-eight days. A pregnancy lasts at least ten months (including recovery). That's a lot to stay on top of. How do you plan to stay conscious throughout all those changes?

Pregnancy can be a fabulous, once-in-a-lifetime (or more, though most of us can count the number of children we'll bear on one hand) opportunity to enter a period of time where every aspect of body and soul shift. You can close your eyes to it and try to keep its disruptions to a minimum. Or you can take a seat front and center to that extravaganza, and who knows what wonders you'll experience.

Start by making a plan for staying tuned in. Make space to explore these complex feelings. This can be a perfect time to begin a journal if you are not already in the habit of keeping one. Line up people you can talk to—who might not necessarily be the same people you usually get support from. Your mother-in-law may not be the most objective listener, for example. But you might thrive on the kinship of other pregnant women also looking for a safe place to explore conflicting new feelings.

Then use the other tools presented in Part Two to explore. Dialogue with your reproductive system; do Dreamagery and invite an image of your baby. These can be effective ways to delve beneath the surface. What are your biggest hopes for this pregnancy? What are your greatest fears? Does your health history impact your current feelings? One survey of pregnant women and their partners who had chosen to end a previous pregnancy because it was abnormal found that they all needed to review the anguish of the experience before they could focus on their current pregnancy.

Keep checking in with your body. Continually notice what your body looks like. Stand naked in front of the mirror. Take pictures of yourself (clothed or unclothed) as your profile changes. The Body Monitoring tool becomes a whole new experience in pregnancy, as everything from the texture of your hair to your skin and your shape transforms before your eyes. The more you do this, the more you will see. Notice what's happening within you, too. In what ways do you feel different? Can you feel the baby move? Guess where its head, buttocks, and feet are?

Check in with your five Centers of Wellness across your pregnancy. It's a great way to be aware of all of the subtle changes that are literally shifting from day to day.

Second, information. At the first prenatal visit, I like to give women an overview of what they can expect. Each trimester is characterized by different commonalities (see "What's Happening Now," page 265). Often I'll hear a woman who has severe morning sickness and fatigue tell me, "I can't do this for nine months!" It's very reassuring to learn that you won't have to—that there are physiological reasons for your distress that will almost always automatically vanish by the second trimester. Having facts can also alleviate anxiety surrounding tests.

- Do a little work to find trusted sources of information. You may elect to receive prenatal care from an ob-gyn, a midwife, a family physician, or some combination thereof, including or incorporating alternative-care providers. These caregivers all have their pluses and minuses. There are also many resources on pregnancy available; compare several and talk to friends to get a picture of whose advice you trust. Cross-check information across sources (the Internet, a book, your doctor) before blindly following it. Old wives' tales and myths abound!
- Be open-minded. The knowledge we have about many aspects of pregnancy changes as new research becomes available. Consider first-trimester nausea and vomiting, which peaks between weeks seven and twelve, for example. There are many basic lifestyle steps you can take to cope, ranging from eating frequent small meals throughout the day to iden-

tifying and avoiding your triggers. Antinausea wristbands, which work by applying constant pressure to acupuncture pressure points, are available over the counter at many drugstores and have been found to be no-risk, low-tech, and effective. There's even stronger evidence for bands that deliver a weak electrical stimulation to the same acupuncture points (e.g., Relief Bands). Some states also sell these in drugstores or they are available over the Internet. Acupuncture itself has been endorsed by a National Institutes of Health consensus panel as an effective treatment for nausea in pregnancy. Many women have success with candied ginger and/or hypnosis. A small fraction of women develop a severe form of morning sickness (hyperemesis gravidarum) that can lead to dehydration, electrolyte imbalances, and more, and requires hospitalization. As you can see, that's a huge range of possible treatments. Investigate all your options.

• Having the right factual information also will inform your daily Center of Wellness choices. We know a lot about how to create the optimal conditions for a growing fetus, and you should take advantage of it. As always, decide how much you need to know. You can read whole books about nutritional needs in pregnancy, or you can rely on a handout from your ob-gyn.

Third, action. The months of pregnancy progress through many choice points. The Feedback Loop can help you meet all of them.

Then, re-reflection. For almost every decision you make during pregnancy, you can (and should) reassess how it's working out. This is true with respect to your choice of a caregiver, which many women are surprised to learn. Goodness of fit between obstetric caregiver and patient is central to a healthy, happy pregnancy, I believe. If you don't like your caregiver as the weeks go on, confront that situation. Discuss it together and decide if another practitioner would be better suited to you. Or if you don't feel comfortable having the discussion, start interviewing other practitioners until you find one you like.

Choice Points in Pregnancy

Just when you're feeling particularly tentative and vulnerable, because of all the changes taking place within and without, you have to make one decision after another. You can't go wrong if you use the Feedback Loop as a way to make your choices consciously. Among the decisions you will face as your pregnancy advances:

- *Prenatal care.* What kind of caregiver do you want (ob-gyn, midwife, family practitioner)? How do you feel about the individual you have chosen? What kind of birth center is that person affiliated with? What type of setting do you prefer?
- *Prenatal testing.* Which tests do you want? How will you proceed based on the findings of those tests? What are your preconceived notions about them?
- *Delivery.* What is your ideal situation around delivery? Who would be in attendance, medically, and whom else do you want to be there? What environment do you want to create? What are your feelings about episiotomy? Labor position? Anesthesia? Alternative approaches, including such things as acupuncture or hypnosis for pain relief?
- *Breast-feeding.* Will you? For how long? Why? Why not?

Those are just some of the medical choices. I'll leave the ones about maternity clothes, baby names, and whether your nursery should be pastels or primary colors up to you, your partner, and the Feedback Loop.

Sex and Pregnancy

The amazing changes related to sexuality during pregnancy can catch even the fairly conscious among us unawares. That's because they tend to be unexpected. As you continue your check-ins and reflections, don't leave out this dimension of your life. What typically happens is this: In the first trimester, nausea and malaise often turn women off completely; they don't want to think about sex. In the second trimester, a sort of hyper sex drive kicks in (thanks to both plentiful estrogen and generally euphoric feelings). You may feel lustier than usual and reach orgasm readily. As raw lust collides with traditional imagery of "pure" or "fragile" motherhood, you may find yourself surprised or even frightened that you don't want to think about your feelings. And in the third trimester, an awkward girth and—for both men and women—fears around hurting the baby often act as a curb on sex drives once again.

That's an oversimplification of the stages, of course. But many couples carry a lot of myth and baggage around their sex lives at this stage. Be aware of those issues rather than burying them. Your relationship will be stronger, your emotional state will be healthier, and you'll have more fun. And no, you won't hurt the baby, even if you have sex toward the very end of your pregnancy. And if you don't feel like actual intercourse, there are a lot of different ways to express your sensuality and your sexuality, so don't close the door. Just tune in to what you're really feeling and wanting, and open the door to creativity!

Cicely's Story: To Amnio or Not to Amnio?

Making choices around prenatal tests can be especially taxing for pregnant women because the stakes are so high. In a nutshell, they must evaluate whether the physical and emotional risk of having the test is greater or lesser than the risks they run in not having the test—and not having the information that it yields.

This was Cicely's second child. Thirty-four in her first pregnancy, she had elected to have amniocentesis, a test in which a needle is inserted into the amniotic sac through the abdomen to withdraw a small amount of amniotic fluid. The fluid contains the fetus's genetic material, which can be used to detect chromosomal defects. It's a great test. But because it is invasive, it carries a 1 in 200 risk of causing miscarriage. It's generally recommended only in three cases: (1) if a mother will be over thirty-five at the time of delivery (since the likelihood of genetic problems rises with maternal age, and at thirty-five the odds are 1 in 200 that amnio might find something, equal to the risk of the test) (2) if there is a personal or family history of genetic problems, or (3) if a screening test indicates a potential problem.

Screening tests aren't foolproof, but they are getting better and better all the time. The two tests that most influence the decision on amnio are ultrasound and the maternal serum screening, usually known as the "triple screen." The name comes from the fact that it's usually three tests from one blood sample: measurement of AFP (alpha-fetoprotein), a substance produced by the baby's liver; hCG; and estriol, an estrogen produced by the placenta. Levels of these hormones that are outside of a normal range can indicate an increased risk of severe birth defects. (There is also a quad screen, which also includes a test for the chemical inhibin-A, an indicator of genetic defects.)

During Cicely's first pregnancy, her age at delivery was the only indication to warrant amnio, but she had very strong and persistent concerns that something might be wrong. That's data, so we went ahead and did the test. Everything was fine.

The second time around, Cicely did not have those same urgent feelings. She was now thirty-six, though, a factor to weigh. "I didn't like having the amnio the first time," she says. "By the end of it, the needle and the procedure were almost as stressful as my worrying. I really don't want to go through that again." We agreed to first have the triple screen and ultrasound, and then reevaluate that choice. The screens indicated nothing amiss. Cicely re-reflected and decided against amnio.

Some women say, "Well, for religious reasons [or other reasons], I would never terminate, so why bother to have the amnio?" That's a valid consideration, provided you take the time to work through the process. Other women who feel equally positive that they would never terminate reflect and decide that they nonetheless want to know in advance if something is wrong, so that they can make preparations mentally as well as practically; they have amnio. You can't really know what you want until you take the time to explore it.

LANDMARK: LABOR AND DELIVERY

Paula, 42:
⁓ *"At a checkup in the middle of my first pregnancy, I heard my husband ask the doctor what labor was like. 'I've heard it's like trying to squeeze an orange out of your rectum. Is that right?' he said. 'More like a watermelon, actually,' my doctor (a man) said, and smiled. I just sat there and pushed my knees together tightly, listening to these two fellows who would never experience the thing firsthand—the way I would in a matter of weeks!"*

Viv, 28:
⁓ *"Isn't there any other way to get it out? I'm serious—can't we just schedule a C-section?"*

Olivia, 27:
⁓ *"I've read all these books, taken Lamaze, talked to my doctor, and asked every mother I know. But I still don't have a feel for what labor is all about. What else can I do? How can I know I'm ready?"*

Frannie, 23:
⁓ *"If I hear one more labor-from-hell story, I'll scream!"*

Childbirth may represent pregnancy's finale to most women, but it's a landmark that you need to start thinking about sooner rather than later. Of all the landmarks on the Fertility Pathway, this one looms on the horizon as the tallest peak, the mother of all landmarks. And yet most women giving birth for the first time cast their eyes away from it—far away. A woman will circle her due date on her calendar and arrange all her plans around it, yet refuse to focus on what that date really implies. She skips right past the great unknown of labor and delivery to think only about the baby who results.

Such feelings are perfectly understandable. The first time around, childbirth is a completely foreign experience. All she knows is that it will hurt. A lot. And it will happen to her.

So here's what you need to do:

First, reflection. Again, start early. Don't wait until your ninth month or even your last trimester to begin contemplating labor.

- Confront your preconceptions about it. What are they? What do you think labor will be like? Consider where those perceptions come from. I'm always laughing louder than anyone in the room at labor scenes on TV comedies. They look really exaggerated, but they're actually more real than you'd think! Labor and delivery *are* unpredictable. And these scenarios (panicked partners, dramatic outbursts, even wisecracking moms-to-be) happen every day. So do the scary stories like those told by your sister's friend, your great-aunt Bess, and all the so-called well-wishers regaling you with horror stories at your baby shower. You don't know how it will unfold for *you*, of course, but you can review what images you've stored up about what you think it might be like.

- Accept the scary-labor mythology and let go of it. The vast majority of the deliveries I've attended have been wonderful, positive experiences. But the stories that inevitably get told are the ones about sixteen-day labors, emergency C-sections, and husbands who hyperventilate and pass out before the pushing starts. Why aren't the women with good labors speaking up? I'm not sure whether it's the human love of drama at work or that the hard-labor camp feels the need to keep talking as part of trying to come to terms with their experience. Don't let the shock of this mythology color your own perceptions too much. Commit to being open-minded about the fact that your labor will be different—even if it's your fourth one—because every delivery is.

- Get clear about what you want the experience to be like. Many women don't want to go there because they believe that they don't have any control over labor. That's a myth. Even in a hospital setting, you have plenty of control. Yes, there are certain aspects of labor that are solely up to your doctors—and God or nature. But that doesn't mean you can't clarify your intentions. (See box.) Share your desires with your partner and your caregiver. Some women commit their thoughts to paper as a birth plan. Know that this is only a plan, which may have to change, depending on the progress of your labor. But that's okay. It's your vision of how you want to bring life into the world that matters. And what ends up happening will be different because of that intention. Realize that you also need to "hand it over"—to God, nature, fate—once the process begins. A birth is like a wedding that way; it will take on a life of its own, and that will be your story. Embrace it for whatever it is.

- Explore your feelings around pain and pain management. What have you heard about various options that colors your opinions in positive or negative ways? What sounds good to you? What sounds unpleasant?

- Keep your options open. What if things don't go exactly as planned? Well, they probably won't. But that doesn't mean your birth experience is "ruined" or lessened. Although there are many things you can do to improve your odds of a good outcome, the labor itself is filled with mystery—in part because you're not the only person involved. Your body and the baby must work in concert. It's a collective experience. (This is your introduction to a concept you will encounter repeatedly in the years to come, which is that you can't completely control your child!) What you can do is become clear about your intentions and do your best to work toward them, recognizing that there will come a point where you have to let the process reveal itself. What happens after that, even if it's an induction, an emergency C-section, or the episiotomy you had wanted to avoid, is just "what is," something you can simply accept as part of your birth story. Honor the mystery and let it reveal itself.

Second, information. Reflection is definitely only half the story when it comes to labor and delivery. I strongly recommend that women learn as much as they need to know about the birthing process. For you, that amount may be different from what it is for your pregnant neighbor, but it should generally be more than you think you need, rather than less. Ideally, that would mean some combination of an extensive interview with your midwife or other labor attendants, lots of book reading, and taking a childbirth preparation class in order to:

- Learn about the different methods for nonmedicated pain management in childbirth and decide whether one feels right to you. Even if you know you'll want drugs, you should be aware that most doctors won't give them until you are in active labor and that there are ways of minimizing pain before drugs are administered. Nonmedicated pain management comprises a whole array of mind-body techniques, breathing exercises, and other methods of pain relief, such as acupuncture, which can be used from the early through late stages of labor. (In China, for example, even C-sections are commonly performed with no anesthesia except acupuncture, and with great success and no significant side effects.) You don't have to commit to one kind of method. Look into them all. A class is a good way to get an overview of options. Lamaze, Bradley, hospital-based courses, and others can all explain the mechanics of labor and introduce you to different kinds of birth experiences. Learn about the different methods for medicated pain management.
- Learn about the pros and cons of giving birth assisted by a doctor or by a midwife, and find out about what doulas have to offer.
- Tour the place where you will give birth. Understand your

Choices for Your Birth Experience

So much is in the setup. If you face the work of labor months before the first contraction, you have less to worry about later. Among the things to consider and explore with your birth team as you shape your desired birth experience:

- Do you want your partner present? Do you want him or her to coach? Do you want anyone else there? What about a doula—a trained labor coach whose job is solely to tend to the mother, not to interface with the medical team, and whose presence often improves outcomes, especially for first-time moms?
- How do you feel about background noise? Do you want the TV turned off? Do you want to bring music? What kind?
- What else about the environment do you envision? Low lights? Fragrance?
- Do you want to keep your glasses on? Wear your own clothes? Which clothes? Think through even the small stuff.
- What kinds of techniques do you want to try to work with during labor? Consider exploring the full range of possibilities, from high-tech pain relief including epidurals to such low-tech mind-body methods as relaxation and breathing techniques, acupuncture and acupressure, and hypnosis. What are your feelings around pain relief? Are some analgesics more appealing to you than others?
- What laboring position do you wish to assume? Lying on your back is the one we're most familiar with, but midwives often encourage women to squat, for greater efficiency and control over the process.

- Are there procedures you wish to avoid if possible, such as inserting an IV line, being confined to bed, or having an episiotomy? Are there procedures you would prefer if possible, such as an internal monitor (after your water has broken)?
- What do you want to have happen immediately after delivery? Do you want your husband to cut the cord? Do you want to begin breast-feeding right away?

Know that it may not be possible for your every wish to come true. There may be limitations based on your delivery, hospital regulations, or other factors. But by stating your intention, you give shape to it.

options there. You also should have some recognition of the stages of labor and what can commonly go wrong. Learn what kind of care there is for the baby in the event of problems.

Third, action. This step is a little different in labor and delivery than for other landmarks. Unless you've been scheduled for an induction or a C-section—and even then—you must wait for the action to begin, rather than initiating it yourself. But if you've done all the prep work, you're far more likely to willingly embrace and accept what comes your way. Moreover, you are apt to have a more positive labor experience. Just as you can choose to experience PMS as a time for self-discovery rather than nothing but cramps and bother, so you can frame the experience of childbirth as a rare opportunity to gain insight into a deeper part of yourself. From the first contractions of labor to the delivery of your baby and the placenta, your body reveals a dazzling array of powers. The female body and soul are at their most raw and magnificent form when a woman gives birth. No matter how often I see it, I'm awed by the transformation I see in the delivery room, when women receive, as one patient put it, "a huge wake-up call to my pride as a woman."

Then, re-reflection. Be sure to reflect on your experience and integrate it into your consciousness. Studies have shown that women often have a driving impulse to relive and retell the birth experience, but the dominant cultural mode is summed up in an old saw: "The world doesn't want to hear about the labor pains; it just wants to see the baby." There is a common tendency to bury your own experience in the collective focus on the newborn baby. Journaling or talking with other mothers can be especially useful. It's essential to process what was wonderful and what was difficult, the joys and the disappointments.

The Mother of All Opportunities

Much of what I've described heretofore concerns how to approach labor consciously, how to prepare and plan in order to lessen your anxiety and fear. What about labor itself? It's difficult to tell a woman how to practice real consciousness about the experience because, as I've said, the experience takes on a life of its own. There are many good tools available to help you manage labor more consciously, such as Lamaze breathing or meditation. Having the preparation isn't enough. In the heat of the moment, you might choose to use them, or you might choose to grin and bear it unconsciously.

However, I can tell you that when women are able to carry awareness right through labor, it can be an incredible thing. If the premenstrual phase of your cycle and PMS are windows to your soul, labor could be said to blow the wall clean away. By paying close attention to your body and soul during labor, you give yourself an opportunity for real insight and an experience of yourself that you are otherwise rarely, if ever, afforded. Women who experience labor and delivery consciously also speak afterward about their profound amazement and exhilaration at what their body seemed to know how to do.

Whatever is most real for a laboring woman is what most gets brought to the surface during labor. I have heard laboring women say astonishing things to their spouses, to their doctors, to their yet unborn children. That's a place where TV's fictional deliveries get it right: The heroine expresses her deepest self at what might seem on the surface to be an unlikely or inappropriate time.

But just as labor can expose the intimacy, gratitude, or joy that's foremost in your soul at that moment, it can also expose darker true feelings. I've heard women swear at their partners or express decidedly unloving thoughts. Afterward everyone laughs and the new mom is sheepish: "You know I didn't mean that! It was just the contractions talking!" Well, that's akin to a woman with PMS discounting the feelings that came to the fore for her right before her period. I would say that hostile feelings toward your partner during labor are something worth exploring later.

Another very common and vivid example of this concerns women who have a history of sexual abuse or rape. Because of the physicality of the baby's body passing through the vagina, something is often triggered in a woman who has not previously processed the abuse. The body remembers. Every labor nurse, doula, ob-gyn, and midwife is familiar with the scene: The laboring mom-to-be has a distinct pattern of being out of control. She has a hard time riding with her sharp contractions; it's difficult to talk to her, and she's very emotional and often physically out of control. She doesn't connect the dots to her past abuse while she's in labor, but that's the underlying issue, laid bare during this time.

Jo's Story: "I Can't Do It!" ⟶

Jo, thirty-four, was midway through an uneventful pregnancy, her first, doing beautifully. I brought up labor and what she was thinking about it. "I don't want to think about it!" she replied immediately.

"Why not?"

"I'm terrified! I don't want to know anything about it!"

I see a lot of women like Jo. I reassured her that plenty of women feel exactly the same way. I asked her what her greatest fears were about the delivery. Right away, Jo admitted that she had never been athletic, and she viewed labor as such a demanding physical event, she was sure her body wouldn't be able to do it.

Although it was clear to me that her body was perfectly capable of childbirth, I knew such reassurances would fall on deaf ears. Jo needed to believe for herself that she was capable. I suggested we try some Dreamagery, inviting an image of labor, to try to get some insights into what was holding her back.

Jo's image of labor was a basketball. (It was an interesting visual, considering her round belly and her description of being poor at sports.) "How do you feel about that?" I asked her.

"I never liked basketball," she said. "I'm not good at it."

I then instructed her to engage the image in a dialogue. What did it want to tell her? The answer: "I know what *I'm* doing; you don't have to do it. Your job is to support me, not be afraid of me."

I encouraged Jo to hold the ball in her imagery. How did it feel? "Strange and unfamiliar," she said.

The image of the ball was simply a way to give voice to her fears. I suggested that she get a real basketball and keep it around, holding it sometimes, as a visual reminder of her conversation and its message. And also that she continue to dialogue with this image, to deepen her awareness of this relationship she had with impending labor.

As labor drew near, Jo still had the same concerns—"Am I tough enough?"—but not the anxiety she once had. That feeling had been replaced by a calmness that said, "Yup, this is unknown, there's a lot about labor that's not in my control, but I accept that."

When the time finally came, she pushed for three hours and delivered a healthy baby girl. "I don't know where my strength came from," she told me with a grin afterward, "but I did it!" I do know where that strength originated: I believe that once her body and her soul were on the same page working together, the labor became more manageable.

Helen's Story: Something Beautiful to Watch ⌒

I love to watch patients like Helen labor. Fortunately, given the nature of my practice, I work with many women who are very conscious in their everyday lives. They bring that awareness gracefully into their pregnancy and tend to have happier and more rewarding labors than anyone else I know.

Helen, thirty-two, had practiced meditation and yoga for years, so relaxation breathing and centering were second nature to her. What's more, she worked to maintain a real awareness of her shifting feelings all through pregnancy. She also was an especially well-informed patient, asking probing questions of me that reflected a good bit of reading without making her overly obsessed with details.

Her birth plan was reasonable, open-minded, and, most important, authentically reflected her nature and her intentions. Helen desired a hospital birth that was nonetheless as low-tech as possible. She wanted her husband with her in the delivery room. She did not want drugs if she could avoid them. She hoped to remain upright as much as possible, and push from a squatting position when the time came. She brought Grateful Dead music to play softly in the background (which I wouldn't have thought would be relaxing, but it worked for her).

Helen paced her room and the delivery floor for several hours, until the contractions began gaining in intensity. Then she stayed mostly in her room, leaning on her husband or rocking in a chair. She was periodically monitored in bed. Throughout, she was very quiet, focused, and calm. During each contraction, she would seem to recede from the rest of us in the room (me, her husband, and the hospital staff) into her own world; she would not respond to conversation until after the contraction ended. She continued in this state throughout active labor, speaking little, in an altered state of consciousness. After about eight hours, I was prepared to offer Stadol to take the edge off her contractions if she felt she needed them, but she seemed in partnership with the pain in a way that was working beautifully.

I could tell by her labor curve when she was approaching transition, and soon the contractions were closer and longer, with several peaks before receding. Yet Helen stayed with each one, being taken to a place outside that room.

Things got hardest when it was time to push, since she had to reposition her body and listen to instructions. She had been laboring for eleven hours and indicated she was too tired to squat, as she'd hoped. But during each push she again found her center and was able to work productively. Her interaction with her husband was especially interesting; he seemed to anticipate her need for back massage or hand holding, and they communicated both deeply and wordlessly.

After an hour of pushing, Helen's robust, black-haired son was born. I left the room feeling I had witnessed something almost sacred, something that I was honored to have been able to participate in and observe. I can only imagine how Helen felt. That's powerful.

LANDMARK: POSTPARTUM

Marianne, 34:
⌁*"I was still in the hospital the day after Ryan was born, and at night after my husband and the visitors had left, I began to cry. I was happy and it had been a good delivery, but I just felt suddenly overwhelmed and weepy. I would have been confused by this if I hadn't been forewarned about it. Instead I just gave in to it and cried myself to sleep. I felt better by the time they woke me up for a feeding early in the morning."*

Linda, 28:
⌁*"I felt so alone. The baby cried constantly. My husband went off to his job and I couldn't even take a shower. My mom was clear across the country—I*

had told her not to come out because we wanted to get used to being parents on our own first. After a week I was crying on the phone for her to come and see me. I was so overwhelmed."

Sharyn, 25:
➤ *"When my doctor asked me what kind of birth control I planned to use now, I just stared at her. Sex was the furthest thing from my mind!"*

Jessica, 29:
➤ *"I didn't know if I would like breast-feeding, so I said I'd give it until my postpartum checkup, six weeks. I was really surprised to discover that I liked it. I love how it makes me feel closer to Jessy. And it's actually pretty easy. Knowing I could change my mind at any time made it easier to take it one day at a time."*

Alexa, 32:
➤ *"I hate breast-feeding—it's a lot harder than I thought, and I'm constantly worrying Taylor isn't getting enough milk. But I'm afraid all the other moms will think I'm copping out if I quit now. All my girlfriends do it—it's like a competition to see who can hang on the longest. It was bad enough when I decided to use disposable diapers instead of a cloth service!"*

Having a baby doesn't end with labor, of course. The first three months of a newborn's life are, for the mother, a time of change as dramatic as each of the previous three trimesters. And yet these changes are routinely discounted by new moms and the people around them. The assumption is that everything goes back to normal—your body, relationship, sexual practices, and so on—except that now you have a baby. But to have that assumption is to be totally unconscious! Delivery was the pinnacle, perhaps, but it was only a point in an ongoing process of change. There is no going back to the baseline of how things were prepregnancy.

The physical changes occur fairly rapidly after delivery and are chiefly—but not completely—in place by about six weeks postpartum. Some consist of returns to the prepregnancy state. Almost instantly, the uterus shrinks back to its former size; the lochia (vaginal discharge) gradually fades in color and amount, and tears or stitches heal. Other changes will persist for months, or even through life. For example, though most hormone levels drop dramatically, they don't return precisely to prepregnancy levels. Estriol, the weakest estrogen, primarily made by the placenta, will continue to exist in your body after giving birth for the rest of your life at levels higher than they were before you conceived. (Even if you give up your baby for adoption, having a baby changes you.) Prolactin, which stimulates breast milk, rises sharply. Breasts swell with milk, and a new mom faces decisions about whether and for how long to nurse.

About seven in ten new mothers have the "baby blues" after childbirth because of the tremendous drop in pregnancy levels of hormones. By the second or third day postpartum, a phase of sudden sadness, moodiness, or anxiety can appear. The feelings that are laid bare are very real and legitimate ones. As with the other landmarks of this pathway, you can choose to fight or bury these emotions, or go into them. Considering the enormity of the changes in your life right now, it only makes sense that this is a time of profound reorientation.

And baby blues or not, there are soul-level changes taking place at this time that are equally dramatic and longer-lasting. The bond between a mother and child can be startling in its intensity. The kaleidoscope of emotions involved in new motherhood rival those of early pregnancy—ambivalence, joy, fear, anxiety, worry—and are heightened by overwhelming fatigue and a new sense of responsibility. Other changed life circumstances only add to a new mother's sense of reinvention: *Who am I now?* The shift from being a working woman to being a mom on maternity leave or home full time is huge, as is the shift from being partners to being parents as well as partners. Modern new motherhood can be isolating, too, thanks to scattered families and a culture that leaves new mothers to fend for themselves at home with little support or care unless it is specially arranged. Against this backdrop, a new mom must make many decisions, large and small, about things she may not have considered ever before, from breast-feeding to aspects of newborn care.

What makes this landmark particularly challenging is that a woman is conditioned to *not* put herself first. With so much focus on her needy newborn, it's easy, almost reflexive, to cast the Feedback Loop aside. This is a mistake on two levels. In the short term it's important to reflect on your postpartum experiences in order to better understand them, and yourself, at this time of enormous transition. Who are you now? What do you need? Reflection is also vital for the long term. You'll be a mother for the rest of your life. Better to start the habit of nurturing yourself rather than ignoring your own needs, right from the get-go. Otherwise it's not just you who will suffer, but your baby and your partner, too.

Key Postpartum Choices

- Will you breast-feed? This decision has a lot of parallels to HRT in perimenopause. It's a choice, not a stance. You don't have to pick one position and cling to it, come hell or high water. Although I am strongly pro-breast-feeding when the circumstances fit, because of the benefits to the baby and the mother, I've seen many patients done a disservice by militaristic attitudes on the subject: *Breast-feed for a full year or you're a failure.* Not true! There's no right or wrong answer here, only a decision about what is truly right for you. Recognize what your circumstances are, and your predispositions. Get information on how to do it. Although it's a natural process, believe it or not, most women do better when they are taught how.

- What kind of birth control will you use now? This decision is very often made unconsciously. A woman will either just do what her doctor suggests (because she's too tired to focus on it), or do what she did before pregnancy (because it's easiest or all she knows), or not do anything (because she just had a baby or is nursing, so what are the odds she'll get pregnant again?). Each of these modes has its perils. A conscious decision takes many factors into account. Are you breast-feeding? Today's low-dose oral contraceptives may be fine for many young and healthy women, while others do better on a progestin-only pill. Does it matter if you have more children right away? Don't count on breast-feeding as a natural contraceptive; there are zero guarantees. By the time your first period resumes, you probably will have already begun ovulating again—which means you can get pregnant. One choice I am not in favor of for postpartum use is Depo-Provera. One of its side effects is depression, and considering that there are enough other hormonal shifts in play now, I don't think it's worth the risk.

Whether you are deciding whether or not to breast-feed, what kind of postpartum birth control to use, or when or whether to go back to work, you can use the Feedback Loop to make your choice a conscious one.

First, reflection. Making space in your life for this process can be a challenge. If you kept a journal during pregnancy, try to keep it up now—even if it's only in bleary snatches or just a few times a week.

How does being a mother feel? Exhilarating? Exhausting? In what ways do you think you have changed? Your personality? Your priorities? Your daily routines?

How does the reality of motherhood compare with your expectations? Harder? Easier? Has your relationship with your own mother been altered in any way? How do you see her differently?

How has your relationship with your partner changed? How do you feel about him or her as a parent? How are your communication styles weathering the transition to parenthood? Your sex life?

How has your relationship to work changed? If you are on leave, what do you miss? What do you not miss?

Second, information. Knowing what to expect from new motherhood can smooth the way. Your doctor will help make sure you're healing properly, but not all ob-gyns make a concerted effort to assess how you're doing psychologically. Be forthcoming at your postpartum checkup even if you aren't asked first.

If you are trying to decide about breast-feeding, seek as much information as you need to know. You have a variety of sources to choose among, including your doctor, the La Leche League, books, Web sites, lactation consultants (often employed by ob-gyns or hospitals), and so on. Learning how it's done (from how to hold the baby to how to position the nipple in the baby's mouth) can make a huge difference in your satisfaction and success. It's also important to feel comfortable with the information you receive. If you feel pressured, that's data, too.

Explore your options for postpartum birth control if you have not done so yet. If you discussed this before delivery, reevaluate. You may need to reassess in light of, for example, a bad laceration that makes the very idea of a diaphragm unappealing. Find out if there is any new information that should change your choice now. (See box.)

Third, action. Take the steps that feel right for you.

Then, re-reflection. This is key! Know that this is a fluid time, and your situation is changing all the time. No decision you make is permanent (except maybe circumcising a son), so take your time choosing, and then revisit and see how it feels.

Postpartum Depression

The majority of new moms experience short-lived bouts of weepiness or anxiety, the so-called baby blues. For a small percentage of these women, depression can linger, manifesting as anger, withdrawal, marked changes in appetite or sleep, panic attacks, or fears or fantasies of harming the baby. This is postpartum depression (PPD), a condition that is easily treated with support and often pharmaceuticals. The hard part is identifying the condition in the first place. Too often women suffer needlessly in silence because they wait until the six-week postpartum checkup and then don't bring up the issue if their ob-gyn doesn't bother to ask. Or a woman is afraid that admitting these symptoms means she is somehow a failure at motherhood. Nothing could be further from the truth!

PPD is real. Getting it is not a sign that you don't love your baby or are a poor mother. It's a chemical imbalance. Be conscious of your state of mind in the postpartum weeks. If you have any questions about how you're feeling, find help. Tell a friend, ask your doctor. The issue is not whether you meet the clinical diagnosis of PPD or not. Sometimes patients think, *Well, if I don't meet the diagnosis, I don't have it, so I don't have to worry about what I am feeling.* Or they think, *If I don't meet the diagnosis, I must be a terrible mom to be having these feelings anyway.*

You don't have to wait until you are sick to get help. Be proactive. This is a stressful time by definition, and help really can make things easier. Consider supports such as having someone check on you daily, help with housekeeping and meals (paid help, if that's an option for you), or joining a mothers' group where you can compare notes with others at a similar stage of parenthood.

LANDMARK: MISCARRIAGE

Sue, 28:
⟶ *"I know a lot of women have miscarriages. I was only nine weeks pregnant anyway. We'll try again in a few months. I'm not really worried."*

Carmela, 22:

⌁ *"After it happened, it seems like people came out of the woodwork to share their miscarriage stories with me. I had no idea it was so common. Until mine, my mother never told me she had had several herself. Somehow hearing all the stories made it easier for me to grieve and move on."*

Kat, 37:

⌁ *"Oh God, not again!"*

Since miscarriage is estimated to occur in up to 40 percent of all pregnancies, it's reasonable to think about it as a normal, if disheartening, landmark you might encounter for reasons having nothing to do with anything you did. Many miscarriages happen so early that a woman is not even aware of having experienced one. Others are more painful on every level.

Some advice when it happens:

First, reflection. Even if a pregnancy wasn't planned or desired, there are difficult issues to deal with when you have a miscarriage. Sometimes women feel guilty, worrying that something they did or didn't do was the trigger. That's rarely the case. Most often, it is the body's way of taking care of pregnancies that were abnormal. A miscarriage after the first trimester, although much more rare, can be especially traumatic because the woman has begun to have a much stronger bond with the fetus. But any miscarriage can be devastating, depending on your circumstances.

- Don't fall into the prevailing culture of denial about miscarriages—the belief that if you don't acknowledge it and don't "dwell" on it, you'll recover from the loss more quickly. Miscarriages can be traumatic, disappointing, frightening, depressing, and painful. To have one represents the loss of an unborn child and all that means to you. Because society does not acknowledge this as a "real" loss makes it all the more important that you do whatever work of mourning you need to do.
- Confront your misgivings and grief rather than brushing it off. Try to pinpoint what is most disturbing or painful to you

about the experience. A nagging fear that you are to blame? That you might have a physical problem and never carry a baby to term? That you've disappointed your partner?

• Seek out support. Women often uncover a huge hidden network of kindred spirits. The majority of women experience a miscarriage at some time. Reach out and you will quickly discover that these women are all around you.

Second, information. Knowing the facts about miscarriage is comforting. Most of the time we don't know why women miscarry. The conventional wisdom, which I share, is that miscarriage is often nature's way of responding to birth defects or abnormal pregnancies. We do know some things for certain. Miscarriage is not caused by intercourse, exercise, or lifting something heavy. When I sit down with a woman who has just miscarried, I listen carefully to her concerns and fears about why it happened. Most women find it tremendously comforting and guilt-easing to have the myths separated from the facts. For example, having one miscarriage puts you at no increased risk for having future problems. I don't usually worry medically until a woman has had three miscarriages in a row; even then, I take her level of anxiety into consideration as information to help determine our next steps together.

Know, too, that a miscarriage can affect both your body and your soul during subsequent pregnancies.

Third, action. The action step following a miscarriage is to decide whether you want to try again or retreat back to the Cycling Pathway for a while. Even if you weren't trying to get pregnant this time, after reflecting you may discover that you actively do want to try to conceive now. Whatever you choose, take your time making this choice because it's usually recommended that a woman wait for one full cycle after miscarrying to allow the body to reset itself (and to make it easier to identify when conception occurs the next time around). But you need to get yourself psychologically as well as physically ready. Your partner should also be mentally ready. This might be one cycle later, or it might be a space of several months or longer.

Then, re-reflection. After you have made a choice about trying again or not, it's very useful to revisit that with regularity. If you're going to try again, does it feel all right? It would be natural to be more tentative, but if you are feeling rushed or uncertain, pay attention to that. Often I see women more zealously practicing conscious conception (see box on page 273) after miscarrying. They have a new sense of urgency that it has to be "tonight;" and then each new cycle without a baby is more discouraging than it once was. That's a normal response. Check in with it so that you have a solid sense of what's causing it. If you have elected to move off the Fertility Pathway, keep checking how that is for you. Are you content? Or are you eager to start again?

Wendy's Story: A Farewell Ritual ⟳

After the miscarriage of her first pregnancy at nine weeks, Wendy was bereft. She and her husband, Carl, had been trying for almost a year to conceive. He was characteristically practical: "We'll just try again. It's a common thing." But Wendy, who at thirty-six was already worried about her age, felt less benignly optimistic. She didn't want to think about future babies. She could only think about *this* baby.

"I couldn't get over it in a way everyone expected me to," she said. "I was supposed to just tuck away my sadness, wait a month, and try again for a baby. But I couldn't stop grieving, and I felt guilty about it."

Rituals can be a useful way to mark an occasion, to honor what might be otherwise skipped over. A birthday party is a ritual. So is a retirement party. We have morning rituals and dinner rituals. I like to light candles at the evening meal, to signal the importance of coming together and shifting focus away from the hum of the day. Wendy decided to use a ritual over her miscarriage to help her move on.

"I wrote down all the names I had been thinking of for the baby," she said. "I cut the list into strips and made a fire in the fireplace even though it was July. Then I burned the strips one by one, saying good-bye to each name. Laura. Wilson. Victoria. David. When all the slips were ash, I sat there cross-legged and sobbed as though I never could be comforted.

"After a while, I was wrung out from crying. My head was throbbing and my nose was all stuffed up. I was disappointed. I thought that the ritual would help me heal.

"It turned out that I had been in too big a hurry. A few days later, I ran into a friend in the parking lot at the mall. She was taking her new baby, Laura, out of the car seat. I was able to say to her, "That's one of my favorite names," without feeling that I was just this side of a meltdown.

"In that little moment I realized that I *had* begun to heal. I just needed time."

CENTERS OF WELLNESS MODIFICATIONS FOR FERTILITY

Follow the general guidelines for good health highlighted in Chapter 8, tweaking them to accommodate the special needs associated with where you are on the Fertility Path. Preconception and the first trimester, for example, share many nutritional needs because at both times the body is working to prepare the optimal home for new life.

This phase of life can be a big opportunity. For many women, this pathway inspires changes across the five centers that had previously seemed out of reach for one reason or another. With the powerful new motivation of desiring a healthy baby, I've seen countless women quit smoking, reform their diets, cut out alcohol, lose excess weight, make more down time for themselves in their busy lives, or take other steps that enhanced their well-being. You now have an incentive like none you've ever had before. Ask yourself, *What do I want to do with it?*

ℬ Movement

You're not sick, you're pregnant (or trying to be), or you've just given birth. So while you want to treat yourself with tenderness, you need not move about as if you are as fragile as an egg. If you're pregnant, your fertilized egg is well protected within you, changing every day on its way from minuscule clump of cells to fully formed fetus.

Postpartum, get your doctor's green light to resume workouts, and let your body be your guide. Rely on the Body Scan to help give you a sense of what you're ready for.

At any point on the Fertility Pathway, choose Movement every day to benefit body and soul. Note: Women in high-risk pregnancies may require special Movement precautions based on their individual situation.

Before conception and early in pregnancy:
- *Be sure to check in with your body every day.* Both trying to conceive and being pregnant can be stressful. The needs of your body and soul may be more unpredictable than ever. You may be on a walking program but wake up one morning to find that your body is better served by gentle stretching. Or you may want to stretch, but your already loose ligaments tell you they don't need too much. Decide what your body is ready for each day, what it needs. The Body Scan and Body Monitoring tools are especially helpful during this time.
- *Evaluate what kind of changes you need to make to your fitness program.* Most routines can be adapted to pregnancy. Some sports, such as scuba diving, waterskiing, or platform diving, need to be abandoned for the time being. Many things fall into a gray area, depending on whether you have been already doing them, the nature of your pregnancy, and other considerations. Give careful consideration to your Movement choices.

Mid- to late pregnancy:
- *Keep moving.* There is evidence that women who are fit have shorter and less painful labors, and recover faster.
- *Monitor the way your body responds during exercise as well as at rest.* Don't make any assumptions about how you'll respond even to activities you're accustomed to. Your tendency to overheat or become light-headed can increase, and as your pregnancy progresses, your center of gravity will shift. The hormone relaxin increases as your pregnancy advances. Its role is to prepare your body for delivery, so that your pelvic bones can separate to accommodate the delivery of the fetus. Its effect is to make all of

the joints in your body feel looser and more flexible. You may begin to notice that you truly do "wobble." Before you can decide how to modify the activities you choose, you have to be keenly aware of these subtle (and not-so-subtle) changes. Be more careful about the activities you choose, and be especially wary about actions that involve balance.

Postpartum:
- *Find the time to do something every day.* Movement benefits your mental outlook as much as your physical recovery. You can do stretching exercises the day after giving birth. Slowly move up to doing small things—a walk to the mailbox, putting the baby in a stroller or front-carrier for a walk around the block. Your body will let you know when it's ready for more.
- *Focus on what Movement does for your inside more than your outside.* There's a temptation to obsess over "baby weight" and your stretched midriff. But losing weight postpartum can take up to a year. Many moms get discouraged and give up. Don't. If you concentrate on how exercise makes you feel—the instant benefit—the visual results will follow.

ℬ Nutrition

Preconception and pregnancy require certain adjustments in your diet. Pregnancy can also inspire new aversions, cravings, and eating habits. Spend time evaluating your current diet and examining, through the reflection and information steps in the Feedback Loop, what the optimal changes are for you now. While there is ample information out there about nutrition in pregnancy, let me highlight some of my special interests:

- *Ask yourself.* Review the questions in the Consciously Female Inventory regarding Nutrition, and those in Chapter 8, but now reframed for your childbearing. Have your eating habits changed? How? Do certain foods repulse you? Do you crave certain foods? How do you feel about gaining weight—apprehensive? Resigned? Eager to experience voluptuousness? Revisit these considerations throughout your pregnancy.

• *Avoid alcohol.* Excessive consumption has been linked to low birth weight, birth defects, and behavioral and developmental problems in the baby. Although there is disagreement about what constitutes "excessive," this is one time in your life when it's safest to simply avoid the stuff altogether.

Before conception and early in pregnancy:

• *Avoid botanicals and rethink your vitamins.* While a prenatal vitamin supplement is highly recommended, avoid botanicals and megadoses of vitamins, as these have not been studied in pregnancy. For example, excessive intake of vitamin A (also found in animal liver and cod liver oil) is toxic and can cause birth defects. Conversely, one vitamin you should be sure to take is folate. Since 1998, the U.S. Food and Drug Administration has required manufacturers to fortify some grain products such as cereal and flour with folic acid, but you shouldn't rely on fortified products alone; most women also need a supplement. The recommendation is for 400 milligrams of folic acid a day. Folic acid has been proved to significantly reduce the risk of open-spine defects such as spina bifida. A Swedish study found that folate also seemed to prevent miscarriage.

• *Minimize or avoid caffeine.* Especially in the first trimester, stick to the equivalent of one cup of coffee or less. More is associated with increased incidence of miscarriage.

• *Try ginger or vitamin B_6 to reduce nausea.* Candied ginger or ginger tea as well as vitamin B_6 have been shown to be effective, especially in combination with an acupressure band.

Mid- to late pregnancy:

• *Go fishing.* Be certain to include oily fish in your diet. Such fish (for example salmon and sardines) provide a great source of omega-3 fatty acids during pregnancy, especially in the third trimester, which are used in the development of the central nervous system of the fetus. Low levels of omega-3s have been associated with a less well developed visual system in young childhood. Reserves of these essential fatty acids get used up in the last trimester, and it's possible that a lack of omega-3s after delivery predisposes a woman to postpartum depression. If you dislike fish, you can get omega-3 from fish-oil capsules. Be aware that some fish contain high levels of mercury and should be avoided or eaten sparingly; check FDA recommendations. (Off-limits fish include shark, sword-fish, king mackerel, tilefish, and some local-waters fresh fish.)

Postpartum
- *Continue following your pregnancy diet.* Even though you're no longer nourishing your fetus, it's important to recognize the first few weeks after delivery as a healing period.
- *Don't sacrifice calories in a bid to shed pregnancy pounds.* You actually need an additional 450 calories a day over your prepregnancy norms to produce breast milk.
- *Concentrate on calcium-rich foods.* Some of the calcium you take in leaves your body in your breast milk.
- *Get enough fluids if you're breast-feeding.* Keep a sports bottle or Thermos of water handy where you usually nurse.
- *Monitor your urine.* If it's dark, you probably need to up your fluid intake.
- *Continue taking your prenatal vitamins.* The extra iron and folic acid may still be needed in a body depleted by childbirth and breast-feeding.

⚘ Mind

We don't always give women the space to express the normal ambivalence of the Fertility years. The message from others and from our culture at large may be that it's wonderful to be pregnant, even when it doesn't always seem that way, for either parent. It's important that every woman be allowed to recognize and express her true feelings, not only the socially appropriate ones.

Making space for actions that nourish the Mind Center's needs is especially important throughout this time of life. Practice one relaxation technique daily to calm your mind and give it nourishing space. You may want to explore this more extensively if you are feeling anxious about conceiving or are having difficulty.

- *Explore your feelings about pregnancy.* Even a woman who has struggled through years of infertility treatments may be quite anxious or even ambivalent when she finally becomes pregnant. And a woman for whom this is a second or third baby, or beyond, will also have new feelings that she might not have expected, because she's at a different place in her life from the last time she was pregnant.
- *Start a journal.* Understand that your feelings will drastically change over time, just like your body. Fertility is a perfect time to begin a private journal if you have not been using one already.
- *Dialogue with your baby.* Whether you're pregnant or hoping to be, the Dialoguing tool is a great way to explore your feelings around pregnancy.
- *Expect a postpartum dip.* The veil between your conscious and unconscious selves is particularly transparent after childbirth, with anxieties and fears surfacing readily. Known as the "baby blues," this condition affects half to three-quarters of new mothers. It sets in within the first few days after giving birth and usually disappears within two weeks. I urge patients to both expect it and put it to their advantage, rather than fearing it and waiting it out. Your whole world has just changed. So what *are* your fears now? That you don't know anything about baby care? That your husband will no longer find you attractive? That you'll never lose weight? That you're just not ready yet? All of these are normal reactions,

and you'll be way ahead of the game if you meet them head-on. Accept that they're there. You may not be in a position to do anything about them yet, between the twin stresses of fatigue and physical recovery. But you will have helped yourself simply by recognizing their normalcy.

ℬ Spirit

- *Join a support group.* Almost every landmark on the Fertility Pathway can be enriched by the right kind of support. Patients in fertility treatment programs, for example, have been shown to optimize their odds for success by participating in formal support groups, such as those sponsored by hospitals or community centers. But, depending on your circumstances, you may find that all you really need is the support and company of friends, family, or neighbors who have gone through something similar or are experiencing it now. There are some great Web sites and chat rooms that may be helpful.

- *Commune with your baby.* Pregnancy is magical in the sense that an opportunity to connect with something larger than yourself is right there within you! Some women choose to name the baby, frame the new superclear ultrasound pictures, and talk to the fetus often. For other women, those things might feel too vivid; they prefer to think of the baby in more of an abstract way, a mysterious life force within. Either way is fine. The important thing is to connect. I'll never forget the woman who told me that she was so busy, she sometimes glanced down with surprise at her midsection, having "forgotten" she was pregnant for hours, even days, at a time. Connecting is good for mother and baby. Preliminary research suggests that the quality of the maternal-fetal relationship may have an impact on outcome. Your relationship with your child really does begin prenatally, whether you are conscious of it or not. By definition, you live in relationship to each other. So I really encourage women to mine that bonding process well before delivery.

- *Arrange pregnancy and labor support.* It comes as a surprise to many women that their partner may not be the best person to act as labor coach. Although you will want that person's love present, not all dads-to-be are naturals at the many things that are needed to support a laboring women. It can be hard for them to see the woman they love in pain. You might want to consider a doula, a professional labor support person. Doulas support the expectant mother during pregnancy, during labor, and after delivery. Doula-assisted labors have been found to be 25 percent shorter, with 60 percent fewer epidurals and half as many C-sections. One interesting study comparing moms who took Lamaze birth preparation and moms who had doulas found that the latter group were more receptive to help, felt more secure, had less emotional distress in labor, and rated their infants as significantly less fussy than did the other group.

- *Arrange postdelivery support.* As much as you thrive on support during pregnancy, you need it tenfold afterward. Unlike the fleeting "baby blues" that are probably hormonally connected, postpartum depression is a more insidious condition that can set in anytime in the year after a baby's birth. Although this condition is not well understood, researchers believe that mothers without the support of close family and friends are most at risk. A recent study at Emory University found that both depressed mothers and their babies have increased amounts of the stress hormone cortisol. Other cultures build a lengthy, supportive recovery time into the experience of having a baby; the mother and child are often housebound and looked after, never left alone, for at least a month. Here, dads go back to work, grandparents are likely to live far away, and the new mom is on her own, expected to cope with her new life with a minimum of mindful transitioning.

- *Reflect on life's larger questions.* The time of creating new life is a perfect opportunity to reflect on life's overarching matters, such as the meaning of life, birth, and death. Reflect on your family relationships, your connectedness or lack thereof, and what your desires are for your baby.

♉' Sensation

Whereas on the Cycling Pathway you might have found yourself in need of extra TLC around your period, during a pregnancy you may be surprised to be in that mode for an extended span of time—say, twelve months! The intensity of your Sensation needs may fluctuate, being highest in the early weeks, in the days leading up to labor, and through to the first postpartum weeks. But they can also remain higher than usual all through the pregnancy. Take heed and act accordingly.

- *Recognize that your environment plays a big role in your level of comfort and calm.* Try to make your environment at work and at home reflect, as much as possible, a comforting and safe message. There's a good reason for the urge to "nest," to fashion a welcoming nursery for the baby—and it has as much to do with you now as it does with the practical necessity of creating a place for the baby to sleep. If that was all that mattered, we'd be tossing blankets in drawers and not obsessing over a Winnie the Pooh theme vs. Noah's Ark.
- *Acknowledge your shifting sexual needs.* Even before conception, anxieties about infertility, or the mechanics of the fertility procedures, can disrupt passion and intimacy. During pregnancy, a woman can go from total revulsion concerning sex (especially if she is having a hard time with first-trimester nausea) to insatiable randiness (midway) to a feeling of "the spirit is willing but the flesh is in the way" (the third trimester). Postpartum, she may encounter issues around recovery, breast-feeding, fatigue, and how she and her partner perceive each other now that they are also parents. Notice

these bumps as they crop up and work with them. Explore how you really feel; assume nothing. Women sometimes think that fertility is their business and are reluctant to share their feelings with their partners, especially around sex. Nothing could be further from optimal.

- *Remember that your Sensation needs will rise during labor.* Pack your hospital or birthing center bag with things that cosset and comfort you—socks that are not just warm but pretty and soft, music that relaxes, something meaningful as well as pleasant to look at for your focal point in breathing exercises.

- *Protect your intimate time with your partner.* A bulging belly and, later, a bawling newborn have a funny way of making sex fall off the priority list. (Hence the old saying, "Three's a crowd.") Find ways to be together, not necessarily sexually, but sensually holding and caressing each other. If sex is uncomfortable even after your doctor gives you the green light, be sure you understand why. Breast-feeding, for example, can cause vaginal dryness that is easily remedied with lubricants.

- *Keep self-cosseting.* A difficult fertility journey can take a long time; don't let up on your sensate needs as the cycle-after-cycle ordeal continues. The same is true during pregnancy and after giving birth. Most new moms notice that there's a 180-degree shift in interest from them to the new baby—not just on the part of outsiders, but sometimes in their partners as well. Be sure to remember yourself, even if it feels like nobody else does. Buy new clothes not just for the baby but for you. Make time for napping and warm baths. Even though you're a mother now, you still have to put yourself first—probably now more than ever—or you won't have the resources to give to others.

Chapter 11

The Transition Pathway

From perimenopause to menopause, as the reproductive system winds down

For is it not possible that middle age can be looked upon as a period of second flowering, second growth, even a kind of second adolescence?...The signs that presage growth, so similar, it seems to me, to those in early adolescence: discontentment, restlessness, doubt, despair, longing, are interpreted falsely as signs of decay....Who is not afraid of pure space—that breathtaking empty space of an open door?

—ANNE MORROW LINDBERGH, FROM "GIFT FROM THE SEA"

The transition from cycling to natural menopause is not sudden. There's no signal moment of drama, like getting your first period. Instead, the disappearance of your menstrual cycles and the conclusion of the reproductive part of your life happens gradually, in fits and starts. The medical definition of menopause is one full year without a period. But from a practical standpoint, when that year has begun can be hard to identify. More recognizable in your everyday life are the first hints of menopause approaching, which can be noticed months or even years before your final period, in the form of erratic cycles and the myriad symptoms of hormonal declines—a phase known as perimenopause. *Peri-* means "around." Perimenopause is the time around menopause.

Perimenopause and menopause itself constitute what I call the Transition Pathway. It's so named because this relatively short time is literally and figuratively a passage from one state (being able to reproduce) to the next (no longer being able to reproduce). Ob-gyns use the same word, *transition,* to describe the stage of labor that occurs when a mother-to-be's cervix is between nine and ten centimeters dilated. Suddenly her contractions and the rate of dilation slow, and it seems as if labor has stalled. But what's really happening during this discrete phase is that the body is preparing for birth. The life stage I refer to as Transition represents a similar bridge between two states, between the dynamic "laboring" days of menstrual cycles and fertility issues and the "rebirthing" a woman experiences when all that is behind her. It is an ending. It represents the closure of a big part of your life. But it's also a time of change, just as puberty and pregnancy are. And as such, it's a gift, a golden opportunity for self-assessment and reevaluation built right into a woman's life cycle.

Maybe that image runs counter to your preconceived vision of menopause and perimenopause as a time of loss, of decline. If so, good! No doubt a woman will face special challenges along the way, not all of them pleasant, from coping comfortably with hot flashes to worrying about waning libido and the empty nest. But if she can listen and respond to her changing feelings and needs, she's more likely to come through this natural transition with a deeply satisfying understanding of who she is now and where she might like to go.

There's some debate about how long this pathway lasts. While it varies from woman to woman, typically it lasts just a few years. Some people think that a woman can be in perimenopause for as many as ten years. That's a pretty long on-ramp. I mark the beginning of perimenopause as the point at which one or more features of a characteristic collection of symptoms begin to be noticed. These include hot flashes, night sweats, irritability, anxiety, loss of libido, irregular bleeding, and fuzzy thinking. (More about all of those shortly.) For most women, these symptoms don't become intrusive until roughly a year or two before actual menopause. There are many gradual changes on the way to menopause, and certainly a woman who's really paying attention can find subtle changes all the time, from her twenties to her forties. When impending menopause really hits, though, it makes a significant enough impact to be unmistakable.

Why? What's going on inside? Let's have a look.

Beth, 48:
⌐ *"If I am going into menopause, I wish it would just happen already. Enough of this stopping and starting."*

WHAT'S HAPPENING NOW: THE CYCLE WIND-DOWN

Menopause is not an aberration but part of a natural plan. The changes that unfold are encoded into your very being. Around her mid-forties, typically, a woman begins to notice that her periods are becoming more variable. They may get longer (or sometimes shorter), with more than usual bleeding (or, rarely, lighter flow). These are the first signs that she has begun to have some anovulatory cycles—cycles in which no egg is released. If an egg is not released from the follicle, the follicle cannot transform as it normally would into the corpus luteum, the tissue that secretes hormones characteristic of the second half of the cycle. If the hormones are not secreted—particularly progesterone—then everything changes. With less progesterone, there is earlier and heavier bleeding. Women ask me all the time why bleeding increases if reproduction is ending. It seems a contradiction, but remember, the bleeding is caused by a lack of the progesterone that would have been secreted if an egg had been released. Then the next month an egg might be released on schedule, and things go back to their "normal" pattern. But what the cycle looks like from month to month is no longer predictable. All usual bets are off.

The average age for menopause in the United States is fifty-one. But it can happen as early as age thirty-five or as late as fifty-nine.

Only a very few lucky women have their periods space out, taper off, and then stop with no other significant symptoms. It would be nice if it happened that way for all of us, but far more typical is for these anovulatory cycles to increase, the time between periods to grow more erratic, and the accompanying symptoms to intensify, due to the disruption in the normal hormonal patterns. During this time, the entire body will be affected, including the brain—so women often experience an inability to concentrate or remember things, which can be very upsetting, since they may interpret these symptoms as a signal of Alzheimer's disease. But in fact they are a perfectly normal and temporary side effect, which will disappear over time.

Another side effect with which many women are only too familiar is hot flashes. No egg also means less estrogen, which causes the classic vasomotor symptoms—hot flashes and night sweats—to begin. Decreased estrogen also causes the bones to lose calcium and weaken, sex drive to decline, and the vagina to become drier.

The erratic anovulatory pattern continues until there are no eggs released at all and no more new cycles begin. Some women skip over this process or have it interrupted by removal of their ovaries along with a hysterectomy, removal of the uterus. This is known as surgical menopause.

Other women experience menopause during their early thirties or, more rarely, their twenties. This is known as premature menopause or, medically, premature ovarian failure. (A funny term, as if menopause is the ovaries "failing," when they are doing exactly what they're supposed to be doing!)

I believe that there's a reason this time is called meno*pause.* Given the forceful connection between the body and the soul, the body is speaking to the soul, encouraging it to get its own needs met. You're at midlife. An enormous part of who you are—your reproductive self—is retiring. So now what?

You can think of perimenopause as a prolonged bout of PMS. You can choose either to override the symptoms or to tune in to them and understand yourself better because of them—just as you were able to make that choice during the premenstrual days of your Cycling Pathway. Only now, instead of the division being between the first half of your cycle and the second half, it's between the first half of your life and the second half. Menopause is a big picture window into yourself. I think it's a gift that we don't just one day stop cycling and the next day

Perimenopause on the Pill

If you are on the Pill or another hormonal form of birth control, the artificial hormones override the pattern described above. You will continue to experience normal cycles because the Pill causes them to be anovulatory and then supplies the hormones to mimic a cycle. So how will you know when you are approaching menopause?

You could come off hormones sometime in your early forties to allow yourself to experience the natural progression of events at the end of fertility. This is the course that I almost always recommend to Pill users.

Or you could stay on hormonal contraception until your late forties, which some women see as a plus because bothersome menopausal symptoms tend to be blunted. But it's important to note that the hormones in oral contraceptives are six times more potent than the typical dosage in hormone replacement therapy (HRT), and we do not know the long-term effects of prolonged use of high-dose estrogen and progesterone. We do know that the risks of the Pill (blood clots, stroke, heart attack) increase as you age. The risks are *significantly* higher if you are a smoker, and therefore in that circumstance this option should not be used.

Some doctors encourage you to stay on the Pill until sometime in your late forties, when they do blood work to assess the level of FSH (follicle-stimulating hormone), which can be checked during the week of sugar pills. If FSH is high, it will mean that you are not ovulating. The thinking behind this conclusion is based on the fact that FSH normally triggers a follicle to release an egg, then declines; if no egg is released, the FSH continues to build in the effort to stimulate ovulation. The resulting high levels of FSH are an indication that a woman is not ovulating. In my own practice I tend not to check FSH levels much, whether a woman is on the Pill or not. I don't see the point. Either she'll present with menopausal symptoms or she won't. Often I see women in the Duke Center for Integrative Medicine who have gone to their regular ob-gyn complaining of hot flashes, low libido, and other symptoms. "She took a blood test and told me not to worry, that I wasn't menopausal yet," such a patient will tell me. "Is that all that can be done?" The doctor has followed the standard protocol, but the symptoms go ignored and a patient is left feeling totally frustrated and disempowered. This situation is frustrating to me, too! I'd rather focus on the experience (the symptoms) than on a test.

How to proceed if you are perimenopausal and on the Pill (or other hormonal contraceptives) is a decision that, like any other, can be made consciously or unconsciously. I prefer my patients to come off the Pill early in their forties. That they get to experience menopause authentically is only part of the reason. They also reduce the risks of being on a high dose of hormones at an age when the risks are increasing. I often see women who are wedded to the Pill because it has served them well for years. Though that may have been true in their younger years, there are many excellent alternatives that would be better for a woman in her forties.

step into menopause. The attendant changes are so big, from having an active reproductive life to having no reproductive life, and with so many potential repercussions, that we all need to take the time to work through this momentous transition.

Embrace that opportunity. Tell yourself, "Okay, I am going to use this time to reflect about what I want the second half of my life to be about." It's easier for some women than for others to shift from viewing menopause as an annoyance to be minimized to seeing it as an opportunity to be heeded. But every woman who makes this transition consciously is better positioned, in terms of her physical, mental, and emotional health and longevity, for the postmenopausal Transformation years.

Important note: You may be on the Transition Pathway, but you can technically have one foot still planted on the Fertility or Cycling Pathway (depending whether you would still like to have a child or not). I've delivered my share of "perimenopause babies" to mothers in their early- to mid-forties who were sure they were no longer fertile. It's rare, but it happens. If you do not want to become pregnant, it's smart to continue using contraception until you are sure you've crossed all the way over to the Transformation Pathway.

LANDMARK: PERIMENOPAUSE

Jess, 48:
⟶ *"I think I had my first hot flash last night. I was in bed and suddenly I noticed my T-shirt was soaked. I'm surprised—I didn't think I would start menopause so soon. But you know what? I'm relieved. I'm done with babies, so I'll be glad to get the whole thing over with."*

Lynne, 52:
⟶ *"Did I know anything about menopause before it hit me? Absolutely not. It was like a stick that smacked me upside the head. Now I wonder, did my mom go through this, too?"*

Martha, 75:
⟶ *"I never really noticed menopause. The whole thing coincided with a very busy time in my life. I was starting to go back to work and get my real estate broker's license. One day I was sitting in a meeting in the mayor's office when I was overcome with a great wash of heat. I wondered if my face was as red on the outside as I felt inside. This happened just a few times. Then, when I was sitting for my exam for my license, I suddenly felt this flood. It was like the last gasp of my period. It was tricky to figure out how to excuse myself from the exam and get to the ladies' room. After that, my periods were done. A dramatic curtain closer!"*

Bess, 54:

⌐"*First it took me longer to climax, then intercourse became uncomfortable because I was so dry, not to mention that I'm gaining weight and still having hot flashes. It makes me think, 'Why bother?' Like nature's telling me I really don't need those parts anymore, so give it up.*"

Ivy, 46:

⌐"*I cannot cope with this roller coaster! Just yesterday I was raging around my house, furious with my kids, the stacks of newspapers, and the fact that my husband never makes any plans for the weekend other than watching sports. But even as I was fuming, I knew that I had that nervous, almost shaky feeling of knowing I was overreacting. My hormones were on the rampage again. I get so sick of this—feeling me-ish one moment and like a raving lunatic the next. How many more years of this can I take? How many more years of it can my family take?*"

When most women think about menopause, they focus on the symptoms first. The disruptions in the menstrual cycle and the altered hormonal rhythms caused when we begin to skip ovulation create certain classic disturbances. These are felt in both the body (hot flashes, night sweats, low libido, vaginal discomfort, sleep disruption) and the mind (forgetfulness, "fuzzy thinking," irritability). Each of you will experience the symptoms of perimenopause and menopause differently. For some of you they are minor nuisances or barely noted; for others, they are completely disruptive to life as you once knew it. The tumult of this transition is not limited to your mind and body. Because you are entering a new passage in life, your soul can experience turbulence, too. (I choose the word *turbulence* deliberately; it doesn't necessarily indicate horrible upheavals, merely "a departure from a smooth flow," as my dictionary says.) Given the connection between your body and your soul, you need to approach menopause on both fronts, recognizing how each reflects the other.

Deciding whether to treat symptoms, and how, is entirely individual. But I like to counsel women to approach the whole experience before they zero in on just one symptom, such as what to do about hot flashes. Most bothersome symptoms can be treated. Your goal should not be to negate every feeling that goes with this transition, though. Your body and soul are speaking to you. Listen. Honor the messages you are being given. Only then can you decide what you want to treat, and how.

Here's a Feedback Loop process for connecting with peri-menopause:

First, reflection. To evaluate the symptoms of menopause in your life, begin by making the space to confront your feelings around this huge transition. Because these topics are normally kept buried in our culture, it can be a challenge to bring them to the surface. But there are many possible outlets: write in a diary; confide in another friend the same age; use the Dialoguing tool to reflect on your relationship with your reproductive system as its functionality comes to an end. There's a reason human beings say good-byes. Closure is a very useful concept. Use Dreamagery to explore further any number of issues that might come up as a result of the other work. Invite an image, for example, of your female soul and ask it how it is changing in response to aging, to menopause itself.

I can't stress how important it is to face this transition wide-eyed and head-on. Not because you will then have no menopause symptoms or feelings of loss, but because blocking your feelings will mean a damming up of energies that will then have no place to go, possibly resulting in even more severe symptoms. If you process the experience through your soul, however, your body may have an easier time. "That sounds so New Age," one patient scolded me. New Age or age-old wisdom, there's no denying the interconnectedness of body and soul. Here are some suggestions for using that connection to help you get through the transition more gracefully and comfortably.

- Reflect ahead. What are your greatest hopes concerning menopause? What are your greatest fears? What's informing these hopes and fears?
- Reflect back. What are your feelings about the end of your reproductive life? Everybody has some kind of reaction. A childless woman might regret that she did not experience motherhood. A mother might wish she had had more chil-

dren—or fewer! Explore what your reproductive years were like. What were your greatest joys? What were your greatest sorrows?

- Reflect on the present. Are you having specific symptoms? How bothersome are they? How do they alter your self-image, if at all? Did you expect your symptoms or did they come as a surprise? Have you shared your experience of them with anyone else, including your partner?

Second, information. Learn what symptoms are part of the natural progression, so that you don't, for example, become needlessly concerned that you're losing your mind when you start forgetting where you put your keys and the names of people you've known for years. Knowing what's normal will help you recognize what's *not*—for example, if you find a suspicious lump or you experience a dramatic change in your weight. Again, know how much *you* need to know. You might feel satisfied after a talk with a trusted doctor, or you might want to surf the Web or delve into one of the many terrific books available about menopause and perimenopause.

Know that good solutions to menopausal symptoms exist within both conventional and alternative medicine. But take time to be sure that your sources are reliable ones. This is an area where information is changing rapidly. The information I've offered in the Landmark below should be a good starting place for helping you assess the risks and benefits of HRT.

Third, action. Once you've weighed both your reflections and the information you've collected, make a decision on how to proceed—knowing, even as you do, that you can change your mind later.

Then, re-reflection. Try your course of action for a month, or two or three, and then evaluate how it is working for you. Have your symptoms improved? No different? Don't be afraid to switch gears if something doesn't seem helpful. Also realize that new research is being done every day around perimenopause. You may decide to readjust your course based on something you hear on the news or something that your doctor suggests. Run it through the Feedback Loop. Reflect, get the facts, and see what you think.

Veronica's Story: Menopause Equals Old Lady ⌒⌐

I once gave a talk at the Canyon Ranch Spa about menopause. Afterward, a tall, slim, blond woman, beautifully groomed and dressed, sidled up to me. In a hushed voice she said, "I enjoyed your lecture. I—I—" She faltered. I nodded encouragingly. Her voice dropped still lower. "I think I am menopausal. Nobody knows. I haven't told my husband or even any of my girlfriends," she said.

Interestingly, this lovely woman had just attended a presentation all about menopause. Naturally, most of the attendees (all female) were peri- or postmenopausal themselves. But when I had asked for a show of hands during my talk about who had experienced symptoms, this woman, Veronica, had not raised her hand. She didn't even want a group of strangers to know.

"I came here because I have gained a few pounds lately and felt a little blue," she confided. "I figured I would exercise them away, get back in shape. But yesterday I injured my foot and the doctor said I couldn't work out for a few days, which is how I happened to come to your talk."

Clearly Veronica had not done much deep reflection on the subject at hand. I asked her what menopause meant to her. She looked at the floor, then admitted, "My greatest fear—getting old."

I casually asked if she had ever explored that fear. I always know that I have struck at the heart of a matter if I see tears welling up in a patient's eyes. Who is it that aptly said, "Tears are the language of the soul"? I suggested to Veronica that maybe her injured foot was a gift. It provided her with an opportunity to explore a central topic in her life that she might otherwise have tried to blow right past with exercise. If she bought a journal at the spa gift shop and spent the next couple of days of recuperation going into her feelings around aging, she might gain some insights. She looked doubtful. "But what if I can't think of anything to write?"

"Just write whatever comes into your mind," I said. It's my standard advice to patients: Just try. Put pen to paper, even if your first words are "I don't know what I have to say about this, but..." Write down your dreams, or a picture of what you want your life to be like as an older woman. Write down your fears, the ones you don't even want to give voice to. If you're intimidated about voicing such innermost thoughts, tell yourself that you can shred it all up afterward so there's no "evidence" to worry about. It's the process that provides the insight.

Normally I don't cross paths again with lecture attendees. But several days later I passed Veronica in a hallway at the spa. She looked different—brighter, looser. "I did what you said," she burst out. "I cried for days. I've been writing like a maniac. Just being able to express it has been such a relief." The release process set in motion by the journal had worked its magic on her. Though Veronica had taken only the first steps toward reconciling her fears about aging, they were important ones. In a culture that values youth and appearance so heavily, perimenopause has become synonymous with "over the hill." (I look forward to seeing how this changes as our society gets older; by the year 2015, fully 50 percent of American women will be menopausal!) Of course, you're only over the hill if you choose to go over it. The reflection process can put you where you are comfortable—right at the center of *you*—not where someone else's clichés about youth or aging would relegate you.

I sensed that Veronica would now be heading in a direction she was a lot more comfortable with.

LANDMARK: HORMONE THERAPY CHOICES

Debbie, 45:
⌐ *"Perimenopause came calling for me early. I was only forty-two and I was bummed. It seemed shameful. I didn't want anybody to know. I hid it from my husband because I didn't want him to start thinking of me as 'old.' I got on hormone replacement therapy as fast as my doctor could prescribe it. No way was I going to let go of my youth and shape without a fight."*

Shelly, 53:
⌐ *"I just heard that HRT is bad! Get me off!"*

Sara, 49:

⌐*"Oh, I just hate the idea of having to take something for the rest of my life. I avoided the Pill and used barrier methods for years, and now here's another pill for menopause!"*

Larkin, 51:

⌐*"I don't know what 'normal' feels like, between taking the Pill and taking HRT. To me this seems like a good thing—I'm free from the concerns about unwanted pregnancy or aging that my mother and my grandmother had. Only I'm a little leery about life after hormones."*

There is so much emphasis on menopausal hormonal therapy that I can hardly blame my patients for viewing it as the central question of the Transition Pathway. Except it's not the most important question. It's quite possibly one of the *least* important things to obsess over, both medically and otherwise!

(A note on nomenclature: The National Institutes of Health changed the name "hormone replacement therapy" to the more accurate "menopausal hormone therapy" to get away from the idea that drugs replaced something missing in order to restore a fountain of youth. But the acronym *HRT* lives on.)

At issue is not whether you need hormones, but what you would gain from being on them vs. what you would gain from *not* being on them. Perimenopause is a great time of life to reevaluate all aspects of your health. Your menopausal symptoms are affected by your nutrition, your exercise, your stress level, your relationships, and even your sexuality—all of the Centers of Wellness that I've underscored through this entire book. The choices you make within your Centers of Wellness are your best resources for handling your symptoms.

And the more you focus on your Centers of Wellness—on your lifestyle choices—the less significant the HRT decision becomes. If you have optimal Movement strategies and optimal Nutrition, for example, you are more likely to be protected against cardiovascular disease and osteoporosis. Yet that protection is part of what millions of women were looking for when they took Premarin (a combination of more than ten different estrogenic hormones) and PremPro (Premarin plus a progesterone,

Provera). That once-standard practice was thrown into disarray when the eight-year federal Women's Health Initiative (WHI) study was halted in 2002 because PremPro was found to actually increase the risk of heart attack and stroke in older women in the first few years, not to mention increasing the risk of breast cancer after prolonged use (more than five years). At the same time, it was found to decrease the risk of osteoporosis and colorectal cancer. (Note: Only the arm of the WHI study including PremPro was discontinued; the Premarin-only study, consisting of women who did not need progesterone because they have had hysterectomies, continues as I write this, meaning that the same level of risk as in PremPro has not as yet been identified. But women who still have a uterus are strongly advised to take a combination of estrogen and progesterone, because estrogen taken alone after menopause is known to increase the risk of endometrial cancer. See "My Pet Peeves About HRT," page 339.)

Should you or shouldn't you? There are many different factors to weigh. If you're just looking at the best way to safeguard against heart disease and osteoporosis, the smart lifestyle choices win hands down. If you need relief from certain symptoms, you'll want to weigh the benefits of HRT against the known risks, while investigating the full range of options within HRT as well as effective alternatives.

Over and over patients sit in my office and say things like, "I need to decide my stance on HRT." Or, "I don't know if I'm for it or against it." Hormone replacement therapy is not like abortion, a moral and political issue on which you may feel like you have to take a stand. Nor is it like a hysterectomy, a major medical procedure that is irreversible. Or like a dissertation that you will be called on to defend. There is no good or bad, no right or wrong, and nothing irrevocable.

Your choices around hormone replacement therapy must be completely custom-made—or I should say, *consciously* made! There might be compelling reasons to consider it. There might be good arguments against. Or maybe you try it for three months and reassess. Here's how to get there:

First, reflection. Explore where you're starting from. Use the tools in Part Two to get at answers to the following:

- What are your preconceptions about HRT? What have you heard about how lifestyle and alternative approaches can help with the changes brought on by menopause?

- What are your needs? This is a big one. If you're not having any symptoms, you may not need HRT. It's not something a woman takes automatically when she turns forty-five or fifty. If you are having symptoms, you need to evaluate exactly what they are, what their severity is, and how they are impacting the rest of your life. Can you live with them a little longer to give lifestyle or alternative methods a chance to work, or are they unbearable?

- What are your other motivations for thinking about HRT? A belief that HRT will ward off the effects of aging? Protection from osteoporosis or heart disease because of your family history? Your doctor's recommendation?

- What are the experiences of people close to you? Has your mom gone on it? Your sister? Did you have a friend who once had breast cancer and is convinced it's because she took it? Whether or not there is any medical evidence for a correlation is irrelevant. What experiences may have affected what *you* believe?

- What are your fears? Heart disease and breast cancer if you take HRT? A miserable menopause if you don't?

- What are your hopes? Immediate relief of symptoms? Never having symptoms in the first place? Getting onto the Transformation Pathway without any drug interventions?

- What are your individual health risks? Do you have a high risk of breast cancer or heart disease (which might tilt you away from HRT, since there appears to be a relationship)? Do you have a high risk of colon cancer or osteoporosis (which might tilt you toward HRT, since there appears to be a protective effect)?

Second, information. Once you have greater personal clarity around HRT—your feelings, your individual risks and needs, your motivations, and so on—you are in a much stronger position to evaluate the medical data. Regrettably, there's still much we don't know. (See box on next page.) Nevertheless, take in as much as you feel you need from a trusted source. Your decision making should start with whether you want to try HRT at all. If you do, then you need to decide what kind.

Get your doctor's input based on your individual profile. Realize, though, that individual physicians may have their own biases. In my practice, for example, I work hard to help each woman make the right decision for her, based on the process I am describing here. But if she elects HRT, I am inclined to suggest bioidentical hormones such as estradiol and natural progesterone. These are different from Premarin and Provera, the hormones studied in the WHI, which are not molecularly identical to the hormones produced by your body. Many women report that the side effects that they were having from PremPro resolved almost immediately when they switched to bioidentical progesterone. "Like a magic bullet," I hear often. And studies indicate that natural progesterone works just as well as the Provera in PremPro, while being better for your lipid profile. But, depending on a woman's needs and history, I might recommend that before trying any form of HRT, she consider the many good alternative options, including simple lifestyle changes (described in the Center of Wellness Modifications for the Transition Pathway, found at the end of this chapter), acupuncture, and hypnosis. Take the time to research avenues outside your physician's area of expertise.

It's in your interest to explore each of these forks in the road. What might each of those forks look like for you from a medical perspective?

Third, action. Take your time before diving into this step. You're much better off combining what you learn in the news or from your doctor with knowledge of and sensitivity to your individual situation. Because this is not an area of medicine where there are absolute indications requiring a specific treatment path, your own sense of what you need and want is just as important as your doctor's recommendations. Don't shirk from that thought, embrace it. When you've made a decision that honors mind as well as soul, you're more apt to feel at peace about your decision and less likely to panic over every new research headline (as happened after the WHI study).

My Pet Peeves About HRT

Since the majority of women I see are peri- or post-menopausal, I've had plenty of opportunity to develop my list of the HRT myths that drive me crazy:

- *The notion that there is just one HRT. Wrong! Hormone replacement therapy* is a general term for a kind of medication, like contraceptives or antihypertensives or antibiotics. There are dozens of variations within HRT—actually hundreds if you consider all of the possible permutations in terms of dosages and delivery. There are pills and patches and creams, combination therapies (estrogen plus progesterone) and estrogen alone. There are many different kinds of hormones with many different strengths. The only forms that have been extensively tested are Premarin and Provera. Despite the fact that the major pharmaceutical firms, which fund many of major research initiatives, make bioidentical hormones as well as the nonbioidenticals, such as Premarin and Provera, thus far most of the research has focused on the latter, which are the most commonly prescribed types. Unfortunately, the 2002 WHI findings about PremPro somehow morphed in the global media into *all* hormone replacement therapy. In fact, WHI addresses just those two hormones. The distinction between bioidenticals and nonbioidenticals may prove to be critical—or not. We just don't know at this point.
- *The perception that we now have all the answers about HRT. We don't!* Despite the crushing amount of coverage the landmark WHI study perhaps rightly received, the fact remains that it provided answers to only one particular question. It told us how women

of a certain age (the average age of these women was over sixty-three) were affected by taking a particular dosage of a particular hormonal combination (.625 milligram Premarin, 2.5 milligrams Provera). That leaves quite a lot of variables unestablished!

Another great unknown is how a woman's lifelong exposure to various hormones interfaces with replacement hormones at perimenopause and subsequent risks. What difference might it make if you have never been pregnant or on the Pill, compared with a woman who has spent twenty years on the Pill and also has borne and breast-fed several children? We just don't know yet.

As Bernadine Healy, the former head of the National Institutes of Health who first organized the WHI study, told *Vogue* magazine, that study "is not the last word on the subject. It's the first."

- *The belief that we can take a one-size-fits-all approach to HRT. We shouldn't.* Although a doctor would never give a thyroid medication to a patient without tracking her levels of thyroid hormone, there have never been studies examining the levels of hormones in perimenopausal women when on a given regimen. But for years, all women of all ages, shapes, sizes, hormone levels, and stages of menopause received the exact same dose of HRT. I think the factors that need to be considered include how much hormone an individual woman actually needs and, since everyone metabolizes medications at a different rate, how her body processes the replacement hormones. Then a realistic analysis could be done of the risks and benefits of hormones at varying levels. It may very well turn out upon further study that the risks are the same regardless of the hormone levels, but it would be great to know that! Likewise, it may be that the rise in heart attacks in women taking PremPro were the direct result of preexisting conditions, because the women in the WHI study were all well past menopause when they began the therapy; I don't know that we can extrapolate from this that starting healthy women on PremPro at a younger age (late forties to around fifty) and keeping them on it for only a few years would yield the same heart risks. It's theoretically possible—but based on the research to date, *we just don't know.*

I am reminded of the early experimentation with oral contraceptives. Proper dosages had to be figured out through trial and error. In the 1960s, the first Pill formulations contained 150 micrograms of estrogen; today they typically contain 20 to 35 micrograms. A similar situation may be at work with HRT. It may turn out that the ideal estrogen dosage is half of the typical Premarin dose. We just don't know yet.

- *The idea that all types of replacement hormones are identical. They aren't!* Premarin and Provera have different molecular structures from human estrogen and progesterone. (Premarin is conjugated equine estrogen, made from *pregnant mare*'s urine, hence the name.)

  Bioidentical estrogens (such as Estrace, Estraderm, and Climera) are synthesized from hormone precursors in yams and soybeans to fit perfectly into human estrogen receptor sites, like a lock and key. They're made to have the exact molecular structure of 17-beta-estadriol, the primary human estrogen produced by the ovary premenopausally. Similarly, bioidentical progesterone, known as micronized progesterone (Prometrium), is synthesized to be an exact match for human progesterone. One difference we already know about is that micronized progesterone used with estrogen has been shown to have a more beneficial effect on HDL cholesterol than Provera. (Note: Bioidenticals are misleadingly known as "natural hormones." *Natural* is one of those loaded words that in fact doesn't necessarily mean better or worse. After all, the mare's urine from which Premarin is made is also a natural substance.)

There are other estrogens and progesterones being synthesized in the labs from "natural" substances that are also not native to the female body—at least not the human female body—including the hormones in birth control pills and hormones made from plant compounds called phytoestrogens (found in soy and ginseng) and phytoprogesterones.

Then, re-reflection. This is the best part. You can change your mind. If you decide to weather out the symptoms, do so for a month or two. Are you still feeling all right? Great. Are hot flashes and irritability getting harder to bear? If you try HRT, how do you feel on it? How significantly are your symptoms improved?

Unfortunately, there is a lack of good data on the various options' safety and effectiveness, which makes it hard for women to make apples-to-apples evaluations. Each type of HRT has relative pluses and minuses.

We don't even know exactly which hormones a women needs. It used to be thought that perimenopausal symptoms were caused by a lack of estrogen only. Therefore a woman was given replacement estrogen; if she still had a uterus, she was also given replacement progesterone to protect against uterine cancer, but no progesterone if her uterus had been removed. Researchers are now beginning to recognize that progesterone may play a role in bone protection and other things, for all women. How much helps or hurts and for whom has not been figured out.

More research desperately needs to be done on all kinds of HRT, especially bioidenticals, which have been comparatively underresearched. In the meanwhile a woman can only absorb the new information as it comes up, and keep factoring it into her personal conscious choice making.

Trudy's Story: New Information, New Choice

Trudy is typical of countless patients I counseled after the 2002 WHI study threw everybody's HRT perceptions into question. She was rightfully concerned about how the news should affect her, as she had been taking replacement hormones for five years.

"Since we have new information, it's a perfect time to revisit why you're on hormones and look again at your decision," I told her. Trudy had started HRT when she was forty-eight and had begun having night sweats, anxiety, and other symptoms. She did well on it and didn't have any bothersome problems now. Nor did she have any family history of breast cancer or cardiovascular trouble, which might have altered her choice.

The first thing I had to point out was that Trudy's replacement hormones were not the same as those studied in the Women's Health Initiative. She was on estradiol (Estrace) and natural progesterone, not PremPro. It's impossible to know what to extrapolate from the WHI study that would be relevant to these particular hormones. Nor was she in the same age group as the women studied. But since Trudy was now on the far side of menopause, at the point where risks started to rise with PremPro, she elected to quit HRT. She decided that for two months before quitting she would begin simple lifestyle steps (taking black cohosh and increased vitamin E, improving her exercise program and her stress-reduction practices) that would help ease any symptoms she might experience when she went off the hormones. Once she was ready to stop, I tapered her off the HRT gradually—you never want to quit abruptly, because it's easier on the body to experience a gentle transition, much like the tapering off of hormones that occurs during natural menopause. I like to see patients stick to an HRT change for at least three months, to get a true picture of what it's like. Often a woman will experience hot flashes or other symptoms in a quick flare-up at first, but they recede. (If not forewarned, patients will call to say, "I just had a night of sweats! Give me the stuff back!")

Trudy did have some hot flashes, but they ended after the first month, and she felt fine. We ramped up her efforts in maintaining her Centers of Wellness and did not resume the hormones.

Chris's Story: New Information, Different Choice ⟶

Another patient was already on PremPro when she came to see me, although I had not been the prescribing physician. When I met Chris, fifty-six, before the study that called the drug into question, I encouraged her to think about the bioidentical Estrace and progesterone, which I generally prefer. She was reluctant because her symptoms had been severe—horrid hot flashes, sleep disorders, and memory problems. "I couldn't think to save my life," she said. The PremPro helped, and she was firm about wanting to stay on it.

After the WHI study came out, though, I worried about Chris. Her sister has breast cancer, and one of the study's findings had been an increased risk of the disease. Her regular exam was coming up, and I was glad.

On the day of her appointment, I talked to her about the potential dangers of PremPro for her, particularly given her history. She had been on it for five years, and that was the point at which the risk for breast cancer for PremPro users rose. Her bone scans were great; she didn't need the HRT for that.

Chris listened. But what she really wanted to discuss that day was depression. She had been laid off. Her husband had made some bad stock trades and they were on the brink of bankruptcy. As if all that wasn't enough, her daughter had been in a bad car accident and now needed round-the-clock care. Chris felt very strongly that she needed stability in life right now more than experimenting with a new HRT. She understood the risks with PremPro but did not feel equipped at this point in time to change. Reluctantly but empathetically, I agreed. I wound up giving her a prescription for an antidepressant that day, along with a number of recommendations for her Centers of Wellness. We agreed to check back in three months to evaluate where she stood.

Greta's Story: An Integrative Approach ⌐

Patients who have faced the question of HRT for the first time after that fateful summer of 2002 bring a different reality to the landmark. Many women already in their fifties and sixties took up HRT with little question, because it was simply recommended across the board by physicians. It was not a difficult choice for a generation raised on the powers of the Pill and eager to hang on to a specific image of youthfulness prized by the culture.

Greta is more typical of a slightly younger generation. At forty-six, she had been surprised to experience her first hot flash. She began to feel a generalized depression. Then there was the drop in sex drive she first wrote off to a stressful career and "bad moods." But the headlines about the risks of HRT when the news about the WHI study came out caused her to be more skeptical about starting hormones than Trudy and Chris had been. "I want help, but I don't want hormones if I don't really need them," she said. "Is there anything else I can try?"

Greta and I explored her starting perceptions around HRT and menopause. One of the tools I asked her to pay special attention to was the Five-Center Review. She thought about her needs within these domains over time, and how she was presently satisfying them. I then gave her my list of lifestyle recommendations to help manage symptoms. Those things that a woman can do easily (diet changes, supplements, exercise, Spirit and Sensation steps) I strongly encourage. There are other things that can significantly help symptoms but require spending extra money, such as mind-body therapy or seeing a practitioner of Chinese medicine. I make those suggestions along with the others and then leave their follow-up to an individual's interest and ability.

Greta enthusiastically revamped her five Centers of Wellness and made an appointment with a psychologist I recommended to try learning self-hypnosis. She also began practicing relaxation tools to use whenever she felt a hot flash. Inspired by her progress, Greta's best friend embarked on a similar journey. The two women then enlisted a third buddy also the same age, and they all began using the Consciously Female approach together. "We call ourselves the Durham Ya-Yas," Greta joked, after the book and the movie about four lifelong friends who supported one another through many transitions and called themselves the Ya-Ya Sisterhood. Greta has not felt she needed HRT yet; one of her friends has and uses the lifestyle approach simultaneously.

Ultimately, success in menopause is not avoiding HRT. Nor is it avoiding every hot flash. Success is making the transition manageable and smooth—and *conscious*.

LANDMARK: FACING HYSTERECTOMY

Audrey, 45:
—"A hysterectomy sounds like something that happens to old ladies! I am just forty-five!"

Ellen, 68:
—"Certainly I am well past having children and all that, but I really worry that losing my 'female parts' will make me less of a woman. I am apprehensive."

A hysterectomy (surgical removal of the uterus) may take place at any time in a woman's life, from her teens to her nineties. In fact, it's the second most common major surgical procedure in the United States (after C-sections). But it's a slightly trickier question when the need arises in perimenopause, requiring special reflection. That's because many of the conditions that point to the need for a hysterectomy will disappear naturally after menopause.

Fibroids are a good example. I'd guess nine out of ten women with fibroids have no problems after menopause, because fibroids are estrogen-dependent. After menopause, estrogen falls and the fibroids shrink. So if you are close to that point in life and can endure any presenting symptoms a little longer, know that the symptoms will soon pass and you will have avoided major surgery.

Waiting it out is not always possible. For example, a woman who is thirty-three and has already had children might develop fibroids that cause significant pain and bleeding. It hurts, she can't have intercourse, and the flow of blood can be quite heavy. No way does she want to live with such symptoms for possibly another two decades until she hits menopause. But a woman in her mid-forties might choose to wait and see.

There's no right or wrong way to proceed. Either course is within the standards of care. Yet it's another choice that deserves to be made consciously. To make the choice unconsciously means you'll probably do whatever your doctor recommends. Many women find themselves in a scenario like this: You're in for your annual exam and mention you've been having heavy periods. Nothing too bad, just different. The exam reveals fibroids, and your doctor recommends a hysterectomy. Two weeks later you're having your uterus removed, and—"while we're at it"—your ovaries are removed, too. Now, your bleeding problem is solved, but let's back up a minute. Having your reproductive organs removed involves general anesthesia, major surgery, and all the risks that go along with them. And that's just the insult to your body. What about your soul? You've skipped right over the multiyear perimenopause process that would have helped you gradually adjust to the end of your reproductive life, and you haven't given yourself the period of reflection that might have helped you process that transition consciously. The result may be that you find yourself feeling suddenly old and resentful of being thrust too abruptly into postmenopausal life.

To make the choice consciously, on the other hand, is to opt for or against surgery with an open mind and an open heart. It's always wise to go into surgery feeling positive about it. That relaxed state has been linked to better outcomes, quicker recovery, and less need for postoperative painkillers.

A route to bring you to that place:

First, reflection. Okay, so you might need a hysterectomy. How do you feel about that? Check in with your five Centers of Wellness.

Journal about it. This is as perfect a landmark as any to have a dialogue with your reproductive system.

- What are your preexisting ideas, if any, about surgery in general and this procedure especially? Do you know anyone who has had a hysterectomy? (Do you even know if your own mother has had one or not?) Have you had prior surgeries?
- What are your thoughts around your uterus? Some women feel strongly that it's a symbol of their feminine self that belongs there till the very end. Others think, "Gee, no more symptoms, no more periods, great!" And what about having your ovaries removed at the same time, even though there are no medical indications for doing so?
- Consider your medical story. How bad are the symptoms? How old are you? When did your mother have menopause— a possible indicator for you? If fifty-one is the average age for menopause, how far off are you? How much longer might you have to endure any symptoms you are having?
- As you should do for any elective surgical procedure, take a few days to imagine going down that pathway. How does it feel? Then live with a different choice for a few days, and compare your responses.

Second, information. Understand your doctor's position regarding the surgery. Understand what's involved, from before surgery to after surgery. Some women like to learn everything they can, practically down to studying the surgical manuals. Others want only a top line from their most trusted source.

Hysterectomies can be done abdominally, vaginally, or as a laporo-scopically assisted vaginal hysterectomy (LAVH). The choice can depend on the size of your uterus, how far it descends down the vagina, the preference and skill of the surgeon, and other circumstances (such as the position and size of fibroids) and the specific indications for surgery. Which approach is your surgeon thinking about? What are the pros and cons of leaving your ovaries in vs. removing them?

Third, action. There's no going back once the organs are out, so take your time getting to this point. If you do choose surgery, give some thought to how you want to mark the closure of your reproductive phase. Think about what the operation and the transition it signals will mean for you. One patient who was deeply affected by the necessity to have a hysterectomy felt that, when she reflected on it, her reproductive organs symbolized creativity and energy in her life. I asked if there was a physical object in her life that represented that same kind of creative force and suggested she might want to use that as a kind of touchstone for such feelings, to help make this transition feel more intentional and less abrupt. She had a special handcrafted necklace that worked for her in this way, and planned to wear it home from the surgery as well as afterward.

Then, re-reflection. If you do decide against surgery, you can revisit that choice if new symptoms present or other circumstances warrant. Give yourself a certain period of time, say three or six months, to re-reflect. If you have had the surgery, reflect on how you are feeling about it and what kind of steps can best support you in your current place.

Lisa's Story: Confronting Fears

Lisa hated the idea of surgery. She hated the idea of losing her "female parts." "I can't believe I'm even in this situation," said the forty-five-year-old mother of one adopted child. She had abnormal uterine bleeding, caused by hyperplasia with atypia, a precancerous condition. Sometimes it just happens. Lisa's choice was to try to manage the condition medically, which can be difficult as it requires high-dose medication and frequent testing to be sure the medication is working, or to have her uterus surgically removed. Lisa's doctor felt a hysterectomy was in order, along with removal of her ovaries. I was the second opinion.

Medically, either route was acceptable. Her hyperplasia was not immediately life-threatening. So Lisa and I explored her strong feelings against the surgery. "I just don't like invasive procedures," she said. As we talked, it emerged that she was more fearful of surgery than of cancer. Her grandmother had died on the operating table during heart surgery. "I couldn't bear to leave my daughter without a mother," she confessed. We also explored how the prolonged bleeding was interfering with Lisa's quality of life and how the idea of a hysterectomy intersected with her ideas around aging. Then we looked at the medical facts. Statistically, Lisa was much more likely to die from uterine cancer than from surgery. If she did not have the hysterectomy, she certainly might live a long and happy life through careful monitoring; on the other hand, the precancer would be there inside her, a constant threat.

Armed with an honest sense of her real fears and of the medical pros and cons, Lisa decided that it made more sense for her to have the hysterectomy.

Anxiety and Depression

There are distinct times in a woman's life when she is most susceptible to feelings of anxiety or depression (either separately or together). These are at puberty, premenstrually, in pregnancy and postpartum, and at perimenopause. The last can be a big one, as even women who have never encountered either condition before may be affected at perimenopause, so it can come as a big shock. All of these times are associated with a dip in estrogen. The estrogen loss (which affects neurotransmitters that regulate sleep centers and improve pain tolerance, among other things) doesn't cause the depression and anxiety, but it makes her biologically vulnerable.

At perimenopause, particularly, the onset of these symptoms can be scary. The characteristic "fuzzy thinking" can be misread as part of the aging process. Feelings about the end of one's reproductive life that are laid bare at this stage, regrets left over from the past, uncertainties about the transition ahead, and fear about what the future holds—specifically, "Is this what the rest of my life will be like?"—can be overwhelming. The Massachusetts Women's Health Study, a five-year longitudinal study of women forty-five to fifty-five, found that having a long menopause (over twenty-seven months) has been associated with an increased risk for depression, probably in response to the prolonged symptoms. Women with prior depression were especially vulnerable.

And yet while most women with severe hot flashes are willing to try a treatment like black cohosh, and a woman with vaginal dryness will use an estrogen cream, many women I see are reluctant to take steps to deal with anxiety and depression, or even to give them a name. There's a stigma around being labeled "depressed" or "anxious."

But these symptoms deserve to be addressed. I urge any woman who is feeling depressed or anxious (or often both) to acknowledge her symptoms and discuss them with her health care provider. Together you can put the problem on the table and explore it. Exercise, for example, is a terrific nonpharmaceutical way to find relief. There are other steps you can take, including support groups, botanicals, and pharmaceuticals. There is no reason to suffer unnecessarily. Yet I often see women who are adamantly against taking antidepressants (Prozac, Zoloft, etc.) because to do so would make their condition more real. They'd rather suffer.

Whether you choose medication or not, or other strategies or not, is ultimately up to you, dependent on your individual needs and feelings. But know that if you're not owning up to anxiety and depression in the first place, you can't make any healing choices.

On a side note, it's interesting that generally in our culture antidepressants are horribly overused and misused. We're medicating people who are just experiencing normal life, not unusual stress. During perimenopause, however, I see women's general openness toward antidepressants and antianxiety medication close down just when the need may be particularly acute.

If you decide to take medication for these conditions, check back in with yourself about your decision after a few months. You might go off the medication (under medical supervision) and see how you feel. Too many people go on the drugs because of changes in their life that are situational, but then the situation changes and they keep on automatically—unconsciously—taking the medication.

CENTERS OF WELLNESS MODIFICATIONS FOR TRANSITION

Lifestyle is huge in Transition! Every Center of Wellness plays a key role in how successfully you will be able to navigate this challenging time, when the signs of life's cumulative wear and tear are growing more apparent. Fortunately, many women find that they have more time to devote to tending their Centers of Wellness now that children are older and careers are established.

Take steps now, if you haven't already, to adopt heart-healthy measures. When researchers at New York's Albert Einstein College of Medicine looked at thirteen thousand women between the ages of forty-two and fifty-two for their future risk of heart disease, it was found that based on their current status, by age fifty-five more than half would need some type of lifestyle change or drug therapy to avoid heart attack or stroke. Perimenopause, the study concluded, was the prime time to make amendments. Waiting until after menopause to take steps to reduce the risk of heart problems may be waiting too long. Remember that heart disease is the number one killer of American women.

∅ Movement

Exercise becomes more important as you get older, not less. The benefits to both body and soul are profound. Weight-bearing exercise (with dietary changes and added calcium) is a no-risk way to provide yourself with more effective protection against osteoporosis. And walking briskly for a total of three hours a week can lower your heart attack risk by one-third—a benefit that will be increasingly important as you move past menopause.

- *Increase weight-bearing exercise.* Research clearly shows that running, walking, or weight training three times a week has a protective effect on the bones as well as the heart and the mind. Aim for five to six days a week for maximum benefit.
- *Befriend your body.* Start a stretching program or meditative-movement program (such as tai chi or yoga) that helps reduce stress while it moves your muscles.
- *Don't suffer.* If your exercise program isn't bringing you joy, ditch it and find something that does. There is a link between exercise, overall fitness, and reduced menopausal symptoms. And there's also a link between enjoying what you are doing and being committed enough to keep doing it.

∅ Nutrition

A generally well-balanced diet is as important as ever, but certain shifts can help you better weather perimenopausal symptoms and position you for strength in postmenopause.

- *Eat more soy.* Soy is the best source of isoflavones, phenolic compounds that are converted by the body into compounds that bind weakly to estrogen receptors. Consuming about 60 grams of soy protein per day may be helpful for short-term (two years or less) relief of hot flashes and night sweats. Consuming more than 90 grams has been documented to decrease cholesterol levels and may protect against bone loss. Can't swallow that much soy? Lentils and chickpeas are other sources of isoflavones.

- *Try black cohosh to reduce menopausal symptoms.* This herb, found in over-the-counter products such as Remifemin, appears to be the most effective herbal medicine out there. In numerous studies of short-term use, at doses of 20 milligrams twice a day it appears a safe and effective way to ease night sweats and hot flashes. Because long-term use has not been well studied, the *Physicians' Desk Reference* suggests use for only six months. But traditionally, this herb has been used over the course of years.

- *Try chasteberry (*Vitex agnus-castus*) for breast discomfort and heavy bleeding.* Although not well studied, this herb (also known as sage tree hemp, monk's pepper, and Indian spice) may inhibit prolactin, a natural hormone that affects the breast. It can also help ease the heavy bleeding of perimenopause by having a progesteronelike effect.

- *Proceed with care.* One-third of women use herbal remedies to treat their menopausal symptoms, but "natural" doesn't necessarily mean better. Obtain herbs only from trusted sources; if you're in doubt, listen to your instincts. There is no good medical evidence showing that wild or Mexican yam cream, ginseng, evening primrose, or the Chinese herb dong quai (when used alone) is effective in treating menopausal symptoms. Some herbs can be dangerous; for example, kava (extract of *Piper methysticum*) can lead to severe liver toxicity and in cases has led to the need for liver transplants, and death.

- *Continue to limit alcohol.* If you cut it out completely during your fertility years, you don't want to go back to the bottle now. Alcohol consumption is associated with breast cancer and memory loss, and cutting back may also help manage menopausal symptoms. Limit yourself to one drink a day or less.

- *Quit smoking.* In the Fertility Pathway, you might have quit out of concern for children you might bear. But if you didn't, quit now—for you.

✍ Mind

With the boundaries between body and soul especially permeable at this stage, you may feel a greater interest in Mind actions than during previous phases of your life.

- *Dialogue with your female soul.* What does that concept mean to you now? The end of the reproductive phase is a ripe time for such explorations because, let's face it, a huge amount of our self-concept as women is tied up in reproductive issues: trying to get pregnant, trying not to get pregnant, being a mother, having periods. Having a "conversation" with your female soul is a way to take your temperature about what being a woman means to you right now.
- *Learn relaxation techniques and use them, if you're not doing so already. If you are, use them more frequently.* Stress is known to increase the intensity, frequency, and discomfort of hot flashes. Whether you choose yoga, meditation, prayer, breathing, or the simple exercises covered in Part Two, really try to make one or more relaxation techniques part of your daily life.
- *Practice deep breathing or another breathing technique when hot flashes come on.* Bringing a focus on breathing has been found effective at triggering the relaxation response, which is generally good for reducing stress, and specifically helpful for reducing the severity of the flash.
- *Mentally reframe your experiences.* Use language that reflects the silver linings, not the thunderclouds, of the menopausal transition. Try to move your focus from the loss of the ability to have children, for example, to the freedom you will enjoy from birth control and from worries about pregnancy. My

friend Diane reframes the experience of a hot flash by calling it a "power surge"!

ℛ Spirit

Your Spirit needs in perimenopause become more important because you are moving toward a time in life that will be regulated less by the rhythms of the body and more by the needs of the soul. The specific actions and daily steps you might choose to take now are not different from those available to you at other times of life, except that you may naturally grow more interested in pursuing them. Seek a mix of time alone and time in communion with others. Don't let uncomfortable symptoms isolate you from the strength that company can provide. This tends to be a time of heightened introspection. Often women find that this time feels right to start a deeper exploration of their spirituality.

ℛ Sensation

Your sensate needs take on a practical dimension in perimenopause. Be aware of what those are and how you can nurture them. For some women, for example, low libido—low sexual desire—appears as a menopausal symptom that can cause continued problems postmenopausally if not addressed now. It can be caused by physical changes (specifically, waning testosterone and plummeting estrogen) as well as soul-level changes (such as perceptions around aging or the inability to reproduce, or some dimension of your current relationship). Low libido, as well as the other effects of perimenopause, therefore make the Sensation Center of particular importance now; you can't afford to ignore it. Note: There is scant evidence that botanicals help libido problems, and while some women find acupuncture effective, this has not been well studied, so you should proceed with that awareness.

- *Go natural.* Natural fabrics, that is. Synthetics can trap body heat, making hot flashes and night sweats feel even worse. Cottons and other fabrics that breathe feel better. Dress in layers to allow you to better regulate your body temperature.
- *Lighten your bedcovers.* Heavy quilts and comforters can trap heat and trigger flashes.
- *Lubricate.* Many women encounter vaginal dryness for the first time in their lives at this stage because declining estrogen levels can affect lubrication. Breasts swell less in response to stimulation and the vagina does not expand as much as before, which can add to discomfort during intercourse. Not surprisingly, this can affect desire, but even if a woman has reached an excited stage she may still not be adequately lubricated. Don't be afraid or embarrassed to try over-the-counter vaginal lubricants (Astroglide, K-Y jelly), even if you have never needed them before; they can make intercourse more pleasurable. Prescription estrogen replacement vaginal creams can also provide relief. Vaginal moisturizers (Replens) aren't the same things as lubricants, though, and aren't recommended for intercourse.
- *Keep expanding sexually.* Another common phenomenon is for couples, especially in longtime relationships, to fall into well-worn sexual habits. They may have explored freely in the early stages of their relationship (often before they had kids) but have now grown a little stale. A woman who is comfortable with exploring new ways to fulfill her and her partner's needs as sexual and sensual beings—while accommodating a changing physiology—brings a huge gift to the relationship. Read some of the excellent sexuality books (see "Readings and Resources") to explore new horizons. Attend a workshop on tantric sex. Take a sex vacation with your partner—where what you do *after* sightseeing is the trip's main purpose.

Sexuality Now and Beyond

Sexuality covers a broad gamut beyond the baby-making years (as, of course, it did during those years). By midlife new levels of personal maturity allow many women to acknowledge and act on needs that previously went unmet. Others begin an unconscious process of "closing down the store." They've internalized the cultural norms that youth is sexy and aging bodies are not. I often see women who confuse the normal symptoms of menopause, such as vaginal dryness (as the vagina gets thinner and has less natural lubrication) or thinned pubic hair and a flatter mons (the pad of tissue under the pubic hair), with "proof" that they are aging and therefore past their "sell-by date" in terms of sex. In reality, this phase of a woman's life can be a time of reclaiming her sensual and sexual self. But you won't be aware of your sexual feelings if you don't spend time making them conscious.

You can bring your feelings about sexuality now to greater consciousness in the same way you approach perimenopause itself:

Because there are no easy fixes to libido problems, exploring your own feelings around sexuality at this point in your life is critical. Probe all of the factors that can affect desire at any age, including schedule, stress levels, birth control method (e.g., hormone-based contraceptives), and the quality of your relationship.

What has changed for you, on both a body level and a soul level? What are your beliefs, whether or not they have ever been articulated, around aging and sex? What are your concerns around the physical changes you are experiencing due to menopause? How do they interface with your concerns around sexuality, if at all? The combination of physical changes as well as fears about no longer being physically or sexually attractive are a potent combination underlying libido problems for many women.

Do you know women who have gone through menopause and are clearly sexual, sensual beings? What images come to mind when you think of women at this stage of life in terms of sex? What are your greatest fears around sex and sexuality at this phase of your life?

How does your partner feel? Is he or she experiencing any age-related sexual changes? How have these affected your relationship? What changes have you made—again either consciously or unconsciously—as a result of these physical changes? Have you changed the frequency of your sexual encounters? Positions? The process? Are you now using products that you didn't use in the past, and if so, how do you feel about that? Does it impact your experience at all?

Libido is only the gatekeeper to a constellation of sexual changes. Learning a little bit about the normal changes in sexual response that begin around perimenopause can help reduce feelings that something is "wrong" with you. Besides problems with lubrication, you may find that the amount of time it takes to respond to stimulation is longer, your breasts don't swell as much in response to stimulation, and your vagina doesn't expand as much as it did before, which can add to discomfort during intercourse. It may take more stimulation to reach orgasm, and when you do, it may be less intense.

You'll then want to learn as much as you can about how these changes can be countered, which may involve sex counseling or relationship work as well as medical solutions. It's important to have a good physician with whom you are comfortable. If your longtime physician doesn't fill the bill, look for another! Although it is rare that the problem is as one-dimensional as a lack of testosterone (the hormone that controls desire), you should have your hormonal levels checked. Testosterone does drop at menopause. Studies have shown that for most women, however, supplemental testosterone does not help, unless there is a significant deficiency.

Remember as you reassess the needs of your body and soul in this center that you are entering a new phase of your sexuality, not the beginning of the end of it.

Chapter 12

The Transformation Pathway

After menopause, the second half of a woman's life

In youth a woman gives up her blood to nurture other life, and in age she keeps it to nurture her own wisdom.

⌐ OLD NORWEGIAN SAYING

Menopause—defined as the complete cessation of menstrual periods for one year—is the dividing line between the Transition Pathway and the Transformation Pathway. I call it Transformation because, from a hormonal standpoint as well as a situational one, the dramatic shift in your reproductive status means a time of significant changes, of transforming.

Transformation is a vast, long pathway. It covers, for the average woman, as long as her time on the Cycling, Fertility, and Transition pathways combined.

At menopause, a very real shift took place. Your reproductive ability ended. That change had repercussions in every dimension of your life, in both your body and your soul. Your monthly cycles stopped, and with them the cascade of hormonal rises and dips. The levels of different hormones circulating within you then stabilized at new levels, affecting every part of your body: your skin, your hair, your bones, your organs, even your brain. You wound up in a different place. You may feel different as a result—physically, emotionally, mentally, sexually. The choices you make every day may change as they respond to different needs. Your focus in life may be shifting as well, as your children grow and become less dependent, or you accept the reality that you will not be able to bear a child. You may discover more time for yourself. You may hear an insistent urge to explore interests long dormant or totally (even unexpectedly) new. Your work, your goals, your activities, and especially your relationships may be in flux, colored by the changes occurring at this time in your life, and your identity, your appearance, and your very sense of your life's purpose may all undergo a transformation as well.

Menopause was part of the design for your life as a woman. Nature intended childbearing to happen when all of the body's systems were at their prime in order to best foster healthy births. When the body reaches a point, usually sometime in the forties, when the aging of the body as well as of the eggs might hinder the odds of healthy procreation, the possibility of childbearing ends. Obviously, modern women don't expire as soon as their reproductive function is over. While the ability to reproduce is a central dimension of being female, it's not the sole defining aspect.

Thus, I would rather shift the emphasis at this pathway away from menopause itself. To define yourself as postmenopausal is physiologically accurate, but why call this part of life by the name of what it's *not*? I often see patients who focus only on the absence or emptiness that the loss of their periods (and their ability to bear a child) represents to them. But that medical reality is only one part of your life. To be sure, the changes that mark the fifties and beyond are not all rosy. I've never met a woman yet who was totally thrilled by every wrinkle. But it doesn't follow that every month of your life without a period is a downer! To the contrary, for many women this stable new place is an opportunity for a second wind and a second (or third or fourth) act, for newfound interests and continued self-discovery.

WHAT'S HAPPENING NOW: POSTCYCLING

What do a postmenopausal woman and a prepubescent girl have in common? Much more than you'd think. These two stages of life are the

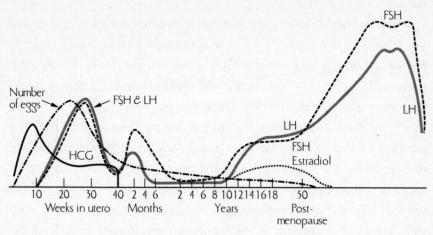

Eggs and hormones throughout the life cycle

two most alike from a hormonal perspective. You started out with very low and stable levels of estrogen and progesterone, with little fluctuation from day to day or week to week. Then after the dynamic years of menstrual cycles and the erratic years of perimenopause, you arrive back at a similar phase of relative stability. It's another cycle, your body coming back around to its beginnings, reproductively.

The key difference: As a preadolescent, you were an unconscious female. Now you are a conscious one (I hope). You have accrued more experience and wisdom and, potentially, deeper insight into who you are as a woman. Another way to think of it: If the Transition Pathway was the transportation, the Transformation Pathway is the destination, the pinnacle.

The other pathways of a woman's life were marked by clear, representative physiological phenomena: PMS, contraceptive needs, pregnancy, postpartum recovery, miscarriage, fertility problems, bothersome menopausal symptoms. All were landmarks of the reproductive system, and all are now behind you. Menopause marked the swan song of the big physical responses to the end of reproduction (hot flashes, low libido, depression, etc.). Once you are past it, most of those have disappeared or stabilized.

But for reasons having to do more with aging than with the end of your reproductive capacity, you can now expect to face an increasing risk of certain diseases and disorders. They are the result of the cumulative effects of habits, exposures, and wear and tear, on top of whatever your genetic vulnerability might be. However, disease is not an inevitable consequence of aging. In the Transformation Pathway, the physical challenges that may now possibly be on your horizon include osteoporosis, heart disease, and arthritis. They are not unique to women, nor will every woman face them. It's possible, indeed, to age without any of them—particularly if you live consciously and fuel your five Centers of Wellness on a regular basis. You can steer away from osteoporosis, never come near stroke or cancer. They are not inevitable physiological landmarks.

Osteoporosis and Heart Disease: Special Risks for the Unconscious

Two conditions warrant special note because they are frequently encountered by postmenopausal women. They're not inevitable events, not part of the inevitable cycle of things, and therefore I can't call them landmarks of this pathway. Rather, they are part of the steady progression of the aging process to which anyone is potentially vulnerable. Because both can be silent killers, women who live unconsciously—without paying attention to preventive steps—are especially at risk.

Osteoporosis

Old bone is continually being replaced with new bone. But after age thirty (when bone mass peaks), that rate of renewal (called remodeling) slows. Especially after fifty, bones begin to lose their density when old bone breaks down faster than new bone is made. Over time, the bones can change from looking like a dense, spongy honeycomb inside to a less dense web of larger holes. These more brittle bones cannot support weight as well and are more vulnerable to breaking. As many as one in two women will experience an osteoporosis fracture in her remaining lifetime. Fifteen percent will have a hip fracture, an especially difficult problem that often shoots a woman down a slippery slope of health problems and is associated with high death rates. As it is, far more women than men get osteoporosis because a woman's bones are smaller and lighter to begin with than a man's. When estrogen drops after menopause, your bones lose the protective effect that estrogen seems to play against bone loss, and the initial disadvantage can worsen as the rate of bone breakdown accelerates.

This problem is not inevitable or insurmountable. Though white and Asian women tend to be at higher risk than African-Americans, perhaps because of a genetic difference in bone metabolism, and osteoporosis can also run in families, a change in lifestyle habits can have a big impact on bone density, even reversing declines. (See "Centers of Wellness Modifications for Transformation" later in this chapter.)

Cardiovascular Disease

Breast cancer may get all the attention and worry, but cardiovascular disease is actually the number one killer of women. One in ten women ages forty-five to sixty-five—and one in three over age sixty-five—has some form of major heart or blood vessel disease. Cardiovascular problems kill more women than cancers of all kinds combined.

Again, your very best protection is lifestyle. A greater consciousness can literally save your life. Movement, Nutrition, and Mind exercises, for example, can go a long way toward lowering your risk. Being aware of your lipid profile (cholesterol levels) and blood pressure is also vital.

As always, this is information you need to check in with regularly. A lifestyle-based program can reverse existing heart disease as well as prevent heart disease from occurring, as research by Dr. Dean Ornish, founder of the Preventive Medicine Research Institute, has shown. Such an approach is truly integrative medicine in action. And Dr. Ornish points out that prevention is especially beneficial for women, who have less access to bypass surgery and angioplasty, and do less well postsurgically than men, yet have been found to reverse heart disease more easily than men.

And finally, you need to be aware of your symptoms, every day. Know your body and what's normal or not for you. Women's heart attack symptoms are not recognized as readily as men's because they can differ. Women may notice, for example, fatigue, shortness of breath, light-headedness, nausea, and confusion before they feel the classic tingling down the left side or crushing chest pain that a man might experience. Sometimes these symptoms are dismissed as "atypical" and therefore not worth the urgent attention given to a man whose complaints match a familiar picture of cardiovascular trouble. Well, that's because "typical" symptoms were based on studies of men! What appears "atypical" in a woman might in fact be quite typical for the female response; we just haven't done enough research yet to give us a good picture of cardiovascular disease in women. But if symptoms like those mentioned above are ignored by a woman or her doctor, her outcome might be more at risk than it should be.

It's incumbent on you, then, to tune in, listen, take any messages you hear seriously—and speak up!

It's not hard to listen to your body now. Your body has more to say, because it can't silently tolerate insult as it did before. This phenomenon is usually first noticed in your forties, and by fifty it is quite clear. I know that after I have spent a night on call, with a full day-night-day cycle on little or no sleep, I feel it much more quickly than I used to in my twenties. Compared to when I was younger, my body now complains more frequently and more loudly, expressing itself in slower reaction times, a crick in my shoulder, and less resilience than I once had. The tools in Part Two all help you heed your body's messages effectively. Because your body is sending you more communications than ever, you need to reply to it with more responses than ever.

Interestingly, as the body-level concerns of the reproductive system fade, soul-level concerns come even nearer to the surface. Previously in a woman's life, the axiom was "as above, so below." What you were feeling in your body was what you were feeling in your soul, whether you were conscious of that kinship or not. Now the reproductive system isn't feeling much of anything on a cyclical basis. But what it is feeling at a soul level (what I refer to often as the "female soul") runneth over. The biological changes brought by the end of one's reproductive life trigger a corresponding wealth of new emotional-spiritual considerations.

The landmarks a woman encounters on the Transformation Pathway, therefore, are chiefly landmarks of the soul. While the exact terrain of this pathway is, as ever, different for every woman, the following turning points almost always loom large. And as ever, you can close your eyes to them, or address them head-on.

LANDMARK: LIFE'S PURPOSE

Bette, 55:
⸏ *"It seems like that part of my life when I was worrying about getting my periods, worrying about getting pregnant, worrying about my kids, all belong to someone else. I remember it in great detail, the way I remember my childhood, but it's in the distance. For so many years, I was always worrying*

about the things related to my reproductive system. Now I worry about the impact I want my life to make on the larger world."

Barbara, 53:
⌐ *"I heard about the empty nest syndrome, but I didn't really understand what it meant until Robbie went away to school. I miss having him around so much! I don't know what to do with myself. I find myself drifting around the house thinking about him, thinking about me. I didn't expect I would be weepy and so out of sorts."*

Pearl, 67:
⌐ *"Stan gets on my nerves. He's retired and I'm retired, but he doesn't know what to do with himself except bug me. I'm busy working on this idea I have for an Internet business. I've finally figured out a nice setup for what to do with myself and now I have to help him figure out one of his own or he'll be the end of me."*

Madelyn, 56:
⌐ *"If you had told me ten years ago that I would be giving a presentation at a national conference in an all-new field, I never would have believed you. It's so different and unexpected. It's great!"*

Having a reproductive life, for better or for worse, shaped a good bit of your life's purpose premenopausally. The most significant embodiment of this for most women is motherhood. Raising a child shapes and re-shapes your life in countless ways—the career choices you make, your interests, your priorities, your stress level. Choosing not to have children gives it another shape, allowing different choices and presenting other realities. So does a fertility quest, whether you became pregnant or not.

Now what? Finding yourself in a new place in life is an ideal time to reinvestigate who you are and what you would like to do with your energy. What is your intention? Stay the course you're already on? Try something different? What's your role in life after your reproductive potential is removed from the equation? For some women, the disappearance of the menstrual cycle raises fears about their value not just to their partners but within the family, the workplace, and the culture at large. Those fears may interfere with the ability to see that the transition also represents a new level of freedom. No more cycles, no more babies (or fear of pregnancy, or expectations for pregnancy), less dependency, fewer mundane daily responsibilities, more seniority and certainty. For many, it's the first opportunity in decades to make choices that are entirely reflective of who she is and what she really wants, whatever that is. We all know women who after menopause go back to school, start their own businesses, travel the world, or embark on profound spiritual journeys. The second half of life seems to be a time when women are most "out there" in the world. It's not coincidence. Rather, it's the confluence of many factors all coming together to raise the questions "Who am I? What is my purpose in life? How do I really want to spend my life?"

You can use the Feedback Loop to make soul-focused decisions, just as you can those that emphasize the body. The possibilities are so varied and individualized that I can't possibly walk you through each one. But let me show you what the process looks like generally.

First, reflection. These questions start from the same place as every choice, with an effort to listen to what's in your soul right now. All of the same tools previously introduced can help. Some women find it especially useful to talk with other women on the Transformation Pathway, comparing notes and drawing inspiration and courage from one another.

- What are your expectations? How do you imagine spending the next decade? How, in the past, have you pictured yourself at fifty, sixty, seventy?
- Who are your role models? If Gram was a cool MD who rode a Harley and traveled the world for Doctors Without Borders, your expectations might be different from a woman whose grandma knit and watched soaps all day in an old-age home. Which role models (within your family or without) appeal to you?
- What do you love? What would it look like if your life was filled with the energy you get from doing what you really love?

- What have you accomplished so far with your life, personally as well as professionally? How does that make you feel? Fulfilled and satisfied? Proud but a little empty? Is who you are externally on a daily basis in tune with who you feel you are inside?
- What have you not been able to accomplish yet? What have you always wanted to pursue but never quite got around to? Are there goals percolating on some back burner that have always intrigued you but been dismissed by the more practical voices in your head (and the more pressing needs of the time)? (See box below.)
- Give yourself permission to think without limitations, then explore without limits. Do not be limited by practicalities. Dream big.

Brainstorming Beyond

Here's a useful and fun exercise for imagining the possibilities for your future. Your brain is wired, out of long habit, to render opinions about its every thought. So while part of you says, "Gee, I might like to do X," another part of you almost instantaneously conjures up all the reasons you *can't* do X. *It's not practical. It's too expensive. Someone might think I'm crazy. Women my age don't do that kind of thing. I've never done it before.* It's hard to get momentum going when you're your own worst critic.

Instead, be aware of that voice. Know that it's active and cautious. Then set it aside. Put on the sky's-the-limit cap that people in business and creative fields use when they brainstorm, following the cardinal brainstorming session rule: No self-censoring. There are no bad ideas. At this stage, everything is viable, nothing is criticized. It's a very freeing rule, because nobody in the room is worried about sounding stupid or impractical. Nobody is interested in what's actually possible, only in the *possibilities,* however off-the-wall.

Your task is to generate as many possibilities as you can for what you might like to do with your life. Set an absurdly high goal, such as fifty ideas. That lets you think wildly; you're not unconsciously pruning and shaping a "good" list of five or ten.

It takes a lot of energy to push beyond the constraints of our culture, the limitations of your experience, and your tendencies to negative thinking. Brainstorming empowers your can-do voice, rather than the more familiar voice that tells you why you *can't* do something.

Then reflect on your list. Which of the ideas really calls to you? Are you more passionate about some things than others? That's important to know. That's data. Rule out nothing at this point. Go on to gather information about several of the ideas that intrigue you most, again, without an eye to plausibility. At this point, you're still in the realm of "what if." Gathering information (talking to people, looking up info online, going to the library, contacting an association, etc.) is not the same as making a commitment. Sit with your reactions and your new knowledge and take one small step toward something. You can always back off if something doesn't feel right. But through successive small steps, you'll move forward. And if you feel moved to begin with a big step, great! Go through the Feedback Loop with it, and if it still feels right, go for it.

Second, information. At this point you may or may not have a plan (or plans) percolating in your head. Zero in on a few ideas that appeal to you. It doesn't matter whether they seem like realistic plans or off-the-wall notions. Perhaps they're a continuation of something you're already doing now, in your career or your personal life. Find out what pursuing or continuing this path would take. Gather information about the degree you always wanted or the trip you've dreamed of.

Assess your health in light of your dreams, too. Are there steps you can take that will give you more energy, more strength, better endurance, a greater sense of fulfillment and balance? Review your Centers of Wellness needs and consult with your physician as needed.

Third, action. Do something. Try something. Sign up for a workshop on starting a business. Find someone who is doing something you might like to try and invite him or her for coffee or have a fifteen-minute phone conversation, to learn more about it. Small steps beget big steps. Or start with a big step if it feels right to you.

Take one small step and see how it feels, and what else it inspires.

Then, re-reflection. Continually check in after each step you take. Do you need to change course or just make a slight course correction? Explore something else?

Kit's Story: A Spiritual Journey

Kit is sixty, a fact that amazes her every single day. She has been married to the same man since her mid-twenties, raised two sons and a daughter, and is now a grandmother (another fact she finds incredible). She is an insurance adjuster but thinks that what she really wants to do is write.

Menopause was a major transition for Kit, which put her in a depressed state for several years. Her physical symptoms had been mild, but a mental fog persisted. She took hormone replacement therapy for a few years at forty-nine, then went off it to see how she did. She felt fine and did not resume the medication. She did continue to feel slightly depressed, however. "I didn't feel old and didn't look old," she recalls. "But I worried that I *was* old."

Much of her life had been defined by being a mother. She was excited about having grandchildren, but it wasn't the same. After a year or so of feeling at loose ends, she began using many the Consciously Female tool kit exercises, especially Dialoguing. The message she heard was that she had been mourning her maternal life and was now ready to explore what it meant to be a postfertility woman today. *Fair enough,* she thought. *What now?*

Not exactly sure where to begin, she took a cultural anthropology course and another in women's history at a local college. Through the college, she joined an educational trip to Hawaii to study the traditional role of women in its native culture, something she never would have considered before.

Gradually Kit realized that she had always had an interest in life's spiritual side that she had not fully explored before. She took more classes and made more study trips, to Mexico, Peru, and other places. At one point she realized that she wasn't interested in acquiring a degree, but she was hungry to learn more. Kit has recently begun working with shamans and other alternative healers to explore her own mental and physical health. "I have a sense I want to do more with this at more of a public level," she says, "but I don't know what that is yet." So she's continuing to work at remaining open and receptive to where that path might lead her.

Trish's Story: About-Face

When she went through menopause at fifty, Trish was unhappily married, a busy physician, and the mother of two teenagers. Twelve years later, she is leading an entirely different life. "I can't say that menopause had anything to do with it, but somewhere afterward I made a transition from being a totally unconscious women to a conscious one who is able to be aware of and value herself as a female," she explains, wonder at her new life still strong in her voice.

Her feelings of dissatisfaction burbled below the surface for years. She had begun to feel she had to go live on her own, but lacked the courage or wisdom to know how to go about it. Then one day at age fifty-two, while mulling her situation, Trish was walking to her hairdresser when she heard an unfamiliar, insistent voice within her telling her she needed to go to Bali. "It was so different from my usual terrified control-freak voice," she remembers. "It was so calm and authoritative."

At the salon, a woman she knew slightly came over to say hello— and mentioned her forthcoming monthlong trip to Bali. Trish couldn't believe the coincidence. "In the space of a half hour, this totally weird, out-of-the-blue idea started to become a plan," Trish says. "I went home and announced to my husband, children, and patients that I was going to Bali for a month."

She did. On her last day there, she was overcome with tears. "I knew that I couldn't simply leap back into my former life," she remembers. And so she didn't. She left her husband and quit her practice. With both children in college, she and her soon-to-be ex-husband agreed to sell their old family home, and Trish downsized into a condo.

Friends and family were baffled—how could she leave everything that had figured so prominently in her life? But Trish felt ecstatic. "While I was away, I had begun to confront my fears of living and of dying. I realized I was in a new story. I call it 'Following the Breadcrumbs,' like Hansel and Gretel. I'm still following their trail, not sure where the crumbs lead."

After much introspection, Trish decided that she had come to believe in the power of what she calls "the feminine energy" within her. "For a long time as a wife and as a physician, and as the mother of older children, I felt that I was using only my male energies," she explains. "Now it's different. I have discovered a luscious, horizontal, and inclusive balance within me of both the male and the female.

"So much of what we understand about being female is caught up with fertility and youth. And when that passes, we have to delve deeper to find our next definition of womanliness, of the feminine. That's what I found in the years after menopause, my own unique sense of the feminine."

Marguerite's Story: Sexual Awakenings

A widow for ten years, Marguerite's sex life had been hung on a peg in the back of her closet for a long time. Even when her husband was alive, she had not explored her sexuality much. "I adored Ben. But we married young, had three children, and fell into traditional ruts," she explained to a Consciously Female group I had started. "Once a week, him on top, me half thinking about what I was going to fix for dinner tomorrow. I was one of those women who didn't understand what the fuss about orgasms was all about, because I hardly ever had one and, truth be told, never expected one."

Now fifty-six, Marguerite fell in love—hard—with James, an architect and widower whom she met when he patronized the plant nursery where she worked. Before long, sex was all she could talk about at our group gatherings. Or rather, it was the framework she'd found for describing her whole life now. Being in love with James totally energized her—the way it galvanizes a woman at any age. But for Marguerite, the sexual dimension of the relationship came as a new and delightful surprise.

"I had never allowed myself to express myself sexually before," she told us one day. "I just did what I thought I was supposed to do. But things feel so different now. Generally, I've grown used to doing what makes me happy and not caring about what other people think, so that attitude seems to have spilled over into my sex life, too." Marguerite confided that she takes the initiative often in the couple's sexual encounters—something she almost never did with her husband. She feels freer now to be creative about where and how their sex play proceeds. Once the passive partner, she's now willing to be the aggressor. James loves this about her and finds it incredibly sexy—which emboldens Marguerite and encourages her further.

Over time, our group began seeing a new, more sparkling Marguerite. The life-affirming nature of her relationship with James had empowered her in other ways. "It sounds strange, but as I explored my sexual self I learned more about my whole self," she explained. "I felt more powerful, more willing to take risks." Six months after they'd met, Marguerite sold the house she'd lived in throughout her marriage and moved in with James. They also began looking for a property that they could renovate and landscape together.

Marguerite's awakening inspired another group member, too. Lynne, a newlywed in her twenties, felt emboldened by Marguerite's tales to become more assertive about her own sexual needs. "I saw how enriched and comfortable Marguerite felt about this sex life that she was totally satisfied with," Lynne told us later, "and thought, 'Gee, why wait until I'm fifty? I need to be brave and try things and have a great sex life I enjoy right from the start of this relationship!' After seeing where it took Marguerite, there's no telling what will happen to me!"

LANDMARK: AGING

Diane, 56:

⟡ *"I'm supposed to be depressed now, old and used up. But I feel freer than I have felt since I was a teenager. I am so much less concerned about what people think about me. I worry much less about other people's agendas. It's as if I finally get to answer the question 'What about me?'"*

Toni, 58:

⟡ *"I am haunted by images of my mother and grandmother as they got older. They were fragile and increasingly irrelevant. I don't want that to be me. I keep shopping for better role models for myself."*

Charmaine, 57:

⟡ *"I am proud of my body, of the fact that I still wear a size six. I exercise for two hours every morning with my trainer. I am in better shape than my daughter. I like when we're mistaken for sisters!"*

Cindy, 64:

⟡ *"I am always startled when I have to tell someone my age. I still think of myself as forty-five."*

Your physical experience of aging is yours alone and depends on many variables, including genetics, lifestyle, and life circumstances. But all women will have in common the experience of facing certain emotional and spiritual issues related to getting older, and this makes it a major landmark on the Transformation Pathway. If there's one thing of which we can be sure, it is this: We are all going to die eventually. Yet our culture at large, and each of us individually, expends an enormous amount of energy repressing that fact. I faced earlier than most people the death of my parents—my mom when I was thirty and my dad when I was thirty-six. I'll always remember being at the bedside of my father and experiencing an enormous amount of anxiety and rage over whether everything was being done for him that could possibly be done. I stayed up nights about the possible impact of doing this vs. that. Wanting the best medical care for a loved one is appropriate, of course, but I took my concern to the extreme. One day a good friend to whom I was railing said to me, sweetly and philosophically, "Tracy, just remember, we all have to die of something." It was one of those revelatory moments. I realized that my fear was not about whether all the right things were being done for my father in life, but about the fact that he would eventually die.

Losing my parents has given me a consciousness of death that has heightened my appreciation of life—when I allow myself to live with that consciousness. That's why I think that death consciousness is important at this age, even though being postmenopausal certainly doesn't mean you're suddenly at death's door. As Joan Borysenko says, "The question is not whether we will die; the question is how we will live." And very often how we live on this pathway is a reflection of our unconscious relationship with death. Face it straight on, make it conscious, and you are more likely to live fully, passionately.

That can be harder than it sounds. Though death is inevitable for all of us, we live in a youth culture. The ideal is frozen at glossy, long-limbed, pert-breasted twenty-five, maybe thirty! This reality is beginning to change as the collective, influential force of the baby boom hits its sixties. We see more silver-haired models in ads and fewer grannies in rockers. Still, the pervasive vibe in this country is that young equals all that is sexy, happening, cool, desirable, and alive.

And so a woman who suddenly finds that her breasts are falling and her vagina is dry gets scared. It's upsetting that cute guys call her "ma'am" now and nobody flirts anymore. She feels threatened by the younger, more vibrant women she sees everywhere, while blinding herself to the sight of all the older, vibrant, cool women who are also out there, and in ever-increasing numbers. Maybe nobody's looking for her advice anymore at work or at home. There are no more noses to wipe. Maybe she looks in the mirror and sees the first hints of her mother's face staring back. Or she can't stop thinking of her grandmother, shut away in a nursing home for years, and wonders if that will be her fate as well.

These perceptions mightily influence the steps we take every day. There's nothing wrong, for example, with plastic surgery and a hypervigilance about weight, provided you make those choices consciously and proceed in a safe manner. Nor is there anything wrong with going gray and worrying (a little) less about your waistline. As with anything else, you can take steps based on a consciousness of your feelings about aging, or you can act unconsciously. In a single day I can see two fifty-something women who both look trim, stylish, and gorgeous, and after a few minutes' conversation it will be clear which one is making the effort because she's running scared from aging and which one is doing so fully engaged with her Transformation-phase life. Maybe you know both kinds of women, too. Which would you rather be?

The Japanese have a word, *shibui,* for a certain type of beauty that only time can reveal. It's felt that a woman's life experiences and personality are reflected in her skin and the lines and marks on her face. A healthy woman is one who can look in the mirror and see *shibui.*

As the musician and cancer survivor David Bailey says, "You don't want to wait until you're dying to begin to embrace life fully."

First, reflection. Explore your feelings around aging. What are your fears? What are your hopes? What does being "old" mean to you? What does it look like?

Explore your feelings around death. Have you ever thought seriously about your own death? What have been your experiences with death? What are your greatest fears? Greatest hopes?

Review your experiences with older people. Who do you admire as a role model? Who is the opposite for you?

How are you feeling now? Use the Five-Center Review, Body Monitoring, and the Body Scan. What do you like about your body now? What do you not like? What do you wish were different?

Second, information. Distinguish between myths and facts around aging. Be careful—there are a lot of assumptions mixed in there. Among them: Older women aren't sexy. Older women can't_____. (Fill in the blank: can't climb mountains, run marathons, get medical degrees, make headlines.) Find sources of information you can trust.

- Continue working with your health care provider. Get an annual checkup to screen for those sometimes silent diseases that begin manifesting much more frequently at this age, especially osteoporosis, hypertension, heart disease, and colon cancer. Find out what kinds of tests are recommended for your age. I give all of my patients a bone density scan at age fifty, to use as a baseline. The U.S. Preventative Task Force recommendation is age sixty. Other tests you need regularly: lipid profiles (cholesterol tests), mammograms, colonoscopies, and Pap smears.

Learn what kind of lifestyle changes are best suited to your health and circumstances. I have seen women make many powerful changes in this phase of their life after learning the compelling evidence about, for example, dietary calcium or the protective benefits of something as easy and basic as walking. Many women have a sense of finally having the time to focus on their health.

Third, action. Whatever choices you face, take care to be proactive, rather than driven along by fear or intertia.

Then, re-reflection. Your choices around aging, including choices about your appearance and your activities, can always change as new information gets factored in.

Jennifer's Story: A Well-Rounded Approach

"I never thought I would be into health like I am right now," confesses Jennifer, fifty-seven. She'd always been moderately active but never focused especially on her health until she experienced an early menopause, in her early forties. That passage proved to be fairly smooth, though, and she continued as before until she was fifty-three, when she developed breast cancer, which was found on a routine mammogram. It was small and localized to the breast, and the treatment she underwent was a mastectomy followed by tamoxifen, a drug that acts like an antiestrogen in the breast and is a standard treatment for many breast cancers.

As a side effect of the drug, however, Jennifer gained forty pounds and began to experience menopausal symptoms such as hot flashes and mood swings. (Tamoxifen not only has antiestrogenic effects on the breast—which is why it is used—but also on the central nervous system. This can cause the vasomotor symptoms associated with menopause, only often much more severely and with very limited treatment possibilities, since hormones are not an option.) The symptoms were bothersome and the weight gain worrisome, since diabetes ran in her family. Jennifer was referred to the Duke Center for Integrative Medicine to help with these problems, since conventional approaches have not been found to be very helpful with these symptoms.

"The breast cancer was a wake-up call!" Jennifer says now. "I think somebody upstairs could have picked something subtler to make me pay more attention to my health, but I'm grateful it all worked out the way it did." What worked out is that Jennifer totally reframed her approach to the second half of her life.

She began focusing not on the weight loss or hot flashes specifically but on her overall attitudes to her Centers of Wellness. Jennifer learned breathing exercises, began swimming and walking short distances, and started Journaling as a stress outlet. Sure enough, she lost only a small amount of weight but felt something kindling within her—a loving attention to her body that had gone ignored for decades.

Over time, Jennifer began to fine-tune her wellness plan and add to it as she felt ready. She joined a gym and opted to work with a personal trainer to learn how to use the weight-training equipment. ("I never thought I'd be a person with a personal trainer," she laughs. "It sounded so Hollywood—but it comes with the price of my health club membership!") Now she works out three times a week doing weights and cardiac work, and keeps exercise balls and weights at home for when she can't get to the gym. "If I don't do it, I feel lousy," she says.

Nutritionally, she added vitamins C and E, began drinking more water, and gradually increased her fiber intake and cut back on sugar. "I don't deny myself much," she explains, "but I have found that a half ounce of fudge satisfies my cravings and then I don't need more."

She began to indulge in weekly massages "more for the stress-releasing benefit to my mind than my body." With her newfound energy, Jennifer became more involved in her local church, taking on leadership roles in programming and the choir that she never considered before. Instead of filling her free time by sitting and eating in front of the TV, she began taking voice and piano lessons, and reading.

"One thing seemed to lead to another," Jennifer explains. "I didn't set out to reform my whole life, but that's ultimately what has happened." Over fourteen months she lost thirty-five pounds and lowered her cholesterol by twenty points. Her hot flashes, which responded to the lifestyle changes she made, particularly the exercise and stress-reduction techniques, waned, although she still has them occasionally.

"I'm enjoying life so much more than before," Jennifer says with a laugh. "Now I call menopause 'the pause that refreshes.'"

Liz's Story: Who's a Matriarch?

I could tell Liz was impatient the minute I walked in the door. Her purse was poised upright on her knees, and her fanny was perched on the edge of her chair. She seemed ready to leave almost before I said hello.

She interrupted my usual new-patient small talk with a tight smile. "I'm new in town. I need a refill of my prescription for my hormone replacement therapy," she explained. Liz wanted me to write the necessary prescription and send her on her way, thank you.

I slipped into my let's-talk-about-your-history mode. Liz was fifty-six and had not had her period in almost ten years. She seemed reluctant to answer my usual intake questions. But she did disclose with a certain pride that since she had begun HRT, she had never missed a day, and she was taking it in such a way that she had never missed a period, either!

I explained that I needed to look at her chart and perform a quick exam before I prescribed anything. And I had a few questions. For example, had she found her menopause troubling in any way, either physically or mentally?

By now Liz looked slightly concerned that she had stumbled onto the wrong doctor for her. She explained that she didn't really know how menopause had felt because the HRT erased her symptoms. "That's just the way I like it. I didn't have to deal with the menopause issue at all."

I shifted the conversation to the rest of her life. Liz had been a widow and was newly remarried to a man with whom she was very happy. Her husband had many children and grandchildren who were around a lot. An overnight matriarch, Liz said she needed to stay as energetic, calm, and "normal" as possible to keep up. "The last thing I need is to have a problem with my hormones," she said.

I shared my impression that she had allowed everything to change in her life—her spouse, her hometown, her extended family—except her perception of herself as a woman. What was she afraid of? I gently asked. Liz thought a moment. "I am not ready to be the village crone. I want to be that youthful woman playing tennis in the TV commercials. I don't want to be the wise elder."

Though she did indeed look like the youthful women in the TV ads, thanks to an excellent diet and vigorous physical exercise, she *was* a wise elder to this large, affectionate network of children, stepchildren, and grandchildren. And I could tell from the proud, involved way she talked about her extended family that she enjoyed the busy role. Taking HRT seemed to symbolize to her that she could still keep up with "the kids."

I explained to Liz that I could find no medical reason not to continue her prescription but that the risks and benefits might be different now from when she began it. I also pointed out that the comfort it provided during her menopause transition was probably no longer necessary, and that while it could give her certain protective benefits against osteoporosis and colon cancer, her sound diet and excellent exercise routines probably gave her all the protection she needed. Meanwhile, the HRT did increase her risk of heart problems and breast cancer. I asked her to think about coming off the medication as an experiment, "to see if it's you or the medication that is doing so well."

She asked to think about it. And then, a few months later, she made another appointment. "I'm ready to try a break from the HRT," Liz said. "A test." Although she might want to go back on it, she was now curious, she told me, to see what it felt like to be her, on the Transformation path. To her surprise, she noticed little difference. She never did go back.

CENTERS OF WELLNESS MODIFICATIONS FOR TRANSFORMATION

Here's your perfect opportunity to nurture your Centers of Wellness like you've never done before. The Transformation Pathway gives a woman both the incentive and the means for optimizing her health across the five centers. You can take many practical steps to reduce the risk factors associated with aging—and you probably have more time to devote to yourself than you've had in years. Take advantage of this unique situation and you're apt to be rewarded with a more robust body and a flourishing soul.

ℬ Movement

If anything, this is a time of life to rev up rather than slow down. Give in to stereotypical imagery of grannies in rockers and you really will find yourself becoming one. The protective effects of exercise in post-menopausal women are plentiful. Some excellent choices now:

- *Walk.* What could be simpler? You don't have to ascribe to the "no pain, no gain" theory of workouts. A massive survey of seventy-four thousand women ages fifty to seventy-nine found that women who walked or exercised vigorously for at least two and a half hours per week reduced their risk of cardiovascular disease by about 30 percent. The more the women exercised, the more benefit they got. But women who spent even a small amount of time walking—more than ten minutes per day—reduced their risk of stroke and heart attack by about 9 percent.

  Walking is also weight-bearing exercise, which helps strengthen bone mass. Exercising more than twice a week has been shown to result in a significant increase in bone density after fourteen months. In comparison, women who do not exercise lose bone.

- *Weight-train.* Like walking, lifting weights is a weight-bearing exercise that protects the bones. A regular strength-training program will also add muscle and increase your metabolic rate, which will make weight loss easier. Many women find it harder to maintain their optimal weight in Transformation because of a slower metabolism. (Note that swimming is a terrific exercise but is not weight-bearing; you need to supplement a swim program with a strength-training one.)
- *Do it for your body as much as your weight.* You might not notice any dramatic weight loss from regular exercise, but you will nevertheless be reaping benefits. Exercise reduces intra-abdominal fat, a hidden risk factor for many chronic illnesses.

ℬ Nutrition

- *Go green.* Greens have always been good for you, but now they are also important to help protect your bones. Eat *at least* four servings per week of calcium-rich green leafy vegetables. Choices include broccoli, collards, cabbage, lettuce, Brussels sprouts, and other kinds of greens. Even iceberg lettuce offers some vitamins A and C, especially in the outer leaves, according to one USDA study, though generally the darker the lettuce the better. Greens also contain vitamin K. A study of more than seventy-two thousand women found that those who consumed the least vitamin K had a 30 percent increased risk of hip fracture compared with those who ate at least the equivalent of a half cup of spinach daily.
- *Increase dietary calcium.* After fifty, you need 1,200 to 1,500 milligrams daily. Switch to calcium-fortified products such as orange juice, breakfast cereal, or ice cream. Other sources: low-fat and nonfat milk, tofu, canned salmon with bones, and the aforementioned greens.
- *Keep eating protein.* In the interests of cutting calories and fat, some women accidentally cut out too much protein. Too little can increase the risk of osteoporosis. The Framingham

Osteoporosis Study found that of men and women ages sixty-eight to ninety-one, those who consumed the least protein had significantly more bone loss than those who consumed the most. Aim for a range of 68 to 83 grams of protein daily. Vegetarians may be at added risk of osteoporosis because vegetable protein sources do not foster bone mineral density the way that animal proteins (meats, poultry, eggs, cheese) do.

- *Focus on fiber.* Older adults who eat just two slices of whole-wheat bread or one serving of high-fiber cereal daily can lower their risk of cardiovascular disease risk by 21 percent, compared with those who consume minimal fiber. Dark breads (wheat, rye, pumpernickel) were found especially useful in one study of 3,588 adults. But check the label to be sure dark bread is actually made with whole grains and not merely darkened with artificial coloring. Fruits, vegetables, and dried beans as well as whole wheat and other whole grains are all excellent sources of fiber.

- *Drink consciously.* Although research has shown that alcohol may have cardiac benefits, that research was done on men. For men, it appears that moderate amounts of alcohol—two drinks a day—raise the level of high-density lipoproteins (the "good" cholesterol). It also helps keep platelets from sticking together, which may help prevent clotting and therefore heart attacks. For women, it's not clear whether there are any benefits, and it *is* clear that consumption of more than one alcoholic drink per day is associated with an increased risk of breast cancer, especially postmenopausally. If you are already a drinker, weigh the risks and benefits of continuing for your individual health profile. If you have a family history of breast cancer, for example, you might abstain on the side of caution. Be vigilant about quantity; only one drink a day is the recommended amount, half of what a male can tolerate, because women get a higher concentration of alcohol in their blood even when they drink the same amount, and are more susceptible to alcohol-related organ damage, according to the

National Institute on Alcohol Abuse and Alcoholism. If you don't already drink, don't start. Sometimes women who have not processed what the end of reproduction means for them turn to alcohol for comfort, avoiding the potentially painful work of emotional processing.

- *Try tea.* Regular consumers of black tea have a reduced risk of osteoporosis. Green tea is a good source of vitamin K and of antioxidants; when consumed daily, it can protect against breast cancer and colon cancer.

- *Quit smoking.* If the desire to avoid lung cancer hasn't been enough of an incentive, here's another one: Studies of twins have found that long-term smoking increases the risk of bone fracture by about 40 percent. A study of more than 116,000 female nurses ages thirty-four to fifty-nine found an increased risk of hip fractures of 20 percent among those who puffed between one and twenty-five cigarettes a day, and 40 percent in those who smoked more than twenty-five cigs a day. Smoking also depletes vitamin C, a deficiency that can lead to brittle bones.

- *Sunbathe.* It's estimated that as much as 40 percent of the population over age fifty is deficient in vitamin D. A seventy-year-old woman would need to drink six glasses of milk a day to get the recommended amount of vitamin D (600 IU) from her diet. Although older skin has a reduced ability to produce vitamin D from sunlight, a combination of regular sun exposure, fortified milk, egg yolks, fatty fish, and possibly a supplement is doable for most women. Use sunscreen to protect skin when you're outdoors, but you can go without it for ten to fifteen minutes (ideally not at midday) for purposes of vitamin D absorption.

- *Review and revise your supplements.* Several nutrients play important roles in preventing the onset of osteoporosis, including calcium, vitamin D, magnesium, vitamin K, and boron. I recommend increasing calcium supplementation to between 1,200 and 1,500 milligrams daily (the total daily recom-

mended); consult your doctor about the best form of supplementation for you. Magnesium is needed for efficient vitamin
D metabolism and helps balance the constipation that calcium
consumption can cause. Take 400 milligrams of magnesium
daily. Vitamin K is needed by the body to activate the primary
protein used for bone synthesis, osteocalcin. If you have been
taking a multivitamin for a long time, read the fine print to see
how much of these various nutrients you are receiving, and
where you need to supplement. Don't rely on supplements to
the exclusion of smart nutrition, though. The very best source
of nutrients at any age is through fresh food sources.

ℬ' Mind

Even though life may not appear to be as stressful on this pathway compared to the others (because by now many women have their routines
and priorities figured out, and fewer drains on their emotions in terms
of child rearing and career building), don't fool yourself. Taking on new
challenges and new adventures and adjusting to the normal changes of
life, both positive and negative, can take a toll. Grown children and mature careers can still vex you almost as much as before.

Therefore it continues to be vital to stay grounded and centered.
Pursue the same Mind steps that worked in previous pathways, or experiment with new ones.

ℬ' Spirit

Your definition of family is liable to look different in the Transformation
Pathway. Children move out. Perhaps parents needing care move in.
Women, on average, outlive their spouses. You might have more time
now for friends than previously. What doesn't change—indeed, what
for many women intensifies—is a need for a connection to things outside yourself.

- *Replace lost connections with new ones.* As loved ones move out of your life, bring new ones in. You may need to make a concerted effort to move past your comfortable routines in order to find these new connections—for example, by joining a group, volunteering in some capacity, or reaching out to friends or relatives whom you know well but are not especially close to yet. A social network is essential to buffering against adversity.
- *Develop a personal definition of spirituality.* For many women this pathway leads to an intensified spiritual journey. For example, you may make a deeper exploration of or commitment to your faith, or explore spiritual traditions different from your own. Spend time thinking about how your spirituality is expressed in your life now, and how you feel about that. Consider more actively pursuing answers to questions of faith that you may have thought about for a long time (or that have come up recently). Studies have shown that people who attend weekly religious services live longer and stay healthier, perhaps because spiritual well-being boosts immune function.
- *Explore death.* Try writing your own epitaph. Rather than a macabre exercise, it's a freeing one that forces you to contemplate your life as a whole, and how you best wish to spend the rest of it.

ℰ' Sensation

- *Think about what brings you sensual pleasure.* Often women in the Transformation Pathway look up for the first time in many years and realize that they have made a habit of putting others' pleasures first. Do you wear the perfume that your partner favors, or do you really enjoy it, too? Are the radio stations set in your car your personal favorites? Who do you dress for? Reevaluate your sensual "greatest hits"—or experiment with new ones—so you don't accidentally fall into ruts or overlook your sensate needs entirely.

• *Give yourself permission to do a Sensation makeover.* Often women will find that the styles of clothes or scents that they reached for in the past don't seem to fit anymore. Explore new looks, fabrics, scents, makeup, activities, sheets, or dishes—all the elements of Sensation in your life.

• *Use it or lose it.* The blood supply to the vagina decreases after menopause. This can cause the tissue to lose elasticity as well as moisture. Regular sex will slow this process, because arousal attracts blood flow. (See the "Sexuality Now and Beyond" box in the Transition chapter for more specific advice about coping with diminished desire, a common problem that begins in perimenopause and can continue to be problematic postmenopausally.)

• *Approach sexual encounters consciously.* Okay, so sights and touches that once immediately aroused you might not anymore. That doesn't mean that you are no longer sexual, only that being "in the mood" often requires more planning ahead. Adapt your encounters to these changes. Arrange the right environment and proceed at a more leisurely pace. Also recognize that some women are perfectly comfortable with being less sexually active. If that's true for you, resist decades of cultural conditioning that there is something "wrong" with this. This is a great example of a situation where it's not wrong if it's right for you, although you and your partner may need to work through this together. Do look for other expressions of your sensual self that might be less sexual. For example, if you decide this is a time when you are consciously choosing to be less sexually active, don't neglect this Center of Wellness entirely. It's still essential to your health, so look for other ways to fuel and express Sensation.

• *Explore ways to express your sensuality and sexuality that reflect who you are now.* I often hear women in the Transformation Pathway describe themselves with adjectives such as *authen-*

tic, potent, honest, gutsy, confident, carefree. What adjectives would you use to describe yourself now—and how do those translate into your sex life and your expressions of sensuality? Think about ways to integrate your new sense of yourself in all aspects of your life.

Readings and Resources

Integrative Medicine

Becker, Robert O., and Gary Selden. *The Body Electric: Electromagnetism and the Foundation of Life.* New York: Quill, 1985.

Dossey, Larry. *Reinventing Medicine: Beyond Mind-Body to a New Era of Healing.* San Francisco: HarperSanFrancisco, 1999.

Geffen, Jeremy. *The Journey Through Cancer: An Oncologist's Seven-Level Program for Healing and Transforming the Whole Person.* New York: Crown, 2000.

Horrigan, Bonnie J. *Voices of Integrative Medicine: Conversations and Encounters.* Edinburgh: Churchill Livingstone, 2003.

Huddleston, Peggy. *Prepare for Surgery, Heal Faster: A Guide of Mind-Body Techniques.* Cambridge, Mass.: Angel River Press, 2002.

Kaptchuk, Ted J. *The Web That Has No Weaver: Understanding Chinese Medicine.* Chicago: Contemporary Books, 2000.

Lerner, Michael. *Choices in Healing: Integrating the Best of Conventional and Complementary Approaches to Cancer.* Cambridge, Mass.: MIT Press, 1994.

Lown, Bernard. *The Lost Art of Healing.* New York: Ballantine, 1999.

Ornish, Dean. *Dr. Dean Ornish's Program for Reversing Heart Disease: The Only System Scientifically Proven to Reverse Heart Disease Without Drugs or Surgery.* New York: Random House, 1990.

Pelletier, Kenneth. *The Best Alternative Medicine: What Works? What Does Not?* New York: Simon & Schuster, 2000.

Weil, Andrew. *Health and Healing.* Boston: Houghton Mifflin, 1998.

———. *Natural Health, Natural Medicine: A Comprehensive Manual for Wellness and Self-Care.* Rev. ed. Boston: Houghton Mifflin, 1995.

———. *Spontaneous Healing: How to Discover and Enhance Your Body's Natural Ability to Maintain and Heal Itself.* New York: Ballantine, 2000.

Living a Conscious Life

Carson, Richard D. *Taming Your Gremlin: A Guide to Enjoying Yourself.* New York: Perennial, 1986.

Christian, Kenneth W. *Your Own Worst Enemy: Breaking the Habit of Adult Underachievement.* New York: Regan, 2002.

Forrest, Steven. *The Inner Sky: How to Make Wiser Choices for a More Fulfilling Life.* San Diego: ACS Publications, 1989.

Johnson, Robert A. *He: Understanding Masculine Psychology.* New York: Perennial, 1986.

———. *She: Understanding Feminine Psychology.* New York: Perennial, 1989.

———. *We: Understanding the Psychology of Romantic Love.* San Francisco: Harper and Row, 1983.

Kabat-Zinn, Jon. *Full Catastrophe Living: Using the Wisdom of Your Body and Mind to Face Stress, Pain, and Illness.* New York: Delacorte, 1990.

———. *Wherever You Go, There You Are: Mindfulness Meditation in Everyday Life.* New York: Hyperion, 1994.

Nhat Hanh, Thich. *Being Peace.* Berkeley: Parallax Press, 1987.

Paulus, Trina. *Hope for the Flowers.* New York: Newman, 1972.

Richardson, Cheryl. *Take Time for Your Life: A Personal Coach's Seven-Step Program for Creating the Life You Want.* New York: Broadway, 1998.

Tolle, Eckhart. *The Power of Now: A Guide to Spiritual Enlightenment.* Novato, Calif.: New World Library, 1999.

Trott, Susan. *The Holy Man.* New York: Riverhead, 1995.

Nutrition Center

Bratman, Steven, and David Kroll, comp. *Natural Health Bible.* Roseville, Calif.: Prima, 2000.

Graedon, Joe, and Teresa Graedon. *The People's Pharmacy Guide to Home and Herbal Remedies.* New York: St. Martin's Press, 1999.

Weil, Andrew. *Eating Well for Optimum Health: The Essential Guide to Bringing Health and Pleasure Back to Eating.* New York: Quill, 2001.

Willett, Walter C., and P. J. Skerrett. *Eat, Drink, and Be Healthy: The Harvard Medical School Guide to Healthy Eating.* New York: Simon & Schuster, 2001.

Movement Center

Brill, Peggy W., with Gerald Secor Couzens. *The Core Program: Fifteen Minutes a Day That Can Change Your Life.* New York: Bantam, 2001.

Gerrish, Michael. *The Mind-Body Makeover Project: A 12-Week Plan for Transforming Your Body and Your Life.* Chicago: Contemporary, 2003.

Krucoff, Carol, and Mitchell Krucoff. *Healing Moves: How to Cure, Relieve, and Prevent Common Ailments with Exercise.* New York: Harmony, 2000.

Nelson, Miriam E., with Sarah Wernick. *Strong Women Stay Young.* Rev. ed. New York: Bantam, 2000.

Spirit Center

Albom, Mitch. *Tuesdays with Morrie: An Old Man, a Young Man, and Life's Greatest Lesson.* New York: Doubleday, 1997.

Borysenko, Joan. *A Woman's Book of Life: The Biology, Psychology, and Spirituality of the Feminine Life Cycle.* New York: Riverhead, 1996.

Dossey, Larry. *Healing Words: The Power of Prayer and the Practice of Medicine.* San Francisco: HarperSanFrancisco, 1993.

Gibran, Kahlil. *The Prophet.* New York: Knopf, 1995.

Koenig, Harold G. *The Healing Power of Faith: Science Explores Medicine's Last Great Frontier.* New York: Simon & Schuster, 1999.

Levine, Stephen. *Healing into Life and Death.* Garden City, N.Y.: Anchor, 1987.

Myss, Caroline. *Anatomy of the Spirit: The Seven Stages of Power and Healing.* New York: Harmony, 1996.

Oliver, Mary. *New and Selected Poems.* Boston: Beacon, 1992.

Remen, Rachel Naomi. *Kitchen Table Wisdom: Stories That Heal.* New York: Riverhead, 1996.

———. *My Grandfather's Blessings: Stories of Strength, Refuge, and Belonging.* New York: Riverhead, 2000.

Rumi. *The Illuminated Rumi.* Translations and commentary by Coleman Barks. New York: Broadway, 1997.

Tarrant, John. *The Light Inside the Dark: Zen, Soul, and the Spiritual Life.* New York: HarperCollins, 1998.

Sensation Center

Anand, Margo. *The Art of Sexual Magic.* New York: Putnam, 1995.

Forrest, Jodie, Steven Forrest, and Steve Midgett. *Skymates: Love, Sex and Evolutionary Astrology.* Chapel Hill, N.C.: Seven Paws Press, 2002.

Holstein, Lana L. *How to Have Magnificent Sex: The 7 Dimensions of a Vital Sexual Connection.* New York: Harmony, 2001.

Saraswati, Sunyata, and Bodhi Avinasha. *Jewel in the Lotus: The Tantric Path to Higher Consciousness.* Fairfield, Iowa: Sunstar, 1999.

Stein, Daniel S., with Leslie Aldridge Westoff. *Passionate Sex: Discover the Special Power in You.* New York: Carroll and Graf, 2000.

Mind Center

Domar, Alice D., and Henry Dreher. *Healing Mind, Healthy Woman: Using the Mind-Body Connection to Manage Stress and Take Control of Your Life.* New York: Henry Holt, 1996.

Moyers, Bill. *Healing and the Mind.* New York: Doubleday, 1993.

Rossman, Martin L. *Healing Yourself: A Step-by-Step Program for Better Health Through Imagery.* New York: Walker, 1987.

Santorelli, Saki. *Heal Thy Self: Lessons on Mindfulness in Medicine.* New York: Bell Tower, 1999.

Siegel, Bernie S. *Love, Medicine, and Miracles: Lessons Learned About Self-Healing from a Surgeon's Experience with Exceptional Patients.* New York: HarperPerennial, 1990.

Wilson, Paul. *The Calm Technique: Meditation Without Magic or Mysticism.* New York: Bantam, 1989.

Cycling Pathway

Dell, Diana L., and Carol Svec. *The PMDD Phenomenon: Breakthrough Treatments for Premenstrual Dysphoric Disorder (PMDD) and Extreme Premenstrual Syndrome (PMS).* Chicago: Contemporary, 2003.

Taylor, Diana, and Stacey Colino. *Taking Back the Month: A Personalized Solution for Managing PMS and Enhancing Your Health.* New York: Perigee, 2002.

Fertility Pathway

Domar, Alice D., and Alice Lesch Kelly. *Conquering Infertility: Dr. Alice Domar's Mind/Body Guide to Enhancing Fertility and Coping with Infertility.* New York: Viking, 2002.

Lieberman, Adrienne B. *Easing Labor Pain: The Complete Guide to a More Comfortable and Rewarding Birth.* Boston: Harvard Common, 1992.

Nilsson, Lennart, and Lars Hamberger. *A Child Is Born.* New York: Delacorte, 2003.

Payne, Nivari B., and Brenda Lane Richardson. *The Whole Person Fertility Program: A Revolutionary Mind-Body Process to Help You Conceive.* New York: Three Rivers, 1998.

Spencer, Paula, and the editors of *Parenting* magazine. *Parenting Guide to Pregnancy and Childbirth.* New York: Ballantine, 1998.

Transition Pathway

Northrup, Christiane. *The Wisdom of Menopause: Creating Physical and Emotional Health and Healing During the Change.* New York: Bantam, 2001.

Vliet, Elizabeth Lee. *Screaming to Be Heard: Hormonal Connections Women Suspect— and Doctors Ignore.* New York: M. Evans, 1995.

Transformation Pathway

Jacobs, Ruth Harriet. *Be an Outrageous Older Woman.* New York: HarperPerennial, 1997.

Tenneson, Joyce. *Wise Women: A Celebration of Their Insights, Courage, and Beauty.* Boston: Little, Brown, 2002.

Weed, Susun S. *Menopausal Years: The Wise Woman Way.* Woodstock, N.Y.: Ash Tree, 1992.

General Women's Health

American Medical Women's Association. *The Women's Complete Wellness Book.* Edited by Debra R. Judelson and Diana L. Dell. New York: Golden Books, 1998.

Angier, Natalie. *Woman: An Intimate Geography.* Boston: Houghton Mifflin, 1999.

Hudson, Tori. *Women's Encyclopedia of Natural Medicine: Alternative Therapies and Integrative Medicine.* Chicago: Contemporary, 1999.

Legato, Marianne J. *Eve's Rib: The New Science of Gender-Specific Medicine and How It Can Save Your Life.* New York: Harmony, 2002.

Northrup, Christiane. *Women's Bodies, Women's Wisdom: Creating Physical and Emotional Health and Healing.* Rev. ed. New York: Bantam, 1998.

Stewart, Elizabeth G., and Paula Spencer. *The V Book: A Doctor's Guide to Complete Vulvovaginal Health.* New York: Bantam, 2002.

Internet Resources

Acupuncture	http://acupuncture.com
	http://medicalacupuncture.org
American Botanical Council	http://www.herbalgram.org
American Holistic Medical Association	http://www.holisticmedicine.org
Consumer Lab	http://www.consumerlab.com
Massage: American Massage Therapy Association	http://www.amtamassage.org
National Certification Board for Therapeutic Massage and Bodywork	http://www.ncbtmb.com
National Center for Complementary and Alternative Medicine	http://nccam.nih.gov
North American Menopause Society	http://www.menopause.org
Office of Cancer Complementary and Alternative Medicine, National Cancer Institute	http://www.cancer.gov/occam
Office of Dietary Supplements at the NIH	http://dietary-supplements.info.nih.gov
U.S. Food and Drug Administration News	http://www.fda.gov/opacom/hpnews.html

Index

breast (*continued*)
344; cancer, support groups, 202;
lump detected, woman's story,
46–47; lumps, 6, 17; monitoring,
145; self-exam, 147–48;
unconsciousness and, 17; well-
rounded approach, cancer and,
woman's story, 379–81
breast-feeding, 290, 304, 306, 308, 317
breathing exercises, 96–97

C

caffeine, 192, 316
calcium, 317, 384; supplements, 193, 255
cancer: birth control pill and, 237;
exercise and reduced risk, 184;
Journaling and, 102; lifestyle choices
and, 76; spiritual needs and, 73. *See
also* HRT; *specific forms of cancer*
cardiovascular disease. *See* heart
disease
centering, xxiii, 96, 195
Centers of Wellness, xxxii, 9, 28;
awareness, 74; Cycling Pathway,
251–61; daily self-check, 74–75;
Fertility Pathway, 313–22; Five-
Center Balance, 181–210; Five-
Center Review, 138–40, 141; health
care and, 70, 74–75; Mind, 9, 70,
72–73, 258–59, 317–19, 387;
Movement, 9, 70, 71–72, 252–54,
313–15, 335, 353, 383–84;
Nutrition, 9, 70, 72, 255–57,
315–17, 335, 384–87; Sensation, 9,
70, 71, 74, 260–62, 321–22, 388–90;
Spirit, 9, 70, 71, 73, 259–60,
319–21, 387–90; Transformation
Pathway, 383–90; Transition
Pathway, 353–60
cervix: "bloody show," 269;
monitoring (self-exam), 145–46;
mucus, antibodies, 215; mucus,
ovulation, 266; ovulation, changes,
266; Pap smear, 216

chasteberry, 256, 354
childbirth, 293–303; choices for the
birth experience, 297–98; conscious
labor and delivery, woman's story,
302–3; delivery choices, 290; doulas
and labor coaches, 79, 80, 296, 297,
320; environment, 296, 297, 298;
Feedback Loop for, 294–96, 298–99;
healing from, 35–36; imagery to
prepare for labor, woman's story,
301–2; labor, 268–69, 286, 293;
labor and being Consciously
Female, xxx; labor, mindfulness in,
11, 299–300; labor, position, 297;
labor, scheduling, 6–7, 15; labor,
unconscious, woman's story, 10–11,
48; Lamaze training, 11, 299, 320;
medicalization, 15–16; medical
procedures, 298; midwife, 296; as
opportunity, 11; pain, 15–16, 17;
pain management, nonmedicated,
296, 297; pain medication or
blocks, 7, 16, 297; sexual abuse or
rape and, 300
children: unconsciousness choices and
childlessness, 19–20, 30–31, 176.
See also childbirth; fertility;
motherhood; pregnancy
chronotherapy, 215–16
colon cancer, 42
commitment, 13, 21–22, 85–110; inner
space (through relaxation), 86,
96–101; physical space, 86, 93–95;
space on paper (Journaling), 86,
101–4; space through talking (one-
to-one or group), 86, 104–9; space
in time, 86, 87–93
communication: group talk, 107–9;
listening skills, 105; one-to-one talk,
105–7. *See also* body
compartmentalizing, 18
complementary and alternative
medicine (CAM), 60–61, 63–66;
infertility therapies, 279;
practitioner, 66; reasons for

choosing, 68. *See also* Integrative Medicine (IM)

conception. *See* Fertility Pathway

conscious kissing, 209

Consciously Female, xxiii; beginning a plan, 211–12; being aware vs. being informed, 27–29; benefits, xxiii, xxxi, 32–55; boosting health goals, 42–44; breathing in, breathing out, 21–23, 68; choices and, xxx, 20, 29–30, 176–81, 216 (*see also* decision-making); commitment and, 13, 21–22, 85–100; courage and, 27; creating a personal framework, xxiv; cyclical nature of a woman's life, 8; daily requirements, 175–212; detecting problems sooner, 38–42; Dialogue and imagery, 149–72; discipline needed, 39; enriching, easing life transitions, 47–50; feeling more alive, living longer, 53–55; health inventory, 112-32; loving vs. critical consciousness, 26–27; making conscious vs. making "right" decisions, 29–31, 177; missteps, learning from, 30; nonjudgmental approach to, 7, 26–27; optimizing health and healing, 34–38; owning your femaleness, 51–53; as patient in health care system, xxx, 56–81; paying closer attention to body and soul, 133–45; plan, 211–12; sparing yourself the "ricochet effect," 44–47; time and, 13; tools to access consciousness, xxxi, 85–172; vs. unconciously female, 7–20; what it means, 5–31

Consciously Female Inventory, 116–30; background of creation, 114; daily life, 122–24; fertility, 118–19, 131, 219; general health, 126; general questions, 116–17; guiding principles, 115–16; menopause, 122; menstruation (periods), 117–18,

131; miscarriage and loss, 121, 132; Movement, 127; never pregnant, 120; Nutrition, 127; pregnancy, 119–20, 132; purpose, 114–15; relationships, 124–25; Sensation, 128–30; Spirit, 128

contraception choices. *See* birth control

cortisol, 197, 198, 221, 320

Creating a Life (Hewitt), 19–20

Cycling Pathway, xxxii, 25, 48, 213–62; benefits to understanding, 216; contraception choices, 235–43; menstrual cycle as central engine, 214–17; Mind steps, 258–59; Movement, 252–54; not choosing pregnancy, woman's story, 226–27; Nutrition, 255–57; PMS and PMDD, choices involving, 229–30; primal cycle, 217–25; Sensation, 260–62; Spirit, 259–60; unplanned pregnancy, 244–51. *See also* birth control; menstruation; PMS

D

Dadaist saying, 137

daily observations, 133–48; Five-Center Review, 138–40, 141; observing vs. interpreting, 137–38; observing vs. obsessing, 136–37; patterns, detecting, 136; watching vs. observing, 136

Dalai Lama, 30

death and dying, 68–69, 388; aging and, 376–78; exercise and reduced risk, 184; fear of, 377–78; Feedback Loop, 378–79; leading causes, 76, 352, 365

decision making, conscious, 29–31, 177; adoption and, 285; brainstorming, 370–71; choices for the birth experience, 297–98; contraception choices, 235–43; Feedback Loop technique, xxxii,

focused, 369–72; postpartum phase, 306–8; pregnancy, 287–89; pregnancy, decision for, 270–74; unplanned pregnancy, 245–47

female gender, 23–26; life-cycle experiences, 107; owning, 51–53; understanding, a woman's story, 52–53

Fertility Pathway (pregnancy and conception), xxxii, 6, 25, 48; adoption and, 285; biological clock and, 270, 274–75; clues to, awareness of, 42; conception, 265–67, 314; conception, conscious, 273–74; Consciously Female Inventory, 118–19, 131; decision for pregnancy, 269–75; harvest of eggs, 15; labor and delivery, 268, 293–303; Mind, 317–19; miscarriage, 309–13; Movement 313–15; Nutrition, 315–17; ovulation, identifying, 219, 265–67, 273; postpartum transition, 269, 303–9, 315; pregnancy, 267–69, 285–93; preparation for parenthood, 265; Sensation, 321–22; single mothers, 274–75; Spirit, 319–21; support groups, 319. *See also* infertility; pregnancy

fibromyalgia, 67

Five-Center Balance, 181–210

Five-Center Review, 138–40, 141

flaxseed, 190, 257

folate, 316

Forrest, Steve, 223

FSH (follicle stimulating hormone), 218, 219, 221, 327–28

Gaudet, Tracy: Andrew Weil and, xx–xxi, xxviii–xix, 96; becoming conscious, xxv–xxvii, xxxi; body and soul check, 134–35; business to-do lists, 89; Dreamagery, 163; as IM practitioner, 70, 76, 113; infertility patients and, 281–84; interviewing patients, 112–13;

menstruation and, xxiv–xxv, xxvi–xxvii, 35; "My Pet Peeves About HRT," 339–42; ob-gyn, as speciality, xxvii–xxviii, xxx; parents' deaths, 376–77; PMS and, 231; Program in Integrative Medicine, University of Arizona, xx, xxviii–xxix, 94; residency, University of Texas Health Sciences Center, xxv; sacred corner, 93–94; shoulder problems, 39–40; time for self-care, 88, 89

"Gift from the Sea" (Lindbergh), 323

glucosamine sulfate, 42, 79

GNRH (gonadotropin-releasing hormone), 221

grief, 45–46; woman's story, 54–55, 310

Grit Your Teeth and Just Get Through It (GYT&JGTI) approach, 17

group talk, 107–9

"Guest House, The" (Rumi), 111

guided imagery (visualization): ovary pain and, 170–72; surgery and, 79; weight loss and, 44. *See also* imagery

H

Hawkins, Maureen, 263

hCG (human chorionic gonadotropin), 219, 267, 268

headache: menstrual cycle and, 214; migraine treatment, 40, 64; relaxation training, 40; unheeded stress and, 32

healing, 69; childbirth trauma, 35–36; consciousness and optimizing, 34–38, 69; injury, 35; lifestyle and, 67–68, 75–77; at soul level, 70; stress and slowed, 36; word derivation, 36

health: balance and, 8; Consciously Female Inventory, 126; consciousness and, 34–38; daily

preparing for childbirth, woman's story, 301–2; safe pregnancy, woman's story, 286; symptoms and, 151; visualization, 152

immune function, 102, 198, 214–15

infertility, 6, 73; adoption and, 285; age, and pregnancy, 271–72, 277; CAM therapies, 279, 284; Dialoguing with reproductive system, 157; grieving and, 282; IVF, 279, 283; outside help, 276–84; women's stories, 281–84

inner self. *See* soul

inner space, 86, 96–101; 4/7/8 breathing, 96–97; mental muscle relaxation, 97–98; progressive muscle relaxation, 98–100

Integrative Medicine (IM), xx, xxix, 58, 59–61; "best of" approach, 59–66; emphasize the whole person, body, mind, and soul, 59, 70–75; healing-oriented, 67–69; low-tech, low-cost, high-touch, 59, 79–81; optimal experience, example, 56–58; proactive, 59, 75–77; self-directed, 59, 77–79

J

Journaling, 42, 47, 86, 101–4, 200; fears of aging, examining, 333–34; Fertility Pathway and, 318; health benefits, 102; labor and delivery, 299; second half of menstrual cycle, 234, 258; unplanned pregnancy and, 245; weight loss and, 44

"Journey, The" (Oliver), 32

Jung, Carl, 151

K

Kabat-Zinn, Jon, 33

kava, 257, 354

L

labor. *See* childbirth

Lamaze, 11, 299

Landmark, xxxii; aging, 376–82; contraception choices, 235–43; decision for pregnancy, 269–75; infertility, help, 276–84; labor and delivery, 293–303; life's purpose, 367–75; miscarriage, 309–13; perimenopause, 329–32; PMS, 227–33; postpartum, 303–9; pregnancy, 285–93; unplanned pregnancy, 244–51

Langer, Ellen, 199

Lao Tzu, 85

LH (luteinizing hormone), 218, 219, 220, 221, 256

lifestyle; changing habitual activities, 87–88; commitment to Consciously Female, 13, 21–22, 85–110; Consciously Female Inventory, 122–24; Cycling Pathway, 252–62; Five-Center Balance and, 181–210; healing and, 67–68; Journaling, 86, 101–4; key factor in development of disease, 75–77; menopause and perimenopause, 338, 352–57; modern sedentary, 72; physical space, 86, 93–95; plan for, 211–12; postmenopause, 383–90; pregnancy, 312–22; relaxation, 86, 96–101; self-care, 86, 87–93; talking, 86, 104–9; well-rounded approach, woman's story, 379–81. *See also* Centers of Wellness

Lindbergh, Anne Morrow, 323

longevity, 7, 53

M

magnesium supplements, 255–56, 387

medicine: Ayurveda, 22, 63; Chinese, 22, 63; complementary and alternative (CAM), 60–61, 63–66 medicine (*continued*)

68; doctor's view of your soul, 20–26; fragmentation of, 60; Integrative (IM), xx, xxix, 58, 59–81; male model, 10–11; Native American practices, 22; Tibetan medicine, 22; Western, xix–xx, 22, 62, 67, 77–78; Western medical education, xxvii, 64–65, 77. *See also* health care for women

meditation, 96–101, 135, 200

men: contrast with women, 23–24, 216; sexual response times, 206–7

menopause and perimenopause, 25, 48; anxiety and depression, 350–52; alternative and nonmedical help for symptoms, 353–57; average age, 325; benefits, 49; bioidentical hormones for, 338, 341; birth control pills, 327–28; Consciously Female Inventory, 122; consciousness, xxiii; Dreamagery and, 163; fears of aging, 333–34; Feedback Loop for, 331–32; fuzzy thinking, 49, 326, 350; hormones, 326; hot flashes, 6, 48, 49, 329–30, 344, 356, 379, 381 (*see also* symptoms, below); HRT, xix–xx, 6, 29–30, 334–45; inner self and, 34, 326, 328–29; integrative approach, woman's story, 345–46; Landmark, 329–30; lifestyle changes, 338, 343, 345–46, 352–57; loss, feelings of, 350, 355, 368; medicalization, 15, 16, 332; Mind, 355–56; Movement, 335, 351, 353; Nutrition, 335, 353–55; premature, 326; relaxation response, 49; sex and libido (Sensation), 356–60; soul dominance, 356; soul turbulence, 330; Spirit, 356; stress and, 355; surgical, 213–14, 326; symptoms, 326, 330–31, 332, 335, 351, 354, 355; trivialization of symptoms, 78; vaginal dryness, 357, 358; wind-down of periods, 325–26, 328–29; women's stories, 330–31, 333–34, 343–46. *See also* Transformation Pathway (postmenopause)

menstruation (periods), 24; accident proneness and, 214; beginning (menarche), 67, 213; birth control pill, 224, 225–26; cessation, birth control pill, 6, 14, 224, 225, 240; Consciously Female Inventory, 117–18, 131; cramps, xxiv–xxv, xxvi–xxvii, 35, 64; digestive system and, 214; dismissal or elimination of, 224; endometrial lining and, 220; first half of cycle, xxvi, 33, 72, 220, 258, 259, 261; follicular phase, 217, 218, 222, 223; food cravings, 256, 257; hormonal activity, 24–25; immune function, 214–15; irregular cycles, 6; length of cycle, 24; luteal phase, 217, 219, 222, 223, 224; menstrual phase, 217, 218, 222; Mind, 258–59; moodiness and work equality, 19, 223–24; moods, 215; Movement, 252–54; muscles and joints and, 214; negative characterization of, 17, 48, 224; nervous system and, 214; Nutrition, 255–57; as opportunity, xxiii; ovulatory phase, 217, 218–19, 222, 265–67; owning hormonal changes, 33; perimenopause, menopause, and wind-down, 325–26, 328–29; primal cycle, 217–25; second half of cycle, xxvi, 33, 163, 214, 220, 258, 259, 261–62; self-awareness and, 48; Sensation, 260–62; sexual responsiveness and, 214; Soul, 222–23, 224, 226; Spirit, 259–60; waxing and waning, xxvi, 225. *See also* Cycling Pathway; dysmenorrhea; PMS

Mind, 9, 70, 72–73; activate the automatic maybe, 199–200; -body techniques, 72–73, 79; center

osteoarthritis, 42, 79, 353, 364–65
osteoporosis, 335

P

pain: acupuncture for, 64, 65; childbirth, 7, 15–16, 17, 296, 297; conventional treatment, 65; unheeded stress and, 32
"paying now, or paying later with interest," 45, 150
Pennebaker, James, 102
perimenopause. *See* menopause and perimenopause
physical space, 86, 94–95
phytoestrogens, phytoprogesterones, 342
Plato, 56
PMDD (premenstrual dysphoric disorder), 37, 229
PMS (premenstrual syndrome), 6, 17, 65, 67, 227–33; identifying, 228–29; insights available, 230; nutrition, 255; perception and, 233–34; Reflection exercise, 230–33, 234; relaxation techniques, 258–59; stress and environmental factors, 232; symptoms as messages, 231; vitamins, 255–56; women's stories, 37–38, 233–34
postmenstrual phase. *See* Transformation Pathway
postpartum phase, 286, 303–9; baby blues, 305, 318; depression (PPD), 308–9, 320; Feedback Loop, 306–8; inner self and, 34; key choices, 306–7; Mind, emotions and anxiety, 318–19; Movement, 315; Nutrition, 317; physical recovery, 304–5; Sensation and, 321–22; Spirit, postdelivery support, 320; weepiness, 6, 303–4
prayer, 197–98, 202
pregnancy, 6, 48, 285–93; abortion, adoption, or having the child, 245–47, 249–51; amnio or not, woman's story, 291–93; bloom of, 268; caffeine, 316; communicate with your baby, 319–20; Consciously Female Inventory, 119–20, 132; consciousness, xxiii; denial of symptoms, 244; Dialoguing, 287; Dreamagery, 163, 167–70, 287; emergency contraception, 247–49; emotions, 318; Feedback Loop and decision making, 245–47; Feedback Loop and medical choices, 290, 291–93; Feedback Loop and staying conscious, 287–89; first trimester, 267; Five Centers and, 71; folate, 316; hyperemesis gravidarum, 289; impact of, 17; inner self and, 34; losses, 6 (*see also* miscarriage); Mind, 317–19; more ready than thought, woman's story, 249–50; Movement, 313–15; nausea, 288–89, 316; never pregnant, inventory, 120; Nutrition, 315–17; perimenopause babies, 329; placenta problems, woman's story, 168–170; relaxin and, 214; reversal of impulse, woman's story, 250–51; scares, 6; screening tests (triple screen), 292; second trimester, 268; Sensation, 321–22; sex and, 291, 321; signs of, early, 267; Spirit, 319–21; support duing, 320; tests, 219; third trimester, 268; as transition, 49–50; unplanned, 244-51; *See also* childbirth
progesterone, 215, 219, 222, 256, 260–61, 267, 325, 343; bioidentical (Prometrium), 338, 341–42, 343
Program in Integrative Medicine, University of Arizona, xx, xxviii–xxix, 94, 112
prolactin, 256, 305, 354
PubMed, 66
"pushing the hold button," 18

Q

Quick Check, 142–43

R

rape, 248–49

Red Tent, The (Diamant), 104

relationships: connections count, 201–2; Consciously Female Inventory, 124–25; infertility, outside help and, 276–84; labor and delivery and, 300; parenthood and, 322; partner's awareness of rhythms of cycle, 262; postpartum phase, 307; pregnancy, decision about and, 271; sex in, 205

relaxation: discipline, 197–98; 4/7/8 breathing, 96–97; meditation and prayer, 197–98; menopause and perimenopause, 355; mental muscle, 97–98; PMS, 258–59; progressive muscle, 98–100; relaxation response, 197–98; training, 40, 49, 96–101

relief bands, 80, 289

reproductive system; Dialoguing with, 152–57; Dreamagery, example of use, 166-67. *See also* hypothalamus; menopause, menstruation

Richardson, Cheryl, 14

Rumi, 111, 138

S

St. John's wort, 256–57

self-care: daily observations of body and soul, 133–48; "extreme," 14; as love, 136; neglect of, 13–14; postpartum, 322; prioritizing, 89; time, creating, 85, 86, 87–93

Sensation (sensuality and sexuality), 9, 70, 71, 74; actions that engage your senses, 208–9; adventurousness, 207; conception choice, 262; Consciously Female Inventory, 128–30; Cycling Pathway, 260–62; daily choices, 182, 205–10; environment, Fertility Pathway, importance, 321; express awareness as a woman, 207, 209; Fertility Pathway, 321–22; Five-Center Review and, 139, 141; hearing, 208; intimacy is a human need, 206; labor and, 322; lack of sex drive, 210; menopause and perimenopause (Transition Pathway), 356–60; menstrual cycle, 214, 222; multilevel nature of sex, 206; ovulation and, 266; permission to live full, Dreamagery exercise, 206; postmenopause, 388–90; postmenopause, sexual awakenings, woman's story, 374–75; postpartum, 321–22; practice conscious kissing, 209; pregnancy and, 291, 321; problems, consulting a doctor, 207; seeing, 209; smelling, 208; strengthen PC muscles, 207; tantric sex, 207, 210, 357; tasting, 208–9; tendency to skip, 206; touching, 208; understand your body's physiology, 206–7; walk, 206

serotonin, 23, 256

sexuality. *See* sensation

sleep, 198–99; Journaling and, 102; mental muscle relaxation, 97–98

smoking, 355, 386

Soul (inner self), 7–8; body's connection with, 34, 56; Dialoguing, 151–57, 355; doctor's view, 20–26; Dreamagery, 161–62; Fertility Pathway, reflecting on life's larger questions, 321; Five-Center Review, 138–40, 141; Five Centers, 70–75; food to soothe, 72; healing, 70; hearing, xxvii; labor and delivery, 299–300; menopause, 326, 328–29, 331, 355, 356; menstrual

story, 373–74; Mind, 387;
Movement, 383–84; Nutrition,
384–87; osteoporosis and heart
disease, 364–67; postcycling,
362–64, 367; power of "feminine
energy," 374; Sensation, 388–90;
sexual awakenings, woman's story,
374–75; soul dominance, 367,
368–75; Spirit, 387–88; spiritual
journey, woman's story, 372–73;
well-rounded approach, woman's
story, 379–81
Transition Pathway (perimenopause
and menopause), xxxii, 25, 67, 213,
323–60; cycle wind-down, 325–26,
328–29; enriching and easing,
47–50; as golden opportunity, 324;
health care and, 62–63, 67;
medicalization of, 67; Mind,
355–56; Movement, 353; Nutrition,
354–55; Sensation, 356–60; sharing
experiences, 107–9; Spirit, 356

U

unconsciously female, xxiii, 7–20;
denial and, 45; disconnecting with
one's needs, 9, 48; health risks of,
32; medicalized, 14–17; politically
driven, 18–20; preoccupied, 12–14;
repression and, 45, 244; unplanned
pregnancy and, 244; willed, 17–18;
women's stories, 8–11, 48
uterine fibroids, 180–81, 346–50
UTIs (urinary tract infections), 9, 207

V

vagina: cultural discouragement from
observing own, 39; cyst, 39;

dryness, 357, 358; epithelial cell
secretions, 214–15; monitoring,
145–46; perineal tears and wounds,
35; rugae, 35
vaginal bleeding, 27, 41
vitamins: A, 384; B$_6$, 255, 256, 316; C,
384, 386; D, 191–92, 193, 386; E,
343; K, 384, 387; supplements, 193,
255–56, 316, 317, 386–87
vomiting, 64, 79, 80
vulvar self-exam, 145

W

walking, 206; postmenopause, 383
water intake, 192, 317
weight loss: consciousness of, 42;
exercise and, 384; imagery,
woman's story, 43–44; Journaling
and, 102; postpartum, 315, 317
weight training, 184–85, 365, 384
Weil, Andrew, xix–xxi, 36, 96;
Program in Integrative Medicine,
University of Arizona, xx,
xxviii-xix
Women's Bodies, Women's Wisdom
(Northrup), xxvi
Woolf, Virginia, 85
women's group, 107–9
work and career: childlessness and,
19–20; hormones and, 223–24;
politically driven unconsciousness
and, 18–20; pregnancy, decision
about and, 271; preoccupied
unconsciousness and, 12–14;
unconscious approach, 90

Y

yeast infections, 6